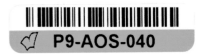

Stuttering

An Integrated Approach

to Its Nature and Treatment

SECOND EDITION

Stuttering

An Integrated Approach

to Its Nature and Treatment

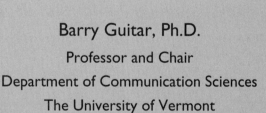

Barry Guitar, Ph.D.

Professor and Chair

Department of Communication Sciences

The University of Vermont

Burlington, Vermont

SANS
TACHE

Williams & Wilkins
A WAVERLY COMPANY

BALTIMORE • PHILADELPHIA • LONDON • PARIS • BANGKOK
BUENOS AIRES • HONG KONG • MUNICH • SYDNEY • TOKYO • WROCLAW

Editor: Donna Balado
Managing Editor: Linda S. Napora
Marketing Manager: Chris Kushner
Production Coordinator: Marette Magargle-Smith
Project Editor: Bill Cady
Copy Editor: Alison T. Kelley
Designer Coordinator: Mario Fernandez
Typesetter: Peirce Graphic Services
Printer and Binder: Quebecor Printing

351 West Camden Street
Baltimore, Maryland 21201-2436 USA

Rose Tree Corporate Center
1400 North Providence Road
Building II, Suite 5025
Media, Pennsylvania 19063-2043 USA

Printed in the United States of America

First Edition, 1991, by Theodore J. Peters and Barry Guitar

Library of Congress Cataloging-in-Publication Data

Guitar, Barry.
    Stuttering : an integrated approach to its nature and treatment / Barry
Guitar. — 2nd ed.
        p.   cm.
    Rev. ed. of: Stuttering / Theodore J. Peters, Barry Guitar. c1991. Includes
bibliographical references and indexes.
    ISBN 068303800-1
    1. Stuttering.   I. Peters, Theodore J. Stuttering. II. Title. [DNLM: 1. Stutter-
ing—therapy.   WM 475 G968s 1998]
RC424.G827   1998
616.85'54—dc21
DNLM/DLC
for Library of Congress   97-41397
                                                                                                                CIP

*The publishers have made every effort to trace the copyright holders for borrowed material.
If they have inadvertently overlooked any, they will be pleased to make the necessary
arrangements at the first opportunity.*

To purchase additional copies of this book, call our customer service department at **(800)
638-0672,** or fax orders to **(800) 447-8438.** For other book services, including chapter
reprints and large quantity sales, ask for the Special Sales department.

Canadian customers should call **(800) 665-1148,** or fax **(800) 665-0103.** For all other calls originating outside of the United States, please call **(410) 528-4223,** or fax us at **(410) 528-8550.**

Visit Williams & Wilkins on the Internet: http://www.wwilkins.com or contact our customer service department at **custserv@wwilkins.com.** Williams & Wilkins customer service representatives are available from 8:30 am to 6:00 pm, EST, Monday through Friday,
for telephone access.

                                                            98 99 00 01 02
                                                        1 2 3 4 5 6 7 8 9 10

Preface

This book is for students of speech-language pathology who seek to know more about the nature and treatment of stuttering.

Since the first edition, co-authored 8 years ago with Ted Peters, a multitude of research studies have been published and many new therapies have been set forth. This revision, however, attempts more than just adding new research findings and including the latest treatment approaches. It is an effort to bring together the latest studies in our field with work in other fields and to develop new views of the etiology of stuttering. To that end, a new chapter (Chapter 4) attempts to integrate findings on the nature of stuttering with evidence from other disciplines to speculate about the neurophysiological substrates of stuttering and the forces that shape its development.

Although the basic division of therapies into fluency shaping, stuttering modification, and integrated approaches is carried over from the first edition, new emphasis is placed on the increasing similarity of approaches as the age/developmental level of the client changes from advanced to intermediate to beginning to borderline stuttering. A new chapter on borderline stuttering illustrates this similarity of approaches, but it also dichotomizes therapies for borderline stuttering as direct or indirect. Where appropriate, new approaches for each level are described, and the author's integrated approach is given in some detail.

In this book, masculine pronouns are used when referring to stutterers, and female pronouns are used when referring to their clinicians. This use of language seems very natural, in that most stutterers are male and most speech-language pathologists are female.

The author hopes that his own experiences as a child who stuttered severely convey a personal perspective on stuttering and that his years as a clinician in public schools in Washington, DC, a hospital in Australia, and a clinic in Vermont provide some authenticity to the therapy sections.

This edition is dedicated to the author's clinician, Charles Van Riper, a recovering stutterer himself, who understood stuttering deeply, and to Van Riper's clinician, Bryng Bryngleson, a nonstutterer whose effectiveness came in part from his desire to understand.

Acknowledgments

I owe much to Ted Peters, my co-author of the first edition of this book; he understood the importance of a logical structure and clear writing. Moreover, his excellence as a clinician still shines through in the therapy sections, particularly those that describe "our own" approach. Dick Curlee, University of Arizona, once again served as outside editor and advisor; wherever the writing is lucid and succinct, he has been at work. My colleague at the University of Vermont, Rebecca McCauley, has helped me immensely with creative ideas for this edition. Nan Bernstein Ratner, University of Maryland, has shown me some of the connections between language and stuttering and provided many imaginative suggestions for the chapter on borderline stuttering and on etiology. I am also indebted to the teachers and students who used the first edition of this book and gave me detailed feedback for this revision.

Many individuals at Williams & Wilkins have been supportive and patient. John Butler, Executive Editor, Donna Balado, Senior Editor, and Tim Satterfield, Vice President & Publisher, Textbooks, kept the faith, despite a few missed deadlines, and encouraged me greatly. Bill Cady, Marette Magargle-Smith, and Alison Kelley have done a superb job on the production of the book. Above all, Linda Napora, managing editor nonpareil, has nurtured this edition page by page and week by week, from the first sentence to the final paragraph, with her combination of cajolery and friendship.

Finally, I thank my wife, Carroll, who has given me abiding support, maintained a constant and valuable interest in my work, and generously slept late on many a summer morning so I could write in solitude by the lake.

Contents

Nature of Stuttering

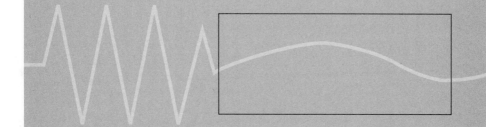

I

Introduction to Stuttering

ABOUT THIS BOOK

Our aim in this book is to teach you to be the most effective therapist for stuttering that you can be. We believe that the best therapy is based on a thorough understanding of the disorder and the principles underlying its treatment. The first five chapters, therefore, are to help you develop an understanding of stuttering. They give you current knowledge about its etiology, onset, and development. They also teach you how stuttering is often unwittingly maintained by the person who stutters, even though he wishes to speak fluently. With this information about the nature of stuttering in mind, the logic of the principles of treatment in later chapters will be clear.

The remaining chapters of the book are devoted to the assessment and treatment of stuttering, which begins with a discussion of the major therapy approaches: stuttering modification, fluency shaping, and an integration of the two. We discuss issues that must be considered in treatment, such as what behaviors the clinician may target and what the clinician's goals for the client may be. We then turn to procedures that may be used to evaluate a client and plan treatment. These procedures are organized by the client's age: preschool, elementary school, and adolescent/adult.

Once you understand how to diagnose and evaluate a person of any age who stutters, then you need to know how to treat that person. We have organized the treatment chapters according to the severity and complexity of the client's problem and the client's age. Thus, we have divided treatment chapters into borderline, beginning, intermediate, and advanced levels of stuttering. At each of these levels, we describe, in detail, fluency shaping stuttering modification and integrated approaches. We hope that as you work your way through these chapters, you will understand more about how the treatment of stuttering is related to its nature. As you develop this understanding, you will be able to choose the treatment approaches that best suit your clients' needs and best match your own clinical style.

We believe that as you grow in experience, you will be able to develop your own innovations in treatment that will derive from your increasing understanding of stuttering and of the individuals with whom you work.

People Who Stutter

Until recently, it was common practice to refer to people who stutter as "stutterers." In fact, some of us refer to ourselves as stutterers and feel some pride in this term. However, we realize that many people prefer not to be labeled "a stutterer." They prefer to be called "people who stutter."[1] They feel, and rightly so, that stuttering is only a small part of their makeup.

Adults who stutter often say that changing the way they think of themselves—as people who happen to stutter but with many more important attributes—was one of the most significant things they did to break the bondage of stuttering. Such experiences serve to remind us that clients are far more than people who stutter. They are people, each with a galaxy of characteristics, one of which happens to be that they stutter. This way of thinking helps us to help not only our clients, but also their families. It helps families listen above the sounds of stuttering to the thoughts and feelings their children are communicating. It helps them see the disfluencies in perspective, as only a small part of the whole child.

The language in this book would grow stale if we used "person who stutters" over and over. So we often refer to "the adult you are working with," "the child," or "an adolescent." We may sometimes find that the word "stutterer" slips back into our writing. But that, too, we feel is acceptable when used occasionally. After all, a stutterer may be someone who is proud that he sometimes stutters and doesn't let it get in the way of his life.

OVERVIEW OF THE DISORDER

This section previews the next few chapters on the nature of stuttering and gives us a chance to reveal our own slant on the disorder. It is intended especially for readers who have not had a course in stuttering, and who may therefore know few details of its nature.

Stuttering is found in all parts of the world, in all cultures and races. It is indiscriminate of occupation, intelligence, and income; it affects both sexes and people of all ages, from toddlers to the elderly. It is an old curse; there is evidence that it was present in Chinese, Egyptian, and Mesopotamian cultures more than 40 centuries ago.

---

[1] Some authors have used the abbreviation PWS for "people who stutter." After polling many people who stutter, both in our own support group and in a National Stuttering Project convention, we have concluded that most people who stutter have a strong dislike for the designation PWS. Thus, we use the more cumbersome but clearly preferable "people who stutter."

What causes people to stutter? Researchers believe there are many influences that determine whether or not an individual will stutter. Neurophysiological, psychological, social, and linguistic factors all probably contribute to its onset and persistence. Stuttering's first appearance in a toddler, for example, may be strongly influenced by constitutional factors, such as a biologically inherited predisposition. Soon, other factors become more important. Stuttering in a young child may become progressively worse in response to family stresses, listener reactions, even the task of learning speech and language. By the time a child is a teenager, learned reactions influence many of the symptoms.[2] By this time, the child has learned to anticipate stuttering and may thrash around in panic when he speaks, trying to escape or avoid it. By adulthood, the fear of stuttering and the desire to avoid it can create a whole lifestyle. An adult stutterer often copes with stuttering by limiting his or her work, friends, and fun to those people and situations that put few demands on his speech.

Figure 1.1 gives an overview of many of the contributing factors in the development of stuttering. In this chapter and the subsequent four chapters, we describe in detail our current understanding of these influences.

Can stuttering be cured? Often, it cures itself. Some young children who begin to stutter recover without treatment. For other young children who stutter, early intervention may be needed to nurture the child's normal development of fluency and prevent the development of a serious problem. Once stuttering has really taken hold, however, and the child has developed many learned reactions, a concerted treatment effort is needed. Good treatment of mild and moderate stuttering in preschool and early elementary school children may leave these children with little trace of stuttering, except perhaps when they are stressed, fatigued, or ill. Most individuals who stutter severely for a long time or those who are not treated until after puberty make only a partial recovery. They usually learn to speak more slowly or to stutter more easily and to be less bothered by it, although some will not improve, despite our best efforts.

Before we delve deeper into the nature and treatment of stuttering, we touch briefly on the personal side of the problem. Some of you may never have had a friend who stuttered or may never have worked with a stutterer in treatment, so we are presenting several examples of what stuttering can be like. Even if you are familiar with stuttering, this section may expand your sense of what stuttering is like for the person who experiences it. These brief sketches portray three individuals who differ widely in age and in their accommodations to stuttering.

CASE EXAMPLES

STUTTERING IN AN ADULT

Tom is a 29-year-old botanist at a state university. He has stuttered since he was 3 years old; his father and brother also stutter. Tom's speech was difficult to understand when he first began to speak, and he remembers his older brother interpreting for him when his parents kept asking him to repeat practically everything he said. Tom was told that his stuttering started as easy repetitions of

---

[2] In the medical literature, the term "symptom" is often used for behavior that signifies an underlying condition: for example, pain in the lower right abdomen may be a symptom of appendicitis. In the stuttering literature, however, symptom has often been used to denote a behavior that is an aspect of the disorder itself, such as multiple part-word repetitions. We use the words "symptom" and "sign" interchangeably to indicate such behaviors.

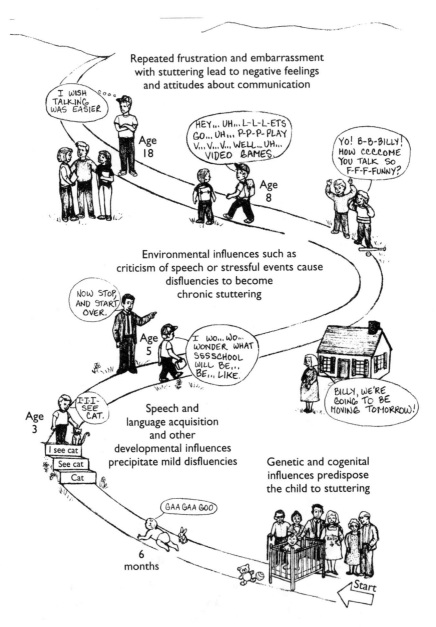

Figure 1.1. Factors contributing to the development of stuttering.

sounds at the beginning of sentences. It gradually worsened during elementary and junior high school. Repetitions kept going on and on, and when he felt stuck on a word, he began to push harder and harder to finish it. By the time he was an adult, Tom stuttered severely, sometimes struggling and contorting his face for what seemed to him like several minutes.

At present, he stutters frequently and with a great deal of tension when talking in a group of people or to someone he doesn't know well. His stutters are particularly long on the first words in a conversation. He is embarrassed and frustrated by his stuttering, especially when he is unable to do what even a child can do easily: just say a single word. During his stutters, Tom knows what he is trying to say, but despite this, he feels his throat clamp shut, and he can't seem to say the word until, after struggling for many seconds, it just pops out.

Tom's stuttering varies. It is usually worse in formal situations, or when a listener is impatient or embarrassed, or when Tom is tired or ill. On the other hand, it is better if he is talking to his wife or children or when he is talking to good friends, especially if there are only one or two of them together. Many times Tom's stuttering is unpredictable, which makes him feel he is woefully out of control.

Tom is very bright; he is nationally recognized for his achievements in botany. But he believes that many people think he is "dumb" as soon as they hear him stutter. This belief may have its roots in elementary school, where he was placed in the lowest reading group because he stuttered severely when reading aloud. He also believes that some of his teachers thought he was dumb because he would often answer "I don't know" when asked questions in class. He knew the answer but couldn't bear the teacher's impatience when he stuttered. Tom's embarrassment about stuttering keeps him from presenting papers at professional conferences. He is also unwilling to teach courses. For these reasons, he has only a research appointment at the university, without the job security offered by a tenured teaching position.

Discussion

Tom's case illustrates some of the hidden dimensions of stuttering. His stuttering consists not only of the contortions he makes with his mouth, but also of the feelings and beliefs that years of stuttering have created in his mind. For example, his misperceptions and fears deter him from even trying to lecture in the classroom, when, in fact, many stutterers handle classroom teaching well.

Tom will probably never stop stuttering, but with treatment he can reduce its severity from a major communication and vocational problem to a minor annoyance.

STUTTERING IN AN ELEMENTARY SCHOOL CHILD

Kendrick is a fifth grader. The speech-language pathologist in his school brought him to our clinic for help in planning his treatment. Like many of his classmates, Kendrick is a study in extremes. He does well in school in every subject that he likes, and poorly in every subject that he hates. Sometimes he stutters severely; other times he is completely fluent. When he stutters, he says he has the sensation of his mouth bouncing out of control as sounds repeat themselves six or eight times. Recently, he has begun to tighten muscles in his throat and blink his eyes in an effort to get words out.

Kendrick talks a lot in class discussions even though he often stutters. He is able to keep his speech flowing in this situation despite frequent repetitions. What really throws him, however, is reading aloud. His teachers call on students to read by going down the rows. Anticipation builds as his turn comes nearer and nearer. He watches the clock, hoping the period will end before he is called on. When it doesn't, and he hears the terrible sound of his name being called, his tongue seems to stick firmly to the roof of his mouth, and he is unable to utter a syllable. The child who sits behind Kendrick takes great delight in this. He usually makes Kendrick's torment greater by bumping his desk against the back of Kendrick's chair and making little stutter-like sounds, which are audible to everyone except the teacher.

Over the past several years, Kendrick's parents and teachers have been at a loss to help him. They have suggested that he think about what he wants to say before speaking or that he slow down and take a breath whenever he thinks he might stutter. He has tried all of their suggestions. Some seemed to work for a little while, but soon stopped, which resulted in feelings of failure and helplessness. Kendrick is regarded as someone with potential for going to college, but there is concern that his stuttering is becoming more severe and that he may begin to withdraw from class participation and become more self-conscious around his peers.

Discussion

Kendrick's stuttering problem is not as severe as Tom's, but it is growing. On the surface, Kendrick's stuttering has changed relatively little since it began. He still repeats sounds, as he did when he was younger, although now he uses a lot more muscular tension to squeeze sounds out. The big change is Kendrick's sensitivity to his stuttering. He has grown more self-conscious about it, since people have noticed it and responded with comments, advice, or impatience. Kendrick is at a crossroad. Proper treatment can reduce his stuttering and make it more likely that he will grow up without a sense that he is handicapped. Without treatment, Kendrick's stuttering is likely to get more severe, and he may feel more and more inhibited about speaking.

STUTTERING IN A PRESCHOOL CHILD

Sally is nearly 4 years old. Her parents contacted us because they were worried about her speech. They were particularly concerned because her uncle had stuttered throughout his childhood, although he has since recovered. Sally is the second of three children; she has an older sister, 7 years old, and a new baby brother, 6 months old. About the time Sally's brother was born, Sally's parents became alarmed when they noticed that she was frequently repeating sounds. The repetitions often went on five or six times before she said the word. Sally continues to repeat sounds, particularly when she is excited or when she is exercising her rapidly expanding vocabulary. Although she usually repeats sounds only three or four times now and her repetitions come and go, Sally's parents are concerned about her speech. Thinking back, they realized that Sally's sister had repeated sounds, but only one or two repetitions each time, and that she had stopped after several months. Sally doesn't seem to mind her repetitions, but her sister does and so do her grandparents. In fact, her grandmother once took Sally aside and gave her some instruction about how to talk.

Discussion

Sally can be treated very effectively if her parents are willing to make some changes in their home. With a clinician's help, they can discover which of the many pressures in their normal family life might be affecting Sally's speech. With several meetings devoted to discussing these factors and how to change them, and some direct work with Sally, Sally's fluency can be increased and she can almost certainly be on her way again, developing normal speech and language.

The three cases provide only glimpses of what stuttering can be like at different stages and for different people. They also echo our earlier comments on the nature of the disorder: stuttering may first appear as occasional, effortless repetitions of sounds, but if it persists, normal childhood experiences such as family stresses and the development of spoken language may increase its frequency and tension. The young stutterer's self-consciousness about his speech difficulty and about listener reactions contribute to his embarrassment and desire to avoid stuttering. This sets the stage for learned reactions that make the confirmed stutterer's problem so complex and treatment so difficult.

DEFINITIONS

Fluency

By beginning with a definition of fluency, we are pointing out how many elements must be maintained in the flow of speech if a speaker is to be considered fluent. It is an impressive balancing act; little wonder that everyone slips and stumbles from time to time when they talk.

Fluency is hard to define. In fact, most researchers have focused on its opposite, *disfluency*.[3] One of the early researchers in fluency, Freida Goldman-Eisler, has shown that normal speech is filled with hesitations (Goldman-Eisler, 1968). Other researchers have acknowledged this and expanded the study of fluent speech by contrasting it with disfluent speech. Dalton and Hardcastle (1977), for example, distinguish fluent and disfluent speech by differences in the variables listed in Table 1.1. The inclusion of intonation and stress in this list may seem unusual. It could be said that speakers who reduce stuttering by using a monotone are not really fluent. But we would argue that it is not their fluency but their "naturalness" that is affected.[4]

---

[3] Throughout this book, we use the term disfluency to apply both to stuttering and to normal hesitancy, making it easier to refer to hesitations that could be either normal or abnormal.

[4] Recent research has examined the effect of unusual patterns on a listener's perception of speech naturalness. See Schiavetti & Metz (1997) for a review.

Table 1.1. Variables Suggested by Dalton and Hardcastle (1977) to Be Useful in Distinguishing Between Fluent and Disfluent Speech

1. Presence of extra sounds, such as repetitions, prolongations, interjections, and revisions
   If a speaker says "I-I-I nnnnneed to have uh my uh, well, I-I-I should get mmmmmy car fixed," he sounds disfluent.
2. Location and frequency of pauses
   If a speaker says, "Whenever I remember to bring my umbrella (pause), it never rains," he sounds fluent. But if he says, "Whenever (pause) I remember to bring (pause) my (pause) umbrella, it never (pause) rains," he sounds disfluent.
3. Rhythmical patterning in speech
   English is typically spoken with stressed syllables at relatively equal intervals; in general, stressed syllables are followed by several unstressed syllables. When this pattern is deviated from markedly, as in cerebellar disease, when the speaker stresses all syllables equally, the speaker sounds disfluent.
4. Intonation and stress
   If a speaker does not vary intonation and stress and is therefore monotonous, he may be considered disfluent. Abnormal intonation and stress patterns may also be considered disfluent.
5. Overall rate
   If a speaker has a very slow rate of speech or if he has bursts of fast rate interspersed with slower rate, he may be considered disfluent.

Starkweather (1980, 1987) has suggested that many of the variables that determine fluency reflect temporal aspects of speech production: such variables as pauses, rhythm, intonation, stress, and rate are controlled by when and how fast we move our speech structures. So, our temporal control of the movements of these structures determines our fluency. Starkweather has also noted that the rate of information flow, not just sound flow, is an important aspect of fluency. Thus, a speaker who speaks without hesitations, but slowly, might not be considered a fluent speaker.

In his description of fluency, Starkweather also included the effort with which a speaker speaks. By effort, he means both the mental and physical work a speaker must do to speak. This is difficult to measure, but it may turn out to be a judgment that listeners can make reliably.

In essence, fluency can be thought of simply as the effortless flow of speech. Thus, a speaker who is judged to be "fluent" appears to use little effort when speaking. However, the components of such effortless speech flow are hard to pin down. As researchers analyze fluency more carefully, they may find that the appearance of excess effort may give rise to judgments that a person is stuttering. Whereas other elements, such as unusual rhythm or slow rate of information flow, may result in judgments that a person is not a fluent speaker, but is not a stutterer either. We discuss aspects of fluency again when we relate dimensions of fluency to various therapy approaches.

Stuttering

GENERAL DEFINITION

Countless writers have tried to capture the essence of stuttering in a few sentences. The following definition is yet another attempt; it borrows most heavily from Andrews and Harris (1964) and Wingate (1964) but adds some of our own distinctions. Stuttering is characterized by an abnormally high frequency or duration of stoppages in the forward flow of speech. These stoppages usually take the form of (*a*) repetitions of sounds, syllables, or one-syllable words, (b) prolongations of sounds, or (c) "blocks"[5] of airflow or voicing in speech. Individuals who stutter are usually aware of their stuttering and are often embarrassed by it. Moreover, they often use excessive physical and mental effort to speak. Children who are just beginning to stutter may not seem bothered or aware of it, but they often show signs of physical tension and increased speech rate, which suggests they are reacting, at least minimally, to their speech difficulty.

Another approach to defining stuttering involves specifying what it is not. For example, an important distinction must be made between the stuttering behaviors just described and normal hesitations. Normal children who are developing speech and language often show repetitions, revisions, and pauses—which are not stuttering. Neither are the brief repetitions, revisions, and pauses in the speech of most nonstuttering adults, when they are in a hurry or uncertain. In Chapter 5, we describe the differences between normal disfluency and stuttering in more detail to prepare you for the task of differential diagnosis of stuttering in children.

A distinction should also be made between stuttering and certain other fluency disorders. Disfluency resulting from cerebral damage or disease, disfluency resulting from psychological trauma, and cluttering (rapid, unintelligible speech) all differ from stuttering that begins in childhood. These disorders may be treated somewhat differently, although some of the techniques we use with stuttering are also useful with other fluency disorders. These disorders are discussed briefly in Chapter 7.

CORE BEHAVIORS

We have adopted the term "core behaviors" from Van Riper (1971, 1982), who used it to describe the basic behaviors of stuttering: repetitions, prolongations, and blocks. These behaviors seem involuntary to the person who stutters, as if they are out of his control. They differ from "secondary behaviors" that the stutterer acquires as learned reactions to the basic core behaviors.

Repetitions are the core behaviors observed most frequently among children who are just beginning to stutter.[6] They are simply a sound, syllable, or single-syllable word repeated several times. The speaker is apparently "stuck" on that sound and continues repeating it until the following sound can be produced. In children who have not been stuttering long, single-syllable word repetitions and part-word repetitions are more common than multisyllable word repetitions. Moreover, children who stutter frequently repeat a word or syllable more than twice per instance (Yairi, 1983; Yairi & Lewis, 1984).

Prolongations of voiced or voiceless sounds also appear in the speech of children beginning to stutter. Often they appear somewhat later than repetitions (Van Riper, 1982), although both Johnson and associates (1959) and Yairi (1997a) reported that they may also be present at onset. We use the term prolongation to denote those stutters in which sound or air flow continues, but movement of the articulators is stopped. Prolongations as short as half a second may still be perceived as abnormal; in rare cases they may last as long as several minutes (Van Riper, 1982). In contrast to our use of the term, other writ-

---

[5] We use the word "blocks" to denote stuttering behavior in which the speaker stops the flow of air or voice. This differs from its historical usage wherein writers would have been indicating any moment of stuttering.

[6] Reviews of the stuttering behaviors reported by parents at the onset of the disorder can be found in Bloodstein (1995) and Van Riper (1982). Yairi's (1982) study details the behaviors that were reported by parents as the first signs of stuttering in a group of ten 2- to 3-year-old children. These findings suggest that part-word repetitions and, to a lesser extent, whole-word repetitions and sound prolongations are the most common first signs of stuttering.

ers include stutters with no sound or airflow, as well as stopped movement of the articulators, in their definition of prolongations (e.g., Conture, 1990; Van Riper, 1982; Wingate, 1964).

Repetitions and sound prolongations may also be part of the core behaviors of more advanced stutterers, as well as of children just beginning to stutter. Sheehan (1974) found that repetitive stutters occurred in the speech of every one of a sample of 20 adults who stuttered. Indeed, 66% of their stutters were repetitions. Many of their stutters were also prolongations, although how many is not clear, because Sheehan's definition of prolongations may differ from our definition.

Blocks are typically the last core behavior to appear. However, as with prolongations, some investigators (Johnson & associates, 1959; Yairi, 1997a) have reported the appearance of blocks at, or close to, stuttering onset. Blocks occur when a person inappropriately stops the flow of air or voice, and often the movement of his articulators as well. Blocks may appear at any level of the speech mechanism—respiratory, laryngeal, or articulatory. There is some evidence and much theorizing that inappropriate muscle activity at the larynx characterizes most blocks (Conture, McCall, & Brewer, 1977; Freeman & Ushijima, 1978; Kenyon, 1942; Schwartz, 1974).

As stuttering persists, we often see blocks grow longer and more tense. Tremors often become evident.[7] These rapid oscillations, most easily observable in the lip or jaw, occur when someone has blocked on a word. He closes off the airway, increases air pressure behind the closure, and squeezes his muscles particularly hard (Van Riper, 1982).[8]

People who stutter vary considerably in how frequently they stutter and how long their individual core behaviors last. Research indicates that an average person who stutters does so on about 10% of the words while reading aloud, although individuals vary greatly (Bloodstein, 1944, 1987). Many people who stutter mildly do so on less than 5% of the words they speak or read aloud, and a few with severe stuttering stutter on more than 50% of their words. Durations of core behaviors vary much less. Stutters average around 1 second in duration and are rarely longer than 5 seconds (Bloodstein, 1944, 1987).

SECONDARY BEHAVIORS

People who stutter don't enjoy stuttering. They react to repetitions, prolongations, and blocks by trying to end them quickly if they can't avoid them altogether. Such reactions may begin as random struggle but soon turn into well-learned patterns. We divide secondary behaviors into two broad classes: escape behaviors and avoidance behaviors.[9] We make this division, rather than follow the traditional approach of dealing with secondary behaviors individually (as, for example, "starters" or "postponements"), because our treatment procedures are focused on the principles by which secondary behaviors are learned.

The terms "escape" and "avoidance" are borrowed from the behavioral learning literature. Briefly, escape behaviors occur when the speaker is stuttering and attempts to terminate the stutter and finish the word. Examples are eye blinks, head nods, or interjections of extra sounds, such as "uh." These are often followed by the termination of a

---

[7] These tremors may differ from the physiological oscillations associated with stuttering reported by Fibiger (1971) and Denny & Smith (1992), or they may be the visible result of such oscillations when the underlying tremor process has been ongoing for several seconds.

[8] You can duplicate these tremors by trying to say the word "by" while squeezing your lips together hard and building up air pressure behind the block. Imagine this happening to you unexpectedly when you were trying to talk.

[9] Detailed descriptions of these behaviors and the learning processes responsible for them are described in Chapter 5.

stutter and are thus rewarded. Avoidance behaviors, on the other hand, are learned when a speaker anticipates stuttering and recalls the negative experiences he has had when stuttering. To avoid stuttering again, he often resorts to the behaviors he has used previously to escape from moments of stuttering—eye blinks or "uh's," for example. Or, he may try something new, such as changing the word he was planning to say.

In many cases, especially at first, the avoidance behavior prevents the stutter from occurring and provides emotional relief that is highly rewarding. Soon the avoidance behavior becomes a strong habit and is resistant to change. The many subcategories of avoidances (e.g., postponements, starters, and timing devices such as hand movements timed to saying the word) are described in Chapter 5.

FEELINGS AND ATTITUDES

A person's feelings can be as much a part of the disorder of stuttering as his or her speech behaviors. Feelings may precipitate stutters; conversely, stutters may create feelings. For example, a person who stutters on his name may feel deep shame for being unable to do something that seems so simple to others.

In the beginning, a child's positive feelings of excitement or negative feelings of fear may result in repetitive stutters that he hardly notices. Then, as he stutters more frequently, he may become frustrated or embarrassed because he is aware that he can't say what he wants to say as smoothly and quickly as others. These feelings then make speaking harder as frustration and embarrassment increase the effort and tension that holds back speech. Feelings that result from stuttering may include not only frustration and embarrassment, but fear of future stuttering, shame about stuttering, and hostility toward listeners as well.

Attitudes are feelings that have become pervasive, part of the person's beliefs. As a person who stutters experiences more and more stuttering, for example, he begins to believe he is a person who generally has trouble speaking. Adolescents and adults usually have many negative attitudes about themselves that are derived from years of stuttering experiences. Often, a person who stutters projects his attitudes on listeners, believing that they think he is stupid or nervous. Sometimes, however, listeners may contribute directly to the person's attitudes. Research has shown that most people, including classroom teachers and even speech-language pathologists, stereotype people who stutter as tense, insecure, and fearful (Turnbaugh, Guitar, & Hoffman, 1979; Woods & Williams, 1976). Such listener stereotypes can affect the way individuals who stutter see themselves, and changing a client's negative attitudes about himself can be a major focus of treatment.

The three components of stuttering—core behaviors, secondary behaviors, and feelings and attitudes—are shown in Figure 1.2. The core behavior is the individual's block on the B in "Boston." The secondary behaviors consist of postponement devices such as "uh," "well," and "you know," and the substitution of "The Big Apple" for "New York." Feelings and attitudes are depicted as the individual's thoughts that he won't succeed in saying the word fluently and his belief that listeners will think he is dumb because he stutters.

BASIC FACTS ABOUT STUTTERING AND THEIR IMPLICATIONS FOR THE NATURE OF STUTTERING

In this section, we cover some of the best-known "facts" about stuttering. These are replicated research findings that pertain to the occurrence and variability of stuttering in the population and in individuals. As we discuss these findings, we will note what they sug-

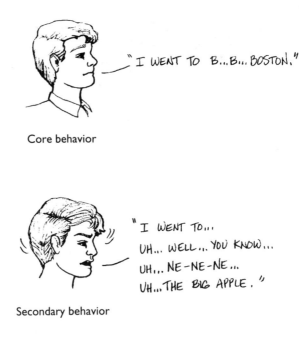

Core behavior

"I WENT TO B...B... BOSTON."

"I WENT TO...
UH... WELL... YOU KNOW...
UH... NE-NE-NE...
UH...THE BIG APPLE."

Secondary behavior

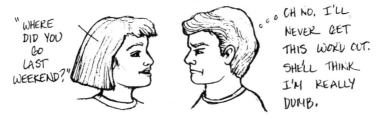

"WHERE DID YOU GO LAST WEEKEND?"

OH NO, I'LL NEVER GET THIS WORD OUT. SHE'LL THINK I'M REALLY DUMB.

Feelings and attitudes

Figure 1.2. Components of stuttering: core behaviors, secondary behaviors, and feelings and attitudes.

gest about the nature of stuttering. Thus, as you read the rest of this chapter, you will become increasingly aware of our perspective on the nature and treatment of stuttering.

Much has been made of the "heterogeneity" of stuttering; many authors have suggested that stuttering is not one disorder, but many. Researchers have made various divisions of the disorder, such as Van Riper's (1982) four "tracks" of stuttering development, and St. Onge's (1963) triad of speech-phobic, psychogenic, and organic stutterers. Our approach is to focus on the majority of people who stutter: those whose stuttering begins during childhood, without an apparent link to psychological or organic trauma. This most common type of stuttering has been called "developmental stuttering," because symptoms usually emerge gradually during a period of rapid speech and language acquisition. We simply call it "stuttering." To denote similar fluency problems that are associated with psychological problems, brain damage, retardation, and cluttering, we refer to their assumed etiology, such as "disfluencies associated with brain damage."

Onset

Our information about the onset of stuttering initially came from parents' recollections of an event that had begun some time in the hazy past. More recently, researchers have been able to interview parents and to record children soon after onset, giving us a clearer picture of the different ways stuttering manifests itself when it begins (e.g., Yairi, 1997a). It may start as a gradual increase in the frequency of repetitions and prolongations that are common in children learning to talk. It also may begin suddenly with disfluencies that are striking in terms of their frequency and duration, as well as the amount of physical tension the child shows when stuttering.

When it begins, stuttering may be sporadic, appearing for a few days or weeks, then disappearing, then coming back. Or, it may disappear altogether after several months. Sometimes, stuttering may persist consistently from its onset.

Researchers generally agree that the onset of stuttering may occur at any time during childhood between the beginning of multiword utterances (around 18 months) and puberty (11 or 12 years). It is *most likely* to occur between ages 2 and 5 years (Andrews et al., 1983). Because of this characteristic onset, stuttering seems not to be a disorder simply of making sounds, but a problem related to using spoken language to communicate. Its onset often coincides, as mentioned before, with a period of rapid expansion of speech and language skills.

Prevalence

The term "prevalence" is used to indicate the extent to which a disorder is widespread. Information about the prevalence of stuttering tells us how many people currently stutter. Accurate and up-to-date information on the prevalence of stuttering is difficult to obtain. The research literature reports many methodological differences among studies, which can result in wide differences in estimates of prevalence. For example, the prevalence of stuttering probably varies considerably with age, and not all studies measure stuttering in the same age groups. Moreover, definitions of stuttering may vary from study to study. Some studies may include relatively normally disfluent individuals in their count; others may exclude them.

Beitchman and associates (1986) assessed the prevalence of speech and language disorders in kindergarten children, using a representative sample. They retested children who failed the initial screening and a random sample of children who passed. The prevalence of stuttering in this sample of kindergarten children was 2.4%. Although this is a finding from only one study, the care with which the data were collected increases its credibility.

Bloodstein (1995) summarized the results of 37 studies of school children in the United States, Europe, Africa, Australia, and the West Indies. These studies showed that the prevalence of stuttering throughout the school years is about 1%. Andrews and associates (1983) came to the same conclusion: about 1% of the school children worldwide are likely to be stutterers at any given time. If the 2.4% prevalence among kindergartners is valid, considerable recovery must take place between kindergarten and the upper grades.

There appear to be no reliable prevalence data for stuttering in adults. However, both Bloodstein (1995) and Andrews and associates (1983) suggest that the prevalence of stuttering is lower after puberty. If so, the prevalence for adults would be less than 1%.

Incidence

The incidence of stuttering is an index of how many people have stuttered at some time in their lives. Like the data on prevalence, incidence figures are not clear-cut because different researchers have used different definitions of stuttering and methods for obtaining their data. Some researchers only report stuttering that lasted 6 months or more, not wanting to include shorter episodes of disfluency. Others report any speech behaviors that informants or parents considered to be stuttering. Estimates of incidence, when reports of informants and parents are considered, are as high as 15%—a figure that includes those children who stuttered for only a brief period (Bloodstein, 1995). When only the cases of stuttering that lasted longer than 6 months are included, incidence appears to be about 5% (Andrews et al., 1983). We think the latter estimate may more accurately reflect the chronic disorder we call stuttering, but the former illustrates how close perceptions of normal disfluency and stuttering may be.

Incidence figures tell us something else about the nature of stuttering. The difference between incidence (5%) and prevalence (1% in school-age children and less in adults) suggests that most people who stutter at some time in their lives recover from it, and we know that prevalence declines after puberty. Thus, unless treatment alone is responsible for such remissions, some aspect of growth or maturation allows many individuals to recover from stuttering.

Recovery Without Treatment

Studies suggest that a large number of people who stutter stop stuttering without professional treatment (Andrews & Harris, 1964; Bloodstein, 1995; Yairi, 1997a). Some of our information about how many people recover from stuttering is based on retrospective reports of adults who say they used to stutter but overcame it without treatment. This information is likely to be somewhat unreliable. For example, some adults who were surveyed may have been told by their parents that they stuttered even though they were no more disfluent than most children. Moreover, some may still have stuttered when they were surveyed, but did not report it. Bloodstein (1995), who reviewed these retrospective studies and their weaknesses, found a recovery rate of 36% to 79%.

The longitudinal study by Andrews and Harris (1964) avoided many of the problems of self-reporting by following up on a group of children from onset of stuttering to their teenage years. They reported a recovery rate of 79%, but this figure included children who stuttered for only brief periods of time. The recovery rates from all studies varies from 23% to 80% (Andrews et al., 1983). The lower rates may reflect the fact that, if children who stutter are observed for only a few years, fewer will have had a chance to recover.

Longitudinal studies of early childhood stuttering by Yairi and colleagues (Yairi & Ambrose, 1992a; Yairi, Ambrose, & Niermann, 1993; and Yairi, Ambrose, Paden, & Throneburg, 1996) indicate that recovery rates for this age group range from 65% to 85%. Children in these studies were diagnosed within 1 year of onset and were categorized as stutterers by parents and two speech-language pathologists. Many recovered within 12 months of onset. Several factors were associated with recovery: earlier age of onset, higher phonological and language skills, higher nonverbal intelligence, recovery of relatives who had stuttered, and gender.

In summary, there appears to be no well-established or widely agreed-upon percentage of stutterers who will recover without treatment. Current estimates depend on many factors—the accuracy with which stuttering is differentiated from normal disfluency, whether the study is retrospective or longitudinal, and the size of the group studied, among other things. In general, we can say that between 50% and 85% of children who stutter recover with or without professional treatment, most before puberty. Factors that may be related to recovery include: a less severe stuttering problem (some studies dispute this), some change in the way the stutterer is speaking (especially slowing speech rate), recovery among relatives who stuttered, good phonological, language, and nonverbal skills, and being female. We now consider the latter variable, the sex factor, in more detail.

Sex Ratio

Studies of the sex ratio in stuttering were first published in the 1890s and have been published every decade since. With this steady stream of information, we ought to have reliable data on this phenomenon. In fact, we do. The results from studies of people who stutter at many ages and in many cultures put the ratio at about three male stutterers to every one female stutterer. There is strong evidence, however, that the ratio may increase as children get older. For example, Yairi (1983) reported that of 22 children who were 2 and 3 years of age and whom parents believed were stuttering, 11 were boys and 11 were girls.[10] In a larger study of 87 children between 20 and 69 months, Yairi and Ambrose (1992b) found a male:female ratio of 2.1:1 overall, although the 20 youngest subjects (under 27 months) showed a 1.2:1 ratio.

Bloodstein's (1995) review indicated that the male-to-female sex ratio is about 3:1 in the first grade and 5:1 in the fifth grade, confirming the hypothesis that the sex ratio increases as children get older. The nearly even sex ratio among very young children who stutter and the gradually increasing proportion of boys who stutter may be a consequence of girls beginning to stutter a little earlier (Yairi, 1983; Yairi & Ambrose, 1992b) and recovering earlier and more frequently (Andrews et al., 1983; Yairi & Ambrose, 1992b; Yairi, Ambrose, & Cox 1996). Thus, females who stutter and don't recover by adulthood may be an interesting subpopulation to study. They may have inherited a stronger predisposition to stuttering or been subjected to strong environmental pressures on their speech, or both (Andrews et al., 1983). Alternately, they may lack the "recovery factor" that most young female stutterers appear to have.

Variability and Predictability of Stuttering

Another important piece of background information about stuttering is how it varies, yet is surprisingly predictable in its occurrence, despite the fact that it seems so inconsistent and so idiosyncratic. This predictability is an important clue to its nature. As we trace the research on stuttering's variability, we will see how this information reflects changing theoretical perspectives on the disorder.

Before the 1930s, stuttering had been commonly regarded as a medical disorder. Lee Edward Travis, the first person to be trained as a Ph.D. to work with speech and hearing disorders, set up a laboratory at the University of Iowa in 1924 to study stuttering from a neurophysiological perspective. He hypothesized that stuttering was the result of anomalous or inefficient cerebral organization. To Travis and his fellow researchers, the variability of stuttering behaviors was seen as part of an organic disorder, and an unimportant part at that. Far more relevant to their research were the stutterer's brain waves, heart rate, and breathing pattern. But in the 1930s, psychologists at Iowa and elsewhere began taking a keen interest in behavioral approaches to the study of human disorders. This enthusiasm spilled over into research on stuttering, and scientists who had been try-

---

[10]Note that these stutterers were not diagnosed by expert clinicians but by parents. Thus, this 1:1 sex ratio must be accepted tentatively. However, other researchers have also reported sex ratios close to 1:1 in preschool stutterers (Glasner & Rosenthal, 1957).

ing to understand the neurophysiology of stuttering gradually began trying to fathom the social, psychological, and linguistic factors that govern its occurrence and variability (Bloodstein, 1995).

ANTICIPATION, CONSISTENCY, AND ADAPTATION

Much of the early research into behavioral aspects of stuttering focused on how stuttering varies in predictable ways. Researchers found, for example, that when stutterers were asked to read a passage aloud, many could forecast—with surprising accuracy—which words they would stutter on.[11] Researchers also discovered that when stutterers read a passage aloud several times, they tended to stutter on many of the same words each time (Johnson & Inness, 1939; Johnson & Knott, 1937). They found that when people who stutter read a passage repeatedly, their stuttering usually occurred less and less often through about six readings (Johnson & Knott, 1937; Van Riper & Hull, 1955).[12] These findings, called anticipation, consistency, and adaptation, respectively, changed some assumptions about the disorder. Stuttering, it seemed, was not simply a neurophysiological disorder. It had characteristics of learned behavior.

These studies not only changed existing views of stuttering, they also opened the door to new treatment possibilities. If much of stuttering is learned, it can be unlearned. The challenge was to determine how much is learned and how to help people who stutter develop new responses. Many of the treatment approaches we discuss later in the book were developed using this orientation.

LANGUAGE FACTORS

One member of the group of Iowa researchers, Spencer Brown, pushed investigations of the predictability of stuttering into the realm of language. In seven studies completed over a stretch of 10 years, Brown found that stuttering varied lawfully with seven grammatical factors during reading aloud.[13] He showed that most adults who stutter do so more frequently (*a*) on consonants, (*b*) on sounds in word-initial position, (*c*) in contextual speech (versus isolated words), (*d*) on nouns, verbs, adjectives, and adverbs (versus articles, prepositions, pronouns, and conjunctions), (*e*) on longer words, (*f*) on words at the beginnings of sentences, and (*g*) on stressed syllables. Evidently, stuttering is highly influenced by the language the stutterer uses.

Later investigators applied Brown's hypotheses to the speech of children who stutter.[14] They discovered that stuttering in elementary school children follows the same linguistic rules as stuttering in adults, but that stuttering in preschool children is different. Stuttering in these very young children occurs most frequently not on noun, verbs, adjectives, and adverbs, but on pronouns and conjunctions. It occurs not as repetitions, prolongations, or blocks of sounds in word-initial positions, but as repetitions of whole words

[11]Johnson & Solomon, 1937; Knott, Johnson, & Webster, 1937; Milisen, 1938; Van Riper, 1936.

[12]These studies were usually carried out by giving the stutterer a passage and asking him to read it aloud. If the experimenter were studying consistency, for example, he would have his own copy of the passage on which he would mark every word the stutterer stuttered on. Then he would ask the stutterer to read it again, and the experimenter would again mark the words stuttered on in the second reading. From this he could calculate the percentage of words stuttered in two (or more) readings.

[13]These findings were reported in the series of papers Brown published from 1935 to 1945 (Brown, 1937, 1938a, 1938b, 1938c, 1943, 1945; Brown & Moren, 1942; Johnson & Brown, 1935). However, only four of the factors (phonetic type, grammatical class, sentence position, and word length) are usually cited as "Brown's factors." The remaining three are brought out in the excellent discussion of Brown's work in Chapter 3 of Wingate's *The Structure of Stuttering* (1988).

[14]Bloodstein (1995) gives an excellent summary of this work.

in sentence-initial positions. This led researchers to hypothesize that, in its incipient stage, stuttering is located at the beginning of syntactic units (sentences and phrases), as if the task of linguistic planning and preparation was a key ingredient in the recipe for disfluency.[15]

FLUENCY-INDUCING CONDITIONS

One of the researchers at the University of Iowa, Oliver Bloodstein, wrote his Ph.D. dissertation on "Conditions Under Which Stuttering Is Reduced or Absent" (Bloodstein, 1948, 1950). In studying the speech of stutterers in 115 conditions, Bloodstein found that, in many of these conditions, stuttering is markedly decreased. Some of these conditions are speaking when alone, when relaxed, in unison with another speaker, to an animal or an infant, in time to a rhythmic stimulus or singing, in a dialect, while simultaneously writing, and when swearing. In later studies, additional conditions that were found to reduce stuttering included, among others, speaking in a slow prolonged manner, speaking under loud masking noise, speaking while listening to delayed auditory feedback, shadowing another speaker, speaking with reinforcement for fluent speech. Various explanations tried to account for the impact of these conditions. Most are compatible with the idea that stuttering has a substantial learned component and is affected by external stimuli such as communicative pressure. Recently, however, new explanations have appeared,[16] reflecting a new trend of thought about stuttering. It has been suggested that "reduced stuttering is associated with conditions in which the neurophysiological demands of speech motor control and language formulation are reduced" (Andrews, Howie, Dozsa, & Guitar, 1982). For example, conditions such as speaking in time to a rhythmic stimulus reduce the demands on both linguistic and motor systems to generate the prosody for speech; whereas speaking slowly reduces demands because language formulation and motor coordination are easier at a slow rate. Some studies suggest that reduced demands may be needed because the brain organization for motor speech and language functions of adults who stutter may not favor rapid processing.

AN INTEGRATION OF FACTORS

Modern research on stuttering has taken a long and complex journey from Travis's laboratory at Iowa in the 1920s. Yet in many ways, its origins have not been forgotten. Travis's view of stuttering as a neurophysiological disorder has reappeared with a new sophistication that incorporates a better understanding of speech and language production and acknowledges a learning component.

This updated view is essentially the model of stuttering presented in this book. We see stuttering as a disorder of neuromotor control of speech, influenced by the interactive processes of language production and intensified by temperament and complex learning processes. Neuromotor control of speech is disordered because inheritance or injury has resulted in an inefficient or unstable cerebral organization. The neuromotor control of these children begins to show disruption as their language development in preschool years requires planning and production of larger and more complex syntactic units. Children who do not spontaneously recover and become persistent stutterers are those who

---

[15]Excellent reviews and theorizing about the language component in stuttering can be found in Wingate (1988) and Bernstein Ratner (1997).

[16]Among many who have proposed new explanation of fluency-inducing conditions are: Andrews, Howie, Dozsa, & Guitar (1982); Martin & Haroldson (1979); Perkins, Rudas, Johnson, & Bell (1976); and Wingate (1969, 1970).

learn maladaptive responses to disruptions. This learning is influenced by biological temperament, developing social and cognitive awareness, and the response of the environment to the speech of these children.

The next few chapters expand on this theme and prepare you to use this information in diagnosis and treatment.

SUMMARY

Stuttering appears in all cultures and has been a problem for humankind for at least 40 centuries. It is characterized by a high frequency or severity of disruptions that impede the forward flow of speech. It begins in childhood and usually becomes more severe with age unless the child recovers with or without formal treatment.

Core behaviors of stuttering are repetitions, prolongations, and blocks. Secondary behaviors are the result of attempts to escape or avoid core behaviors, which include physical concomitants of stuttering, such as eye blinks, or verbal concomitants, such as word substitution. Feelings and attitudes can also be important components of stuttering, which reflect the stutterer's emotional reactions to the experience of being unable to speak fluently and to listener responses to his stuttering. Feelings are immediate reactions and include such emotions as fear and embarrassment. Attitudes crystallize more slowly, from repeated stuttering experiences associated with negative feelings. An example is a stutterer's belief that listeners think he is stupid when they hear him stuttering.

Stuttering begins in childhood, some time between 18 months and puberty, but most often between ages 2 and 5 years. Its first appearance may be either a gradual increase in easy repetitions of words and sounds or a sudden occurrence of multiple, tense repetitions, prolongations, or blocks. Prevalence of stuttering is about 1%. Incidence is about 5%. Recovery rate without professional treatment is between 50% and 85% of children who ever stuttered. The larger percentage probably reflects children who were very mild stutterers or who stuttered for a very brief time. The male-to-female ratio is about 3:1 but may be lower, perhaps 1:1 in very young children who start to stutter. More girls appear to recover during childhood, increasing the proportion of males with the disorder after puberty.

Many persons who stutter are able to predict accurately which words in a reading passage they will stutter on (anticipation). In addition, most tend to stutter on many of the same words each time in repeated readings of a paragraph (consistency). On the other hand, stuttering frequency decreases for most stutterers when they read a passage over many times (adaptation). Stuttering occurs more frequently in certain grammatical contexts. Research has also revealed that a variety of conditions reduce the frequency of stuttering. Their effects may be attributable to changes in speech pattern, reductions in communicative pressure, or both. Research on these fluency-inducing conditions has recently suggested that stuttering may be decreased by reducing the demands on speech motor control and language formulation.

STUDY QUESTIONS

1. What are the differences between "core" and "secondary" behaviors in stuttering?
2. When stuttering is defined, what other kinds of hesitation must it be distinguished from?
3. What are some feelings and attitudes persons who stutter might have, and why do they have them?

4. What is the age range for the onset of stuttering (the youngest and oldest ages at which onset is commonly reported)?
5. What is the difference between "incidence" and "prevalence"?
6. What problems do researchers encounter when they try to determine how many stutterers recover without treatment?
7. Why does the ratio of male-to-female stutterers change?
8. In what ways is stuttering predictable? In what ways does it vary?

SUGGESTED READINGS

Bloodstein, O. (1993). *Stuttering: The search for a cause and cure*. Boston: Allyn & Bacon.
This book is part history and part analysis, written with charm and clarity. Bloodstein covers early treatments for stuttering, the burgeoning of research the 1930s, 1940s, and 1950s, and more recent findings in the realm of neurophysiology. His own orientation on the learning-environmental basis of stuttering comes through, but he gives good coverage of other possible factors as well. Bloodstein is particularly good at conveying the excitement that accompanies research.

Jezer, M. (1997). *Stuttering: A life bound up in words*. New York: Basic Books.
A compelling, sensitive book about the frustrating and sometimes funny things that happen to someone growing up with a severe stuttering problem and learning to cope with it.

Johnson, W., and Leutenegger, R. (1955). *Stuttering in children and adults*. Minneapolis: University of Minnesota Press.
These authors have compiled the research papers from one of the most productive research efforts ever applied to stuttering. These studies, conducted between 1930 and 1950 at the University of Iowa, uncovered many of the basic facts we have about the variability and predictability of stuttering. The first chapter, "The Time, the Place, and the Problem," gives a historical perspective on this research.

Shields, D. (1989). *Dead languages*. New York: Knopf.
This is a novel about a young boy who stutters. It conveys the feelings associated with being a stutterer in a world that prizes spoken language. It is recommended for students who would like to understand a child who stutters.

Wingate, M. (1988). *The structure of stuttering: A psycholinguistic analysis*. New York: Springer-Verlag.
Wingate builds a logical case for the explanation of stuttering as a neurological disorder whose overt symptoms are the result of dyssynchrony in utterance planning and assembly. It reflects current thinking that stuttering has an important language component.

2

Constitutional Factors in Stuttering

ROLE OF HEREDITY

A well-known fact about stuttering is that it often runs in families. For many years, researchers debated about what this meant. Some suggested that stuttering must be inherited because it passed from generation to generation. Others disagreed, noting that political beliefs often run in families, too, but they aren't inherited. Stuttering is learned, they argued, in response to a critical attitude toward disfluency that has been handed down from one generation to the next. A child whose parents were critical of his normal disfluencies would grow afraid and would "hesitate to hesitate." This would start a spiral of more hesitations leading to greater fear, and so on.

For many years researchers aligned themselves with one side of this argument or the other. In the past two decades, a version of the genetic hypothesis has become widely accepted. In part, this may be due to strong new evidence about heredity in stuttering, but it is probably also due to a less deterministic view of heredity. Stuttering, asthma, migraine, and certain other disorders are seen as the result of both heredity *and* environment, acting together, with elements of chance thrown in (Kidd, 1984).

In this chapter, we review three approaches to heredity and stuttering: family studies, twin studies, and adoption studies. These different ways of gathering evidence all suggest that stuttering is partly attributable to heredity. The insights we gain from these studies are vital to us in counseling individuals and families about the risks for passing on stuttering and the prognosis for recovery in children who show signs of disfluency.

Family Studies

Researchers gather evidence of the inheritance of stuttering by looking at family trees of stutterers. They interview family members to find out who, if anyone, among the stutterer's relatives also stutters. At the same time, a control group of nonstutterers is formed of persons matched with the stutterers for age, sex, and other important characteristics. Researchers construct family trees for the control group also and compare the two groups to determine whether stutterers have more stuttering relatives than do nonstutterers. They also search for patterns of occurrence of stuttering (such as those reflecting mendelian types of inheritance) that will rule out nonhereditary explanations such as imitation and family attitudes.

Early Studies

One family study to provide evidence of genetic transmission of stuttering was an interim report on an ongoing study of 1000 families in Newcastle, England. Gavin Andrews and Mary Ann Harris, with the help of genetic researchers Roger Garside and David Kay, investigated the family histories of 80 stuttering children (Andrews & Harris, 1964). They found that (a) stutterers had far more stuttering relatives than did nonstutterers, (b) males in this group were more at risk than females for developing stuttering, and (c) females who stuttered were more likely to have stuttering relatives than were male stutterers. Their results supported a model of stuttering that could be transmitted by either a single gene or a combination of several genes contributing different factors (such as a factor affecting speech timing and a factor affecting tremor proneness).

A geneticist at Yale University, Kenneth Kidd, and his coworkers followed up the British study by looking for familial patterns of stuttering in the United States (Kidd, 1977; Kidd, Kidd, & Records, 1978; Kidd, Reich, & Kessler, 1973). They first reexamined the Andrews and Harris (1964) data, combined with evidence they gathered themselves, and used statistical models to predict the pattern of inheritance. In this and subsequent studies they were able to predict with remarkable accuracy which relatives of stutterers would also stutter. For example, males were more likely to stutter than females; females who stuttered were more likely to have relatives who stuttered. Kidd (1984) concluded that these patterns are best explained by an interaction between the environment and a combination of several genes.

Recent Studies

Research by Ambrose and associates (1993) supports some of these earlier findings, but also differs in important ways. Using the families of 69 very young children who were near the onset of stuttering, Ambrose and associates examined the frequency of stuttering in their relatives. They found that two thirds of these children had relatives who stuttered and that, as in earlier studies, more male relatives than female relatives stuttered. Unlike past studies, however, the researchers found that male and female children had similar chances of having relatives who stuttered. This differs from the findings of Andrews and

Harris and of Kidd and coworkers (1978), which suggested that females who stutter are likely to have more relatives who stutter than are males who stutter.

The differences in these studies may be the result of the differences in subjects' ages and the persistence of their stuttering. Andrews and Harris's subjects were children with a wide age range of onset (up to 11 years old); Kidd and coworkers' subjects were adults who still stuttered. On the other hand, the subjects of Ambrose and associates (1993) were very young children, all close to the age of onset, many of whom recovered from stuttering quickly.

The reason why Andrews and Harris and why Kidd and his colleagues found that female subjects have a higher proportion of stuttering relatives may be because females in these studies were older, with persistent rather than transient versions of the disorder. So they may thus have carried higher "genetic loadings" for stuttering, which means their relatives were also more likely to have received or passed on more of such genetic material. On the other hand, Ambrose and colleagues' very young female subjects often recovered quickly from stuttering and thus may have been less genetically loaded and have fewer relatives who stuttered.

The differences in the subjects studied suggest that these experimenters may have been focusing on different levels of chronicity. The findings of the studies of Andrews and Harris and of Kidd and associates, whose subjects were children of all ages and adults, may be more relevant to persistent stuttering because of the greater percentage of subjects who had stuttered for several years. On the other hand, the data from Ambrose and associates (1993), gathered from children whose stuttering had just begun, may apply to both persistent and transient stuttering, because some of these children were shown to recover quickly and others did not.[1]

Another difference in the three studies is in the genetic models that best describe their data. Ambrose and associates (1993) found inheritance patterns that most neatly fit a model of genetic transmission by a single gene. The data of Kidd (1984) supported a model of transmission by several genes, each of which may be contributing to different factors. This disparity might again be accounted for by differences in subjects. The single-gene model might best fit data that includes very young subjects, many of whom recover (more than 80% of subjects recovered in Ambrose and associates' study). Their stuttering may be a somewhat less complex form of the disorder. Those subjects whose stuttering persists into adulthood (as in the study of Kidd et al., 1973) may inherit additional factors that increase the likelihood that stuttering will be chronic. Their inheritance may best fit a polygenic multifactorial model.

Critical Reviews of Genetic Research

In a recent chapter reviewing genetics of stuttering, Felsenfeld (1997) noted several limitations of the studies mentioned in the previous paragraphs. First, no matched control groups of nonstutterers were used in many of these studies. The studies relied instead on incidence figures from other studies, making the comparison of the incidence of stuttering between families of stutterers and nonstutterers less valid. Second, the data in the first two studies, which reported more stutterers in the families of female stutterers, may be affected by the tendency of females who stutter to be overly sensitive to the presence of the disorder in other family members, as has been shown in other research.

---

[1] A recent study by Janssen, Kloth, Kraaimaat, and Brutten (1996) using adult stutterers found, as did Ambrose, Yairi, and Cox (1993), no greater incidence of stuttering in relatives of females who stutter than males who stutter.

The study by Ambrose and associates (1993) questioned parents of subjects to determine whether other family members stuttered, removing such sensitivity as a possible bias factor. In a recent critical review of the genetics of stuttering, Yairi, Ambrose, and Cox (1996) detailed methodological problems that have plagued many of the past genetic studies. These problems include inadequate definitions of stuttering when interviewing subjects about their relatives, lack of personal interviews of the relatives who were identified, exclusion of relatives beyond first-degree family members, and inaccurate counts of relatives who recovered early.

Yairi, Ambrose, and Cox (1996) suggested that future studies may want to examine subgroups of stutterers, the influence of inheritance on recovery, characteristics of family members who don't stutter, environmental factors that may interact with genetics, and how clinical practice can use data from genetic studies to focus early intervention on those who are less likely to recover without treatment. It is noteworthy that Yairi, Ambrose, Paden, and Throneburg (1996) also identified several variables, which seem to be associated with recovery from stuttering in their sample. Among the characteristics of those who recovered were (a) good scores on tests of phonology, language, and nonverbal skills, (b) family members who had recovered from stuttering, and (c) early age of onset of stuttering.

In summary, despite the small number of studies and their limitations, family studies have provided strong evidence that many stutterers appear to inherit a predisposition for stuttering. Research has not shown what that predisposition is or exactly what physical differences exist in stutterers that may give rise to the symptoms of stuttering.[2]

Twin Studies

The genetic transmission of stuttering can also be investigated by comparing the incidence of stuttering in fraternal and identical twins. Identical twins (also called monozygotic twins) have identical genes. Fraternal twins (dizygotic) may share only half their genes, like any other siblings. Greater similarities in the traits of identical twins compared with those of fraternal twins are generally attributed to inheritance. Twin studies of stuttering have shown that stuttering occurs more often in both members of identical twin pairs than in both members of fraternal, same-sex twin pairs (Andrews et al., 1990; Howie, 1981; Luchsinger, 1944; Seeman, 1937). To use the vocabulary of genetics, there is higher "concordance" for stuttering in identical twins than in fraternal twins. This supports the hypothesis that stuttering is inherited. But it doesn't reveal what is inherited. How does a gene (or several genes) affect a child's speech so that stuttering results? No one is sure. Later in this chapter, we present several "educated guesses" about how an inherited difference might result in stuttering.

In addition to evidence of genetic factors in stuttering, twin studies demonstrate that heredity does not work alone. In one of the twin studies previously cited, although there was higher concordance for stuttering among identical twins, some pairs were discordant (Howie, 1981). In 6 of 16 identical twin pairs, one twin stuttered, but the other didn't. This finding means that environmental factors, as well as genetic factors, are at work to

---

[2] Genetic differences between stutterers and nonstutterers may be extremely subtle and not evident in the child at birth. Researchers have found, for example, that heredity may govern the extent to which an individual may be classically conditioned to fear. Such genetically determined tendencies appear only when environmental conditions are right for learning a fear-induced response.

   Cox (1988) has speculated that the inherited predisposition may be something that interferes with or slows brain maturation, perhaps momentarily, during the preschool years, since onset and recovery seem to be so tied to cognitive, motor, and linguistic development.

create stuttering, at least in some individuals. Remember that environmental factors include prenatal and neonatal physical stress, common in twins, which can cause brain damage. These and perhaps other environmental influences must have interacted differentially with genetic predisposition to produce stuttering for one twin but not the other in these six cases.

An estimate of the relative proportions of genetic and environmental influences was suggested in a later study involving 3810 unselected twin pairs (Andrews et al., 1990). Analysis of these data suggested that 71% of the variance (the probability of whether or not one would stutter) is accounted for by genetic factors, and 29% is accounted for by the individual's environment (including factors influencing the fetus, as well as factors after birth). We hope that future research will reveal the critical aspects of the environment that have this effect. Many environmental factors—which can be influenced by early treatment—have been under scrutiny for some time and are discussed in the next chapter.

In general, researchers who conduct family studies and those who conduct twin studies agree that inheritance plays an important role in stuttering, as does environment. Stuttering is likely to be the result of one or several inherited (or congenital) factors and several environmental factors, which interact in different combinations and proportions for different individuals (see, e.g., Cox, Seider, & Kidd, 1984; Felsenfeld, 1997).

Adoption Studies

One of the most powerful ways to examine the relative contributions of genes and the environment to stuttering would be to look at the families of stutterers who were adopted soon after birth. Greater occurrence of stuttering among the biological relatives of adopted stutterers would support a genetic hypothesis. Greater occurrence of stuttering among adoptive relatives would support an environmental hypothesis.

Because the birth records of adopted children are difficult to obtain, studies of adopted stutterers are rare. Bloodstein (1995) has reported on a sample of 13 adopted stutterers whom he interviewed about stuttering in their adoptive families (information on their biological families was not available). Bloodstein found that 4 of the 13 stutterers reported having relatives who stuttered in their adoptive families, which is slightly higher than would be expected by chance. This small sample, without data from biological families, supports the possibility that environmental factors may have an effect.

Felsenfeld (1997) reported some preliminary data on a small sample of adopted children who had speech disorders (primarily stuttering) and for whom data were available from *both* adoptive and biological families. These data suggested that a history of stuttering in the biological families was slightly more predictive of disorders in these children than was stuttering in the adoptive family.

In short, the evidence suggests that both genetic inheritance and environment are factors in determining whether or not a child will stutter.

Summary

Studies of the families of persons who stutter indicate that relatives of stutterers are at greater risk for stuttering than are relatives of nonstutterers. Females appear to be more resistant than males to stuttering, but relatives of female stutterers might be more likely to stutter. Twin studies show higher concordance for stuttering in identical twins than in fraternal twins. Some identical twin pairs, however, are discordant, which shows that environmental influences are active in some cases. There are only preliminary findings from stutterers who have been adopted, but they suggest that both heredity and environment may be important.

Some unknown factor appears to be inherited, creating a predisposition for stuttering. There may be several predisposing factors, which can act singly or together. Environmental factors may be needed to trigger stuttering in children who have this predisposition. In some cases, the predisposition may be there, but a facilitating environment may nurture fluency and these children never develop stuttering.

DIFFERENCES BETWEEN STUTTERERS AND NONSTUTTERERS

Pinpointing inherited and congenital predisposing factors in stuttering is difficult. To find the cause of a disorder, a researcher must be able to manipulate the conditions that create it. For example, some of the causes of cleft palate have been discovered because researchers selectively bred animals to produce cleft palates. In doing so, researchers were able to identify some of the etiological influences that produce clefting. But communication through spoken language does not occur in animals, which eliminates their use in studying factors that would disrupt such behavior. And obviously, selective breeding or surgery to create stuttering is not an option in humans. Therefore, researchers have turned to indirect approaches. They compare groups of stutterers and nonstutterers on tasks that might be related to speech fluency. If they find, again and again, that these groups perform differently in certain tasks, they may have a clue about the disorder.

Such indirect research is complicated because the differences that are found might be a *result* of stuttering, not a cause of it. For example, in a study of how quickly subjects can say a word that is flashed on a screen, the results might show that stutterers are slower than nonstutterers. This difference, however, might be the result of stutterers saying words more slowly to keep from stuttering. Even if a difference were not the result of trying not to stutter, it might be only a distantly related factor that has no functional relationship to stuttering: some stutterers may have slower reaction times but it is clear that slower reaction times do not cause stuttering. If they did, may of us would start stuttering as we grow older. It's like finding that basketball players have larger shoe sizes than gymnasts. Shoe size doesn't determine who is better suited for each of these sports, but height may be a determining factor. And both shoe size and height are related to one's genetically determined bone size.

Another problem with the indirect approach to studying the nature of stuttering is that comparisons of groups of people who stutter and people who don't often show much overlap, even though the group performances might be statistically different. For example, in an experiment to test motor coordination, some of the people who stutter may show coordination as good as the average person in the group of nonstutterers. And some of the people who don't stutter may demonstrate the same level of coordination as the average person who does stutter. These overlaps remind us that we are typically not looking at factors that are necessary or sufficient by themselves to create stuttering in a person.

In the following section we review findings from studies that compare stutterers and nonstutterers. The literature has many inconsistent research findings that turn up when scientists try to repeat each others' experiments to verify their results. One study finds a difference, but another study reports that it isn't there. Sometimes conflict between the findings of two studies may occur because there are small differences in the way the studies are done. For example, one study may use a 1000-Hz tone for a stimulus, and another study may use a recording of the word "go." Despite these conflicts in results, there are certain areas of agreement. In the following sections, we summarize findings in several important areas in which stutterers and nonstutterers have been compared. In many cases, researchers agree that an important difference between stutterers and nonstutterers has been found.

Intelligence

Several early studies of stutterers' intelligence showed that they were close to the test's norm or only slightly below it (Berry, 1937; Darley, 1955; Johnson et al., 1942; Schindler, 1955; West, 1931). These studies were plagued by lack of control groups of nonstutterers in some cases and by highly selected groups of subjects in others.[3] The slightly lower intelligence quotients (IQs) of the stuttering group, found by a few studies, were usually dismissed as a result of stuttering, not the cause of it. Researchers assumed that stutterers might often be reluctant to give a correct answer because they were afraid of stuttering.

Other studies, using both verbal and nonverbal IQ tests, have shown conflicting results. Andrews and Harris (1964) and Okasha and colleagues (1974) found that IQ scores of children who stuttered were slightly but significantly lower than in children who didn't. The Andrews and Harris study, however, is plagued by the fact that a number of the children in their sample were retarded, which would have depressed the mean IQ of the stuttering group. A study of school-age boys who stuttered and matched fluent controls found that the groups were not significantly different in intelligence (Nippold, Schwarz, & Jescheniak, 1991). Another recent study found that nonverbal intelligence was slightly lower among children who stuttered than a matched control group and that higher nonverbal intelligence seemed to be associated with greater chances of recovery from stuttering (Yairi, Ambrose, Paden, & Throneburg, 1996).

One might guess that, if there is a connection between fluent speech and intelligence, it is because fluent speech relies on intact cognitive functions such as language, sensory-motor processing, memory, and perception. Thus, those who have evident deficits in cognition might be more prone to stuttering. Indeed, Van Riper observed that among those who are mentally retarded, the less intelligent have a higher incidence of stuttering than the more intelligent (Van Riper, 1982).

In summary, there may be slight differences in the average verbal and nonverbal IQ scores of groups of people who stutter and groups who don't stutter. These differences may be related to artifacts of the testing situation or to differences in sample characteristics, or they may be the result of subtle differences in cognitive functioning such as language processing, sensory-motor skills, or perception.

Before leaving this section, we should note that the differences found between stutterers and nonstutterers are based on IQ tests that were designed to measure "general intelligence." This is the unidimensional mental attribute used in the controversial book *The Bell Curve* (Herrnstein & Murray, 1994). A more modern view of mental ability, originating from the work of Thurston and Guilford, and recently elaborated by Howard Gardner (1983), is the concept of "multiple intelligences." Recently, Stephen Jay Gould (1996) examined the genius of Charles Darwin, one of the most famous of all stutterers,[4] and

---

[3] The studies of Darley (1955) and Johnson et al. (1942) were conducted with children from the University of Iowa community. This sample is unlikely to be representative of the general population, and so it doesn't tell us much about the disorder of stuttering per se.

[4] A description of Charles Darwin's stuttering can be found in his son's essay, "Reminiscences of My Father's Everyday Life" (Darwin, 1950).

concluded that his mental powers were best described as "a substantial set of largely independent attributes" rather than the traditional general intelligence. Perhaps if tests
made use of more modern concepts of intelligence, no differences would be found between stutterers and nonstutterers.

School Performance

Studies have shown that stutterers perform slightly below average in school. Stutterers
are more likely than their nonstuttering peers to be a grade behind, and their achievement test scores are lower (Schindler, 1955). At least two factors may contribute to stutterers' poorer school achievement. One is their difficulty in talking, simply because of
stuttering. Many stutterers, including the author during his school days, would answer "I
don't know" to a teacher's question rather than risk stuttering. The other factor is a deficit
in language-related skills, as shown by various standardized tests (Williams, Melrose, &
Woods, 1969). Consider how much of school involves reading, as well as both oral and
written verbal expression. In such a verbal environment as this, both of these factors
would put some stutterers at a disadvantage.

Speech and Language Development

If stuttering arises from constitutional differences in some children, it is natural to ask
whether other speech and language abilities besides fluency are affected. In general, research has found that other speech and language difficulties are more common among children who stutter than those who don't, but the findings are neither simple nor clear-cut.

When assessed on such measures as the ages at which they said their first word and
their first sentence, size of receptive vocabulary, mean length of utterance, and expressive and receptive syntax, children who stutter often score lower than their peers (Andrews & Harris, 1964; Berry, 1938; Darley, 1955; Kline & Starkweather, 1979; Murray
& Reed, 1977; Okasha et al., 1974; Wall, 1980; Westby, 1979; Williams, Melrose, &
Woods, 1969). However, other studies did not find language differences (e.g., Johnson,
1955; Peters, 1968; Seider, Gladstien, & Kidd, 1982).

Children who stutter have also been shown to have difficulty with articulation. In the
clinic, we often observe children in the early stages of stuttering who have multiple articulation or phonological problems and are consequently difficult to understand. Research has repeatedly confirmed the finding that stutterers have roughly two and a half
times the incidence of articulation disorders as that found in nonstutterers (Andrews &
Harris, 1964; Berry, 1938; Bloodstein, 1958; Kent & Williams, 1963; Williams, Silverman,
& Kools, 1968). Nevertheless, a smaller number of studies have found no differences in
articulation ability between children who stutter and children who don't stutter (Ryan,
1992; Seider, Gladstien, & Kidd, 1982).

Two excellent critical reviews of the research on language, phonology, and stuttering
have emerged. In the first review, Nippold (1990) suggests that research does not clearly
support the hypothesis that children who stutter are also likely to have language or articulation difficulties. Rather, she suggests that there may be subgroups of children who stutter who have language or articulation problems related to their stuttering. Bernstein Ratner (1997) concurs and notes that the differences that have been found between groups
of children who stutter and children who don't stutter have been very subtle. She suggests
that future research should use more sophisticated tests of language and phonology and
should look for subgroupings, not only in children, but also in adults who stutter.

These findings about deficits in articulation and language performance at least in some children who stutter can be interpreted in several ways. Some authors have suggested that children who have difficulty with articulation or language will start to believe that speaking is difficult. Their anticipation of difficulty is hypothesized to lead to hesitation and struggle, and then to stuttering (Bloodstein, 1995, 1997). An alternate view is that stuttering, language disorders, and articulation errors all come from a common deficit, which might be passed on genetically. Because circumscribed areas of the brain are responsible for speech and language-related functions, delayed development of (or damage to) these areas may result in language, articulation, or fluency problems in any combination. Small differences in how the brain processes such functions could tip the balance toward any of these disorders.

Another view is that articulation or language disorders may somehow make recovery from stuttering more difficult. This is reflected in the findings of Conture, Louko, and Edwards (1993), St. Louis (1991), and Yairi and associates (1996), whose studies suggest that those children who stutter and also have phonological or language differences are more likely to persist in stuttering.

Anxiety and Autonomic Arousal

The average listener may think that someone who stutters does so because he or she is nervous. Scientists, following up on this impression, have used such terms as "negative emotion," "anxiety," or "autonomic arousal" to specify the emotional states that may cause or accompany stuttering. Researchers have asked whether people who stutter are more anxious than people who don't stutter, and have used measures of physiological arousal such as heart rate, skin conductance, and cortisol secretion to answer those questions. The results of four studies (Caruso, Chodzko-Zajko, Bidinger, & Sommers, 1994; Miller, 1993; Peters & Hulstijn, 1984; Weber & Smith, 1990) indicate that people who stutter are not more anxious than people who don't stutter. Both stutterers and nonstutterers show high levels of autonomic arousal when they have to speak or read aloud, which does not support the belief that stutterers are more nervous or more anxious than nonstutterers.

Several studies of autonomic arousal have shown that higher levels of arousal are associated with more disfluency (Caruso et al., 1995; Miller, 1993; Weber & Smith, 1990). It may be that, although most speakers show increased arousal when they have to speak, only the speech production system of those who stutter is vulnerable to the effects of high arousal.[5] In addition, arousal and stuttering may be chained together so that arousal makes stuttering more likely; when stuttering occurs, it precipitates even greater arousal, which in turn precipitates more stuttering. Thus, effective therapy may need to help an individual maintain fluency under stress as well as reduce the arousal that stuttering itself elicits by providing tools to cope with stuttering.

Sensitivity

A number of authors have speculated that persons who stutter may have been born with an especially sensitive temperament (e.g, Bloodstein, 1987, 1995; Conture, 1991). Such a temperament might trigger distress and increased physical tension in a child when he

---

[5] It is evident, however, that many nonstutterers are more disfluent under stress. White and Collins (1984) have shown that nonstutterers sometimes think people who stutter are nervous because the nonstutterers recognize that they themselves become disfluent when they are nervous.

is disfluent. On the other hand, a placid temperament in an equally disfluent child might allow him to ignore the disfluencies and promote recovery.

Data on sensitivity in people who stutter are meager. In a study using questionnaires, Oyler (1992) found that adults who stutter were more emotionally sensitive than adults who didn't stutter. However, hypersensitivity in adults could be the result of many years of stuttering. Greater sensitivity in children who stutter has been reported in two studies. Fowlie and Cooper (1978) reported that mothers of children who stutter viewed their children as more sensitive than did mothers describing children who do not stutter. Oyler and Ramig (1995) found that parents of children who stutter rated them as more sensitive than did control parents rating their nonstuttering children. Unfortunately, both of these studies used school-age children, whose sensitivity could have been influenced already by their stuttering.

Future studies should assess children just beginning to stutter, comparing their sensitivity with that of a matched control group to determine to what extent sensitivity is associated with the onset of stuttering. Measures of sensitivity should not be limited to parent reports, but should include observation of behavior (see Calkins & Fox, 1994; Kagan, Reznick, & Snidman, 1987). The further question of whether sensitivity may be related to recovery from stuttering can be addressed via longitudinal studies to see whether those who fail to recover have higher scores on various measures of sensitivity and those who recover have lower scores.

Sensory-Motor Coordination

REACTION TIME

Many studies interested in stutterers' sensory-motor coordination have measured how fast stutterers can push a button when they hear a buzzer or how rapidly they can say a word that is flashed on a screen. These reaction time tasks assess a person's sensory (input) and motor (output) systems working together, mediated by a central processor. The first experiments compared vocal reaction time in stuttering and nonstuttering adults and found that adults who stuttered were slower in starting and stopping a sound such as "ahhh" when they heard a buzzer (Adams & Hayden, 1976; Starkweather, Hirschman, & Tannenbaum, 1976).

Gradually researchers broadened their focus. They discovered that stutterers were slower in reacting with respiratory (exhalation) and articulatory movements (lip closing) (McFarlane & Prins, 1978; Watson & Alfonso, 1987). They found that stutterers were slower than nonstutterers whether they are responding to an auditory or a visual signal (e.g., Cross & Cooke, 1979). They found that children who stutter also have slower reaction times (Cross & Luper, 1979, 1983; Cullinan & Springer, 1980; Maske-Cash & Curlee, 1995; Till, Reich, Dickey, & Sieber, 1983).[6] And they discovered that adults who stutter are slower in "tracking" a tone that goes up and down in pitch (Neilson, Quinn, & Neilson, 1976; Nudelman, Herbrich, Hoyt, & Rosenfield, 1987).

In summarizing the many and varied findings in this area, De Nil (1995) pointed out that of about 44 studies of voice reaction time, 75% showed that people who stutter were significantly slower than people who don't stutter, and most of the other studies showed trends in that direction. Furthermore, when investigators used linguistically meaningful

---

[6] These studies actually found that significant differences from nonstuttering children were found only in children who stuttered *and* had language, articulation, or learning problems. This was confirmed in a further study by McKnight and Cullinan (1987). Maske-Cash and Curlee (1995) found that both a stuttering-only and a stuttering-plus-other speech and language disorders group were both slower than control children, but the children with other disorders were slower than the stuttering-only children.

stimuli to test reaction time (words or sentences, rather than isolated sounds), 80% of the studies found significant differences between stutterers and nonstutterers. Thus, the extra time stuttering speakers need to respond may be, in part, related to increased demands of linguistically meaningful stimuli.

Trying to understand what this may mean is easier if we can picture three stages involved in speech reaction time responses. Figure 2.1 shows that the person's first task in a reaction time experiment is to perceptually analyze the stimulus (usually an auditory or visual cue). The second task is one that most persons would hardly be aware of—"planning" or "preparing" the response. This involves selecting the sounds and words and placing them in the proper sequence, a task we do every time we speak, but we do it automatically without being conscious of it. The third task is executing the response. This means sending commands from the brain to speech muscles in the right sequence and having the muscles carry out those commands. In Figure 2.1, these tasks are done in "parallel" fashion. That is, the brain is working on parts of each task at the same time.

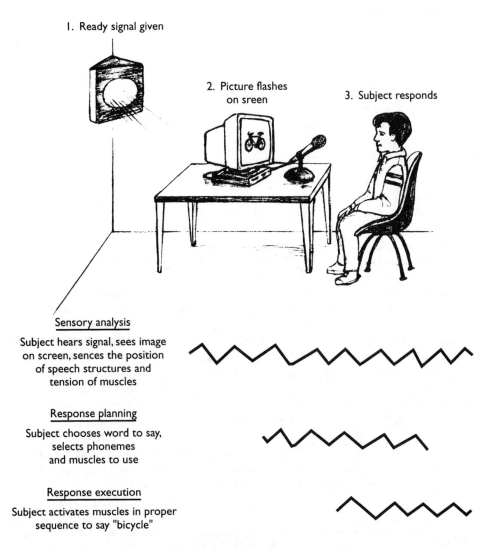

Figure 2.1. Processing stages in a reaction time task.

Models of the way humans process information and respond are based on the view that we have a finite supply of neuronal resources in our brains, and if a task is difficult and requires extra neuronal resources, other tasks have fewer neuronal resources at their disposal and must be done more slowly. Thus, slower reaction times in stutterers may result from difficulties in any or all of the three areas: sensory analysis, response planning, or response execution.

We do not know whether stutterers' apparently slower reaction times arise from a difficulty at one or more stages of sensory-motor processing. Michael Rastatter and Carl Dell (1987) suggested that inefficient language processing during sensory analysis may slow stutterers' reaction times. Megan and Peter Neilson (1991) believe that lack of adequate neuronal resources for "sensorimotor modelling" during the response planning stage may make stutterers inherently slower. Pascal van Lieshout (1995) makes a strong case for stutterers' slower reaction times being a result of slower response execution. He argues that people who stutter inherently lack finesse in verbal motor skills and therefore must use a more carefully controlled form of speech production to remain fluent. This would be like a clumsy driver needing to drive slowly and constantly correct his steering to avoid accidents.

We return to some of these ideas when we present theories of constitutional differences in stutterers. But it is important to note that all of these data and speculations have to be related to the disorder of stuttering. The connection must be made between the deficits that cause slower reaction times and the symptoms of stuttering. How does it happen that a speech motor system that responds slowly sometimes breaks down into repetitions, prolongations, and blocks?

CENTRAL AUDITORY PROCESSING

In their search for a physiological basis of stuttering, researchers have investigated many different parts of the speech and language mechanism, including the auditory system. It is known that learning to speak involves both the motor processes of speaking and the sensory processes of feeling and hearing oneself speak. Some researchers have suspected that stuttering may be the result of errors in how people who stutter hear themselves speak. In exploring this hypothesis, researchers have measured how stutterers' central nervous systems handle various sounds, including speech.

Assessment tools that were developed to detect tumors and other lesions in the auditory system, such as the Synthetic Sentence Identification Test (Jerger, Speaks, & Trammell, 1968), have been applied to adults who stutter with interesting results. Several studies have shown that people who stutter perform more poorly than people who don't stutter on tasks requiring discrimination of small time differences in signals (Hall & Jerger, 1978; Toscher & Rupp, 1978; Kramer, Green, & Guitar, 1987).[7]

One of the tasks that has shown group differences between stutterers and nonstutterers is the Masking Level Difference test. It requires listeners to detect the onset and offset of a tone in the presence of a masking noise. When masking noise is played in the same ear as the tone, there are fewer cues for the listener to use to "filter out" the masking noise and "filter in" the tone. The listener must use very subtle temporal cues to detect the tone, and it is under these conditions that people who stutter, as a group, perform most poorly, when compared to groups of nonstutterers.

---

[7] A review of the research on stutterers' auditory functioning can be found in D.B. Rosenfield and J. Jerger, "Stuttering and Auditory Function" in R. Curlee and W. Perkins' (eds.) *Nature and Treatment of Stuttering*, San Diego: College-Hill Press (1984).

Researchers have speculated that temporal processing of incoming signals is a particular weakness of stutterers who perform poorly on central auditory tests. They have tried to link this weakness to stuttering by suggesting that a single mechanism in the brain may control timing functions for both incoming and outgoing signals (e.g., Kent, 1983). Faulty processing of the temporal dimensions of incoming signals would give rise to stutterers' poorer performance on central auditory tests. Faulty processing of outgoing signals could result in stuttering.

CEREBRAL DOMINANCE

Researchers have also theorized that input and output timing deficits in people who stutter may be related to the cerebral hemisphere of the brain that is dominant for speech. Speakers use both right and left hemispheres of the brain for speech, but the left is usually dominant. This is so, scientists speculate, because the left hemisphere is more specialized for processing brief, rapidly changing signals (like the quick shift of /t/ into /o/ in the word "toe") than the right hemisphere (Liberman, Cooper, Shankweiler, & Studdert-Kennedy, 1967). The right hemisphere is specialized for processing more slowly changing signals, such as music, environmental sounds, and the intonation patterns of speech (Hammond, 1982).

Some experimenters have found that people who stutter are poorer at tests of central auditory processing and have suggested that this deficit occurs because people who stutter do not use their left hemisphere for speech and language functions as efficiently as nonstutterers do. Instead, experimenters suggest that people who stutter use their right hemisphere, which leads to intermittent breakdowns because the right hemisphere is not so adept as the left in processing the rapid transitions that characterize spoken language (Moore, 1984; Moore & Haynes, 1980).

Two reaction time experiments using visual presentations of words as stimuli found groups of adults who stutter to be more right hemisphere-dominant for linguistic processing as well as slower to respond than were groups of adults who don't stutter (Hand & Haynes, 1983; Rastatter & Dell, 1987).

Further evidence of stutterers' apparent preference for right hemisphere processing was gathered by researchers measuring electrical and metabolic activity in the brain (McFarland & Moore, 1982; Wood, Stump, McKeehan, Sheldon, & Proctor, 1980). More recent studies by different research groups using new techniques of brain imaging during speech have confirmed and extended the initial work. Using positron emission tomography (PET scans), De Nil, Kroll, Kapur, and Houle (1995) found that when reading aloud, adults who stutter activated areas in the right hemisphere that were "mirror images" of left hemisphere areas used by nonstutterers for the same task (Fig. 2.2).

It is surprising that these differences persisted even after stutterers became fluent after an intensive treatment program. The right hemisphere activation included not only areas associated with speech-motor planning and execution, but also language-processing areas. Similar findings were reported by Fox and colleagues (1996) in their PET scan studies. They found that, in addition to greater activation of speech motor and language processing areas of the right hemisphere during both fluent and stuttered speech, the adults who stutter showed far less activity than nonstuttering speakers in the left auditory language area. They also reported much greater levels of activation in motor areas of the cerebrum and cerebellum in the stuttering group than in the control group. The fluency-inducing condition in this study (choral reading) was associated with a reduction in the level of overactivation in motor areas for the stuttering group and normal levels of activation in their left auditory areas.

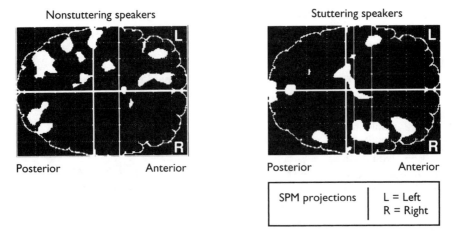

Figure 2.2. PET scans of brains of nonstuttering (*left*) and stuttering (*right*) adults while reading aloud. *SPM,* statistical parametric mapping. (From De Nil, L., Kroll, R., Kapur, S., & Houle, S. (1995). Silent and oral reading in stuttering and nonstuttering adults: A positron emission tomography study. Paper presented at the Annual Convention of the American Speech-Language-Hearing Association, Orlando, Florida, December.

Braun and associates (1996) found, in their PET study of people who stutter and controls, that when disfluent, stuttering subjects did not activate the left hemisphere areas that controls did. Instead, left hemisphere activity was absent and present in homologous areas of the right hemisphere, or activity was seen in both hemispheres.

The results of these brain imaging studies are striking in their confirmation of earlier research that compared groups of adults who stutter with groups of adults who do not stutter on various tasks and measures. Differences in stutterers' auditory processing, language development, speech motor reaction time, reaction time to linguistic stimuli, and delay in tracking auditory stimuli with speech motor responses all may be related to the organization of speech, language, and auditory functions in the brains of those who stutter.

The implication is that people who stutter may be using a less effective part of the brain for processing speech functions—at least when they are stuttering. Richard Curlee (personal communication, 1990) and Douglas Cross (Cross, Sweet, & Bates, 1985) have suggested another interpretation of the increased activity of the right hemisphere during stuttering. They note that right hemispheric activity is usually associated with emotional expression (e.g., Sackeim & Gur, 1978) and that the findings of greater right hemisphere activation during stuttering could correlate with emotionality during stuttered speech.[8] This suggestion also has implications for the onset of stuttering in childhood, when many functions, presumably including speech and emotion, appear to have greater bilateral representation. Fluency may be especially vulnerable to emotional disruption then because of "crosstalk" or interference between speech and emotional expression.

A more specific formulation of interference by right hemisphere negative emotional overflow has emerged from the laterality studies of William Webster (1990, 1993). Webster found that adults who stutter were slower than adults who don't stutter at simultaneous tapping of two different rhythms using their right and left hands. He also found that,

---

[8] Although much of the earlier literature suggests that emotions were functionally localized to the right hemisphere, more recent work (e.g., Calkins & Fox, 1994; Kinsbourne & Bemporad, 1984) has indicated that positive approach-oriented emotions are lateralized to the left hemisphere, whereas negative, avoidance-oriented emotions are lateralized to the right.

unlike nonstutterers, adults who stutter showed no right-hand advantage in the tapping task. Generalizing from hand-tapping to speech, he speculated that stutterers, like non-stutterers, can use their left hemisphere for control of speech and language processing and other sequential motor tasks. But unlike nonstutterers, Webster suggested, stutterers have weaker or more vulnerable left hemisphere speech-processing functions. Attention or neural resources may be easily diverted from left hemisphere processing by either emotional activity in the right hemisphere or momentary right hemisphere processing of speech. This would lead to a breakdown in the sequential motor planning for fluent speech.

Webster (1993) speculated that the supplementary motor area (SMA) of the brain, which is involved in directing hemispheric traffic and regulating speech motor organization, may be at fault and allow this misappropriation of neural resources in stutterers. This same area has been implicated in the brain imaging studies of Pool, Freeman, and Finitzo (1987) and Pool et al. (1991) and the lip and jaw coordination studies of Caruso, Abbs, and Gracco (1988).

STUDIES OF FLUENT SPEECH

Reaction time responses, such as lip closing or saying "ahhh," are relatively indirect measures of speech. Researchers have been able to make more direct assessments by examining the speed and coordination of stutterers' speech movements when they are talking fluently. Even when they are fluent, people who stutter, on average, have longer vowel durations, slower transitions between consonants and vowels, and delayed onsets of voicing after voiceless consonants (Colcord & Adams, 1979; DiSimoni, 1974; Hillman & Gilbert, 1977; Starkweather & Myers, 1979).[9] These results of acoustic studies have been supported by "kinematic" research, which has measured the movements of speakers' speech structures (Alfonso, Story, & Watson, 1987; Zimmerman, 1980). As a group, stutterers have been found to move some of their speech structures more slowly, even in fluent speech, than do nonstutterers (e.g., Zimmerman, 1980).

So what does this mean? Why might many stutterers speak more slowly than other speakers even when they are fluent? Some researchers think that this finding reflects delays in processing incoming and outgoing signals. Stutterers may be unable to process the neural signals fast enough to make the rapid, precise movements used in normal conversational speech, especially at times when they are under the stress of planning a complex sentence or competing with other talkers. Their delays in voicing onset or slower transitions during fluent speech may simply reflect a slower mechanism working at its normal rate. A different view, suggested by more skeptical researchers, is that such delays and slowing movements only reflect the way stutterers have learned to talk to avoid stuttering. They have developed a slow, cautious style of speaking that keeps them from stuttering.

Yet another interpretation is that slower movements are the result of heightened tension in muscles having antagonistic functions for speech production (Starkweather, 1987). For example, increased tension in muscles that move a structure forward (agonists), as well as muscles that hold it back (antagonists), would make movement of that structure considerably slower. Imagine two people pulling a rope in opposite directions.

---

[9] Several sources review both reaction time studies and acoustic studies of stutterers' fluent speech. Woodruff Starkweather, for example, reviews both areas in his monograph *Stuttering and Laryngeal Behavior: A Review,* Rockville, MD: American Speech-Language-Hearing Association (1982). He also reviews these studies in Laryngeal and Articulatory Behavior in Stuttering: Past and Future in Peters and Hulstijn (1987). More recent studies can be found in H. Peters, W. Hulstijn, and C.W. Starkweather's (Eds.) (1991). *Speech Motor Control and Stuttering,* Amsterdam: Excerpta Medica. An excellent review of this area of research is available in the first section of Van Lieshout (1995).

Even if one were stronger, pulling the weaker one would be slow because of the resistance against the other person pulling.

The slowed movements of stutterers' speech structures would account for not only slow reaction times, but also the longer durations and delays in their fluent speech as well. A number of studies have reported that people who stutter excessively co-contract agonist and antagonist muscles of both the laryngeal (Freeman & Ushijima, 1975; Shapiro, 1980) and articulatory (Guitar, Guitar, Neilson, O'Dwyer, & Andrews, 1988) muscle groups during stuttering.[10] These studies, like Starkweather's (1987) review, have noted that heightened tension in agonist and antagonist muscles appears in the fluent speech of stutterers. This finding has led many researchers to the position that stuttering is not an "all or nothing" event (Adams & Runyan, 1981; Bloodstein, 1987). Sometimes, stutterers may speak freely, without a trace of excess tension. At other times, they may have excess tension whose effect isn't heard by listeners as stuttering. At still other times, muscle tension may be so great that both the person who stutters and listeners are acutely aware of stuttering. This continuum of fluency reflects the subjective impression of many stutterers, including the present author.

Summary

There is substantial evidence that, as a group, people who stutter differ from people who don't on cognitive, linguistic, motor, and perceptual tasks. Cognitively, children who stutter seem to score a little lower on standardized tests and do a little more poorly in school. Linguistically, some stutterers—perhaps a subgroup—may have slight delays in language or articulation development. For some, subtle language problems may persist into adulthood. People who stutter have slightly slower motor reaction times, especially when language processing is involved in the reaction time task. Perceptually, stutterers have been shown to score slightly lower on tasks of central auditory processing, perhaps more so when fine discrimination of temporal information is needed.

When scientists have looked "upstream" from measures of performance at the periphery, they have found in electroencephalographic and computer imaging studies of the brain that stutterers' brains show clear differences from brains of nonstutterers. Nonstutterers tend to activate predominantly left hemisphere brain structures when they are speaking or reading; stutterers show less left hemisphere activation and more activity in the same areas of the right hemisphere. Some of these studies have shown differences in parts of the brain that may be important for cognitive, linguistic, motor, and perceptual processing. Thus, the results of brain imaging studies seem to parallel the results of performance on reaction time tasks and linguistic assessments.

What do these differences between stutterers and nonstutterers mean? Are they signs that a constitutional predisposition causes stuttering? We don't know the answers to these questions yet, but it is unlikely that any of these differences directly cause stuttering in everyone who stutters. Research reveals that many persons who stutter don't show such differences, and many nonstutterers do. Thus, it is not necessary to have such differences to be a stutterer, and having such differences is not sufficient to make one a stutterer.

One explanation, mentioned earlier, is that the differences in brain function and task performance may be simply the result of some general differences in brain development that allow stuttering to begin. That is, they may be causally unrelated to stuttering. An-

---

[10]Note, however, that like most findings, this evidence is disputed by other studies. Caruso (1988), McClean, Goldsmith, and Cerf (1984) and Smith (1989, 1995) have reported absence of co-contraction of opposing muscles during stuttering.

other possibility, which we suggested in the section on speech and language differences, is that some of these differences may give rise to communication problems such as language or articulation difficulties or a high level of normal disfluency, which, through the frustration and failure they engender, produce stuttering. Thus, these brain changes may be causally, but indirectly, related to stuttering.[11] These are, of course, speculations. The differences between stutterers and nonstutterers remain intriguing clues that await a unifying theory relating them to stuttering.

SPECULATIONS ABOUT CONSTITUTIONAL FACTORS IN STUTTERING

There are no formal theories of stuttering, with carefully delineated postulates, hypotheses, and corollaries. Instead, researchers have developed explanations of stuttering, usually based on models of other disorders or extrapolated from current understandings of normal speech production. They have pulled together current evidence to explain stuttering from a particular point of view, guide further research, and, in some cases, influence how stutterers are treated. These explanations change every few years, as more data come in and as new models in related disciplines are developed. Doubtless, the explanations of stuttering we summarize in this section will be superseded by others in a few years.

We have chosen several contemporary views of constitutional factors to discuss briefly in the following text. Although these views differ, they are not mutually exclusive. Linked together, they provide us with some interesting notions about what might be inherited and how that might result in stuttering.

Stuttering as a Disorder of Cerebral Localization

Although normal speakers use both right and left halves of their brains for speech and language, evidence suggests that, for most people, the left hemisphere is dominant for language, in the sense that it handles the segmental information in speech and language. Studies of normal subjects have demonstrated this with a wide variety of techniques.[12] Studies of brain-damaged patients have also confirmed left hemisphere dominance for language, finding that far more speech and language disabilities result from left hemisphere damage than from right hemisphere damage.

Stutterers may deviate from the pattern of left hemisphere dominance, according to the cerebral dominance theory of stuttering developed at the University of Iowa in the 1920s. In an atmosphere of intense scientific curiosity and collaboration among researchers, Samuel Orton, a neurologist, and Lee Edward Travis, a psychologist and speech pathologist, observed that many stutterers seemed to have been left-handers whose parents changed them into right-handers (Travis, 1931). This change, they suspected, led to a conflict of hemispheric control of speech in which neither side was fully in charge of the midline anatomical structures used for speech. In turn, it was hypothesized that this created neuromotor disorganization and mistiming of speech, which led to stuttering. The treatment was simply to switch stutterers back to being left-handers. As

---

[11]The reader is encouraged to read Chapter 10, Inferences and Conclusions, in Bloodstein (1995) for a full description of this view.

[12]Among the methods that have demonstrated left hemisphere dominance for language are brain wave and blood flow studies, electrical stimulation of the brain, measures of response to linguistic stimuli delivered to each half of the brain, and anesthetization of each hemisphere with sodium amytal.

you might guess, this simple treatment was fruitless. Furthermore, evidence was never found that most stutterers were originally left-handers. Consequently, the original cerebral dominance theory of stuttering languished for many years. But in the 1960s, data started to trickle in suggesting that stutterers may not, after all, have normal left hemisphere dominance for language. In the 1970s and early 1980s, more studies were published supporting this finding.

In 1985, a new version of the cerebral dominance theory of stuttering was proposed. Two neurologists, Norman Geschwind and Albert Galaburda, published a theory that suggested that many disorders, including stuttering, dyslexia, and autism, are the result of a delay in left hemisphere growth during fetal development and consequent right hemisphere dominance for speech and language (Geschwind & Galaburda, 1985). The delay in left hemisphere development in these male-related disorders was thought to be caused by a male-related factor. Geschwind and Galaburda hypothesized that the delay might be the result of fetal exposure to excess secretion of the hormone testosterone in utero. So far, no evidence has been found to support their hypothesis about testosterone,[13] but their theory is still of great interest.

Geschwind and Galaburda's theory suggests that a delay in left hemisphere development may affect speech and language for the following reasons. Various structures that evolve in the left hemisphere during embryonic development appear to be especially suited for speech and language functions. As these structures develop, specialized nerve cells, which are destined to sprout the neural connections for speech and language processes, disperse from their point of creation in the "neural tube" (where the central nervous system is formed). These nerve cells normally migrate to areas in the left hemisphere that are appropriate for their function. But if development of left hemisphere structures is delayed, cells in the right hemisphere may develop the functions usually developed in the left hemisphere, for which they may be most suited. These right hemisphere structures and the organization of their connections may give rise to inefficient "networks" of neural activity for processing of speech and language.

Because the brain is relatively plastic, especially during the first years of life, the child's experiences modify these neural networks. Thus, some children who have atypical or "anomalous" brain structures and functions may reorganize their neural networks to process speech and language more efficiently. They may thus outgrow stuttering. But other children may not be able to develop more efficient networks. For them, repeated experiences create well-worn traces in the fabric of the neural networks. These well-worn traces result in thoughts and behavior that become more and more difficult to change as they get older.

Although speculation about atypical cerebral localization in stutterers has received some support from research, especially from the recent PET studies reviewed earlier, the details about how stuttering behaviors result from abnormal localization is another question, requiring other theories.

Stuttering as a Disorder of Timing

Several authors have concluded that the known facts about stuttering point toward a disorder of timing. For example, Van Riper (1982, p. 415) has suggested, "when a person stutters on a word, there is a temporal disruption of the simultaneous and successive pro-

---

[13]Neilson, Howie, and Andrews (1987) presented data that don't support the testosterone hypothesis. Animal experimentation has shown that when one member of a twin pair is male and the other a female, the female is likely to have some male traits perhaps because of the presence of testosterone. Looking at a sample of stutterers in twin pairs, they found no evidence that stuttering would be more likely in females with a male co-twin.

gramming of muscular movements required to produce one of the word's integrated sounds. . . . " Building on Van Riper's view, Raymond Kent (1984) marshalled several lines of evidence to support a hypothesis that stuttering arises from a deficit in temporal programming. He speculated that this deficit is the result of inappropriate localization of some speech and language functions in the right hemisphere and is manifested in an inability to create the precise timing patterns needed to perceive and produce speech efficiently. Like a conductor of a symphony orchestra, who must regulate when each section plays, as well as the speed or beat of their playing, the timing patterns for speech may determine the rate at which we speak and the order of movements to produce sequential sounds. Like an orchestra conductor integrating the timing of several sections, the brain must coordinate complex timing relationships for phrases, syllables, phonemes, and segments.

The inability to perform precise timing functions consistently, Kent suggests, may stem from the fact that a stutterer's left hemisphere is not as well developed as the right hemisphere. Because the left hemisphere is specialized for processing brief, rapidly changing events, such as those needed for fine motor control of verbal output, a person who stutters may be disadvantaged when trying to process at the speed or frequency required for normal speech. This central timing function, Kent points out, must not only regulate left hemisphere aspects of speech production, but must integrate timing of rapid left hemisphere-generated speech segments with the slower prosodic elements of speech.

Kent also notes that emotion may play an important role in disrupting timing in the speech of someone who stutters. As we indicated earlier, the right hemisphere is thought to be heavily involved in the expression of certain emotions. The stutterer's deficit, then, may be that his timing functions for speech are arranged so that they are (a) not as efficient as those of a nonstutterer and (b) vulnerable to interference by right hemisphere activity during increased emotion. How this deficit causes the repetitions, prolongations, and blocks we hear in the beginning stutterer's speech is not dealt with in this theory.

Stuttering as Reduced Capacity for Internal Modeling

Another theory of constitutional factors in stuttering has been advanced by researchers studying motor control of speech and other movements. Megan and Peter Neilson have suggested that the repetitions of beginning stutterers are the result of a deficit in their ability to create and use "inverse internal models of the speech production system" (Neilson & Neilson, 1987). This rather complicated sounding theory can be easily understood if we go back to an assumption about how children learn to speak.

During their first year of life, infants store up perceptions of the speech sounds they hear around them. They also play with speech sounds and learn what movements make which sounds. In other words, their brains construct both a store of the speech stimuli they hear and will try to produce when they speak and a model of the relationship between their motor movements and the sensory consequences. This might be called a sensory-motor model for speech or an inverse internal model of how speech is produced. It is an "inverse" model because it inverts the sensory targets into the motor commands needed to hit them. As infants learn to produce the sounds they hear, they constantly use and refine their sensory-motor model for speech. They plan a word or sentence on the basis of what it should sound like (the target), then they load their sensory-motor model and generate motor commands based on the target they are trying to hit.

This process of learning to speak is like learning to drive a car. At first, keeping the car on the road requires your constant vigilance. But as you learn the relationships between turning the wheel, stepping on the accelerator, and going where you want, the linkage becomes automatic, even when driving a stick-shift vehicle in stop-and-go traffic. Moreover, the linkage is refined as you encounter different driving conditions and different cars—cars, for example, with loose steering wheels and sticky accelerators. Drivers establish a sensory-motor model for driving. Children develop a sensory-motor model for speaking.

Figure 2.3 depicts a schematic of how the brain may transform desired sensory (perceptual) targets into motor commands for speech. In the figure, the desired output (the word or phrase, for example, that a child intends a listener to hear) is fed into the inverse internal model of the speech production system. Here, the desired output enters as sensory code (its expected auditory and kinesthetic results), is "inverted" by the model, and exits as movement code or motor commands. Experience, practice, and vocal play have helped a child learn to make these inversions or transformations. Moreover, this internal model is continually updated as a child learns more and as a child's system changes with age. The motor commands exiting the internal model are sent to the muscles of the speech production system, whose constructions produce the movements that result in a planned utterance; feedback of the process and its output is sent to the modeling circuitry. Retracing our steps for a moment, when the motor commands are sent to muscles, a copy of these commands (called "efference copy" by motor physiologists) is also sent to the modeling circuitry. Here, the efference copy is transformed into hypothetical output (a model of what the output should be, based on these commands). This hypo-

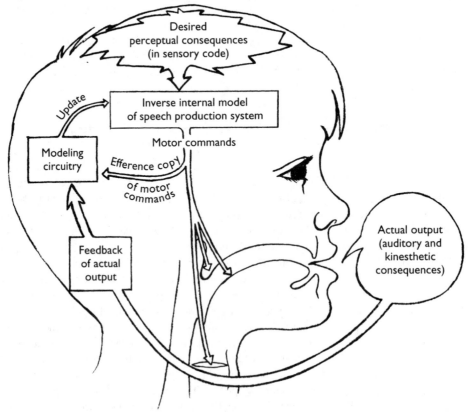

Figure 2.3. Schematic of the inverse internal model theory of speech production.

thetical output is then compared with the feedback of the current positions and movements of the speech mechanism and, if necessary, the inverse internal model updates its ongoing motor commands so that the desired output is more accurately produced. These components of the speech production process are assumed to use the corticocerebellar structures and pathways commonly described in neural models of speech output (e.g., Neilson & Neilson, 1987; Neilson, Neilson, & O'Dwyer, 1992).

The Neilsons and their coworkers have used the inverse internal model of the speech production system to understand the performance of stutterers in experiments (Neilson, Quinn, & Neilson, 1976) that tested their ability to track an auditory tone that changed unpredictably. In one ear, subjects heard a changing "target" tone, and in the other ear, they heard a changing "cursor" tone, which they could regulate with a hand-held device. Their task was to track the pitch of the target tone with the cursor tone. The Neilsons' experiments showed that stutterers were poorer than nonstutterers at tracking an auditory tone that went up and down in pitch. Stutterers were still poorer than nonstutterers after practicing the task. These results suggested that stutterers might have some weakness in learning the relationships between the sounds they want to say and the movements required to produce them. They have difficulty in making sensory-to-motor and motor-to-sensory transformations, but this impairment doesn't always produce stuttering. When circumstances don't call for a large amount of the brain's functional capacity in speech and language areas, stutterers can compensate for their slight weakness. On the other hand, when a large portion of its functional capacity might be allocated for language tasks such as choosing new words or making complex sentences, the impairment cannot be compensated for, resulting in more repetitions. As these researchers have put it, "whether one will become a stutterer depends on one's neurological capacity for these sensory-to-motor and motor-to-sensory transformations and the demands posed by the speech act" (Andrews et al., 1983).

How do these intermittent deficits in available brain capacity result in the symptoms of stuttering? This theory attempts to account only for the core behaviors of early stuttering—repetitions and prolongations. According to the theory, repetitions and prolongations are the result of inadequate transformations of sensory targets, transformations that should generate the motor commands for speech. A speaker with reduced capacity may begin to speak, but is often unable to plan and carry out the rest of his utterance without disruption. The repetition or prolongation may occur while the speaker is pushing ahead with speech while his brain is still planning the following syllables and how to link them with the initial sound.

Stuttering as a Language Production Deficit

Many researchers have been intrigued by the influence of linguistic factors on stuttering. For example, stuttering often begins when a child enters a period of intense language development. Similarly, stuttering is most frequent when language load is heaviest—in longer utterances, at the beginnings of sentences, and on longer, less familiar words. These factors have prompted several theorists to propose that stuttering reflects an impairment in some aspect of language production. We use the term "language production" because these theorists believe the problem is not in the motor execution of speech, but rather in the planning and assembly of language units (such as phonemes) that occur before speech production.

Herman Kolk and Albert Postma (1997) have developed a "covert repair" hypothesis to explain stuttering. They believe that both stuttering and normal disfluencies are the result of an internal monitoring process that we all use to check whether what we are about to articulate is exactly what we mean to say. Perhaps this would be clearer if we imagine for a moment that language production is like a factory making bicycles (Fig. 2.4). The factory must monitor the quality of its bicycles by checking them at different stages. Some quality checks occur after the bicycles leave the factory, when customers and factory workers themselves ride them and tell the factory if there are any defects in them. In speech and language production, this is like a speaker's auditory feedback—the sound of your own words as you are speaking them.

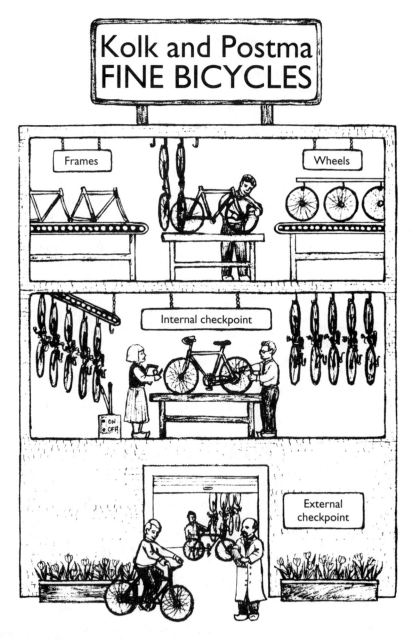

Figure 2.4. Quality control in a bicycle factory as an analogy for part of the language production system in the brain.

The bicycle factory might also use a second quality checking process—one that occurs inside the factory before the bicycles are shipped out. This is like an internal monitoring process of speech and language. Without being aware of it, you check the "phonetic plan" for what you are about to say before you articulate it. This way you can detect potential semantic, syntactic, lexical, and phonological errors before they are articulated. Just as the production line in a bicycle factory would have to be halted when a defect is detected, so speech production is interrupted when your internal monitor detects an error in your phonetic plan. Repairs need to be made before production can continue. Kolk and Postma (1997) believe that the halting of production and the repair process explain the disfluencies in normal speakers and children who stutter.

The most common stuttering disfluencies—repetitions, prolongations, and blocks—all are the result of correcting or "repairing" phonological (rather than semantic, syntactic, or lexical) errors detected in the phonetic plan before articulation. In the case of part-word repetitions, the speaker detects an error in the final part of a syllable (the "p" in "cup"), restarts the phonological encoding process ("cu-cu-") and keeps it going until he successfully encodes the correct phoneme and can produce the entire syllable. Prolongations are thought to occur when the phoneme of a word or syllable prior to an error is a continuant (such as "l" in the word "lips" when the error may be in the vowel). In this case, the continuant is prolonged until the speaker successfully encodes the phoneme following the continuant.

Blocks are thought to result from errors in the initial sound of words or syllables. An error is detected, speech production is halted for repairs, but the speaker may try to plunge ahead, building up muscle tension, unaware of the automatic error detection and repair that is in progress.[14]

Kolk and Postma (1997) suggest that stutterers are more prone to phonological encoding errors because they are constitutionally slower at this task. In various articles, they lay out the evidence supporting this view, suggesting among other things that the benefits of a slower speech rate on stuttering derives from the greater amount of time stutterers need for phonological encoding.

Several years before Kolk and Postma (1997) published their covert repair hypothesis, an innovative language production view of stuttering was offered by Mike Wingate (1988). It was called *The Structure of Stuttering: A Psycholinguistic Analysis.* In this book, he reviewed the linguistic and neurological research on stuttering and proposed that it results from a dyssynchrony of functions in various areas of the brain—left hemisphere, right hemisphere, and subcortical structures. These different areas, Wingate suggested, are responsible for different elements of language planning and production, elements such as consonants, vowels, and prosody.

Wingate hypothesized that when the stutterer produces the initial part of a syllable, consonant and vowel and prosody all must be synchronously blended. If, at this critical moment, some component lags behind, the result is a disruption in speech production that we observe as stuttering. It is as if, in our imaginary bicycle factory, the wheels, gears, and frame all must be put in place at the same time on a high-speed assembly line. If one component is held up, production is halted. How this halt appears in speech as a repetition, prolongation, or block is not explained in Wingate's hypothesis.

Another theory of stuttering as a deficit in language production was proposed by Perkins, Kent, and Curlee (1991). These authors suggest that stuttering results from a dyssynchrony between two components of language production. One component is "par-

---

[14]Details on other types of disfluencies are available in Postma and Kolk (1993).

alinguistic"—a right hemisphere social-emotional system that is responsible for vocal tone and prosodic functions. The other component is linguistic—a left hemisphere segmental system that is responsible for the content of language, its semantics, syntax, and phonology. The two components must be integrated before language is produced. If one lags behind the other, whatever the reason, the resulting dyssynchrony produces disfluency.

Perkins, Kent, and Curlee add to this dyssynchrony two elements that must also be present if the resulting disfluency is stuttering, not just normal disfluency. First, the speaker must experience time pressure, from either an outside source or an inner feeling, which makes him try to continue speaking even though the delay in paralinguistic or linguistic processing has resulted in an incomplete or anomalous speech motor program. Second, the speaker must experience a subjective feeling of "loss of control," arising from not being aware of why he cannot say the word.

In our analogy of the bicycle factory, Perkins, Kent, and Curlee's theory might be characterized as a production line that stops when one of the two major subcomponents of the bicycle are not ready for assembly. Moreover, in this factory the boss demands that the production line move rapidly, and workers panic when the production line grinds to a halt. Frantic workers keep trying to restart production without knowing what the problem is nor how to fix it.

These language production views of stuttering have much in common and account for some of the facts known about the disorder. In the next section, we consider how they and other theoretical perspectives compare in their attempt to explain the constitutional basis of stuttering.

SUMMARY

Research on genetic transmission of constitutional factors in stuttering suggests that a predisposition to stuttering may be inherited. Support for this hypothesis comes from studies showing that, compared with nonstutterers, stutterers are more likely to have family members who stutter. Moreover, male relatives are more likely to stutter than females. Some studies suggest that females who stutter are more likely to have relatives who stutter, but more recent studies with very young subjects have found no such differences between the sexes. Several factors have been suggested as possible predictors of recovery, including family members who have recovered from stuttering. Two models of genetic transmission have been proposed: transmission by a single gene or transmission by several genes, each contributing to several factors.

Research on stuttering in identical and fraternal twins have found that identical twins have higher concordance for stuttering than do same-sex fraternal twins, providing support for the genetic hypothesis. However, many identical twins are not concordant for stuttering, confirming the importance of environmental factors, as well. Results of adoption studies also support both genetic and environmental factors in the etiology of stuttering.

Scientists have compared groups of people who stutter and people who don't stutter on many dimensions in an effort to identify differences between the two groups that would help us better understand the disorder. These studies suggest that groups of people who stutter often have slightly lower performance on unidimensional intelligence tests, particularly those requiring verbal adeptness; their school performance may be slightly poorer; their speech and language development may be a little delayed; they are no more emotionally aroused that nonstutterers, but when aroused, their stuttering increases; their reaction times, movements of speech structures during fluent speech, and tracking performances are slower; their central auditory processing test scores are slightly depressed; and finally, their right hemispheres are more active during speech and language performance than are those of nonstutterers.

Several theoretical models for a constitutional etiology of stuttering have been proposed. Geschwind and Galaburda (1985) hypothesized that normal left hemisphere growth is delayed during fetal development, causing speech and language functions in stutterers to be localized inappropriately. Kent (1983) and Van Riper (1982) suggested that stuttering is the product of mistiming of neuromuscular commands for speech. Neilson and Neilson (1987) suggested that stuttering results from inadequate neuronal resources to make the necessary sensory-to-motor transformations for fluent speech.

Several language production models of stuttering have been proposed. Kolk and Postma (1997) hypothesize that stuttering disfluencies result from errors detected in the phonetic plans for speech and the consequent halting of speech production while errors are repaired. Wingate (1988) hypothesized that faulty integration of the consonant, vowel, and speech prosody in the initial part of a word results in stuttering. Perkins, Kent, and Curlee (1991) attributed all disfluencies to a dyssynchrony of segmental and suprasegmental elements for speech in the development of speech motor programs; if the speaker experiences time pressure to speak and that his disfluency is out of his control, the disfluency is stuttering.

The studies and theoretical views presented in this chapter will soon be superseded by others as scientists continue to gather new data and speculate about their meaning. This is an interim report on some of the constitutional factors that appear to influence stuttering. In the next chapter, we consider developmental and environmental factors that are thought to interact with constitutional factors to create the first symptoms of stuttering.

STUDY QUESTIONS

1. What evidence is there that stuttering is inherited?
2. What do family studies tell us about who is most at risk for inheriting stuttering?
3. Some studies suggest that females are more likely to have relatives who stutter; other studies show that males and females are equally likely to have relatives who stutter. What might explain these two different findings?
4. What studies provide evidence that stuttering is the product of both heredity and environment?
5. Researchers have found many differences between groups of stutterers and nonstutterers. Discuss why we cannot say that these differences "cause" stuttering.
6. What findings suggest that many stutterers have deficits in speech and language functions other than stuttering?
7. Name four findings of differences between stutterers and nonstutterers that reflect a possible speech or language deficit.
8. Name four measures of sensory-motor functioning which have shown stutterers to perform more poorly, to have more errors, or to respond more slowly than nonstutterers.
9. How might delays in speech and language development in stutterers be related to their poorer sensory-motor coordination?
10. Briefly describe three theories of the constitutional basis of stuttering described in this chapter.

11. Do any of these theories suggest why the early symptom of stuttering is repetitions of syllables? If so, which theories?

12. In the Geschwind-Galaburda theory of right hemisphere localization of speech and language, why have these functions migrated to the right hemisphere?

13. In Kent's view of stuttering as a timing disorder, why would right hemisphere localization of speech and language disrupt timing?

14. In the theory of stuttering as the result of inadequate sensory-to-motor transformations, why would learning new vocabulary interfere with fluency?

15. It might be said that theories of stuttering as hemispheric localization problem, as a timing defect, and as a language production problem are all correct? How would you defend this statement?

SUGGESTED READINGS

Andrews, G., Craig, A., Feyer, A.-M., Hoddinott, S., Howie, P., & Neilson, M. (1983). Stuttering: A review of research findings and theories circa 1982. *Journal of Speech and Hearing Disorders, 48,* **226–246.**

This article distills the research about stuttering into a small number of "facts"—those findings that have been replicated by more than one study. Although the model of stuttering at which the authors arrive is controversial, the review is very worthwhile in its summary of a great body of research. It is also worthwhile to read the responses to this article in the commentaries on the subsequent pages of this issue of the journal.

Bloodstein, O. (1995). *A handbook on stuttering,* **5th ed. San Diego: Singular Publishing Group, Inc.**

This book, which we frequently cite in our references, contains a critical review of research in practically every area of stuttering.

Curlee, R., & Siegel, G. (Eds.) (1997). *Nature and treatment of stuttering: New directions,* **2nd ed. Boston: Allyn & Bacon.**

The authors who contributed to this book are working at the forefront of research and clinical work. Their chapters provide detailed information about the nature of stuttering and the theories of its etiology.

Springer, S., & Deutsch, G. (1981). *Left brain, right brain.* **San Francisco: W.H. Freeman & Company.**

This is a clearly written and well-illustrated book about the functions of the right and left hemispheres. Although it is somewhat dated, it is a good introduction to readers who are not familiar with neuroanatomy.

Starkweather, C.W. (1987). *Fluency and stuttering.* **Englewood Cliffs, NJ: Prentice-Hall.**

This book is a useful description of facts about various aspects of stuttering, including the relationship between language and stuttering, differences between stutterers and nonstutterers, and the variability of stuttering. Starkweather takes these facts in each area and relates them to theory in a coherent way.

Van Riper, C. (1982). An attempted synthesis (pp. 415–453). In *The nature of stuttering.* **Englewood Cliffs, NJ: Prentice-Hall.**

Van Riper brings together the information he has reviewed throughout this text and formulates a theory of stuttering as a disorder of timing. A very readable author.

Yairi, E., Ambrose, N., & Cox, N. (1996). Genetics of stuttering: A critical review. *Journal of Speech and Hearing Research, 39,* 771–784.

This critical review of genetic research surveys the evidence for the inheritance of stuttering gathered over the past 60 years and highlights strengths and weaknesses of various studies. It is useful as a guide to past genetic studies and as a source of advice for future studies.

3

Developmental and Environmental Influences on Stuttering

Many factors both within the child and in his environment create the conditions under which stuttering first emerges and then grows progressively worse, stabilizes, or stops. Some of these factors seem to be part of normal childhood development, such as the child's explosive growth of speech and language skills during his preschool years. Other factors may be very common situations that most children take in stride as they grow up; for example, competition with siblings for attention and speaking time in a busy home. These factors, which we call developmental and environmental influences, interact with constitutional factors such as those discussed in Chapter 2. Figure 3.1 depicts the interaction of constitutional factors that predispose the child to stuttering, with developmental and environmental factors, which contribute to the emergence of stuttering during the busy and sometimes stressful years of childhood.

The interaction of constitutional factors with developmental and environmental factors is ongoing, day by day. Like the forces of weather on the surface of the earth, developmental and environmental factors have a gradual, cumulative effect. For most children, there is not a sudden landslide of stuttering, but a more gradual erosion of fluency. The conditions at the onset of stuttering are typically not unusual or dramatic, and the child is usually not under great stress, nor has he just experienced some traumatic event. The ordinariness of the environment when stuttering first appears is reflected in this observation by Van Riper (1973, p. 81):

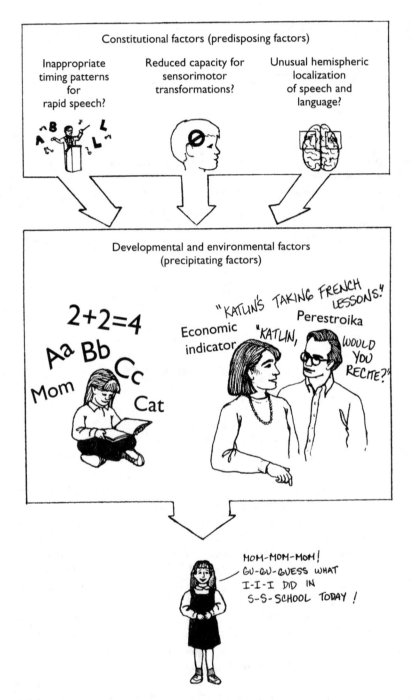

Figure 3.1. Predisposing constitutional factors interact with developmental and environmental factors to precipitate or worsen stuttering.

> *In the great majority of children we have carefully studied soon after onset, we were unable to state with any certainty . . . what precipitated the stuttering. In most instances there simply were no apparent conflicts, no illnesses, no opportunity to imitate, no shocks or frightening experiences. Stuttering seemed to begin under quite normal conditions of living and communicating.*

Because the child's situation is so ordinary when stuttering first emerges, research to determine critical developmental and environmental factors affecting its onset and progression has not produced substantial results. This is a domain of educated guesses and tentative conclusions. Evidence for developmental factors is inferred from the fact that the onset of stuttering almost always occurs when children are growing rapidly, physically and mentally, in their preschool years (Andrews et al., 1983; Wingate, 1983). Evidence for the influence of the environment comes in part from clinical reports of particular stresses sometimes associated with the onset of stuttering and its remission when these stresses are lessened. Environmental factors are also implicated by the higher prevalence of stuttering in those cultures that are more achievement- and conformity-oriented (Bloodstein, 1995).[1] Finally, some sources of evidence for genetic factors in stuttering are also evidence for environmental factors. Studies by Andrews, Morris-Yates, Howie, and Martin (1990), Howie (1981), Kidd, Kidd, and Records (1978), and Yairi, Ambrose, Paden, and Throneburg (1996), for example, indicate that both genetic and environmental influences contribute to the occurrence of stuttering. This evidence, however, does not suggest what these environmental factors might be. Because of the paucity of hard data on specific developmental and environmental factors, this chapter is more speculative than the last. Wherever we can, however, we try to tie speculations to facts.

In the following pages, we divide developmental and environmental factors into separate sections, but they do not operate independently. Rather, they are intertwined in their effects. As an example, consider how much more vulnerable a child may be to pressure for rapid and complex speech in his environment when his speech is still in an early stage development.

DEVELOPMENTAL FACTORS

Our view of how developmental factors affect fluency in children assumes that the brain must share its resources to cope with many demands.[2] Like a computer, the brain can work on several things at once. Like a computer, the more tasks it does simultaneously, the slower and less efficiently it does each one. Unlike a computer, if the tasks are dissimilar (such as driving a car and talking about the weather), there is less interference between them. But if the tasks are similar (such as rubbing your stomach while patting your head), there is more interference between them (Kinsbourne & Hicks, 1978). The problem of shared resources is more acute in children because their immature nervous systems have less processing capacity to share (Hiscock & Kinsbourne, 1977; 1980). Some children are especially at risk for straining their developing resources. They may be delayed in their development and refinement of speech-language skills; yet they have to compete in a highly verbal environment. Or, their language development may surge ahead of their speech motor control skills, giving them much to say, but a limited capac-

---

[1] It has been argued that genetic influences, which also are somewhat responsible for marked differences in cultures, may just as easily explain these results.

[2] This sharing of resources by a limited capacity system is similar to assumptions of the reduced capacity for internal modeling view of stuttering, described in Chapter 2. It is essentially the same as the capacities and demands model of developmental and environmental factors, described later in this chapter.

ity to express themselves articulately. These children may become excessively disfluent as other developmental demands outpace their more limited ability to coordinate the complex movements of rapid, articulate speech.

Here is an example of this competition between burgeoning language and slower motor ability. Several years ago, we evaluated a 4-year-old girl whose uncle and grandmother stuttered. Her parents were concerned because this child had been repeating words and sounds excessively for 1½ years, sometimes up to 20 times per instance. However, her language development was well above average: she began to talk with single words at 9 months and to produce sentences intelligibly at 12 months. Her motor development lagged somewhat behind; she had not walked until 18 months. We think it is possible that her disfluencies emerged as a result of the high proportion of resources used for language (and an urge to express that language) in the face of less advanced capacity for motor activities, including fluent speech. In other words, a disparity between language facility and motor ability may have been an important contributor to her stuttering.[3]

To appreciate how many skills and abilities the child is developing at the same time, look carefully at Figure 3.2. This chart covers only social, motor, and language domains, but it is clear that children must master many different abilities simultaneously. If children are slower in developing one or more areas, their road to maturity may be steep and difficult at times. Let us now look at some of the domains of development and how they might contribute to the onset of stuttering.

Physical Development

Between ages 1 and 6 years, children grow by leaps and bounds. Their bodies get bigger. Their nervous systems form new pathways and new connections. Their perceptual and motor skills improve with practice and maturation. This intensive period of growth is a two-edged sword for children predisposed to fluency problems. Neurological maturation may provide more "functional cerebral space," which supports fluency, but it also spurs the development of other motor tasks, which compete with fluency for available neuronal resources. An example of such competition is the common observation that children learn to walk first or talk first, but not both at the same time. Netsell (1981, p. 25) says of this trade-off: "The practice of walking *or* talking seems sufficient to 'tie up' all the available sensorimotor circuitry because the Toddler seldom, if ever, undertakes both activities at once." Berk (1991, p. 194) suggests that "when infants forge ahead in spoken language, they seem to temporarily postpone mastery of new motor skills or vice versa."

The momentary lags and leaps of motor skill and language development may explain normal disfluency as well as stuttering. If a child is learning new language concepts, which temporarily postpones mastery of *speech* motor skills, the expression of more complex language forms will be impaired until speech motor skills catch up. For reasons we don't yet understand, this may account for the reduced speech intelligibility in some children, disfluency in others, and both problems in still other children.

We would suspect that a significant delay in development of fine motor speech skills

---

[3] Nonstutterers also sometimes find they have temporary disfluency if they need to reorganize motor movements. We have known fluent adults who have suddenly become more disfluent when they have broken their right arm and had to learn to write with their left hand. This anecdotal evidence suggests the possibility that demands associated with neural reorganization for non-speech tasks may increase disfluencies. If speech and language networks in some children are vulnerable to disruption, as is suggested in Chapter 2, moments of growth and neural reorganization may be times when disfluencies begin or become worse.

in a child with a strong urge to communicate and rapidly developing language abilities may set the stage for more serious disfluency. There is some evidence that children who stutter are slower in developing fine motor coordination, but the many conflicting results suggest that this is not a simple issue.[4]

Another time during which physical development may affect speech is when physical growth of the whole body, including the vocal tract, occurs rapidly. This may require a child to learn new sensory-to-motor and motor-to-sensory transformations as he tries to produce an intended sound with a changing speech mechanism. This explanation was suggested by Stark, Tallal, and McCauley (1988) as one of several hypotheses to account for their finding that above-average height and weight are strong correlates of articulation impairment.

Cognitive Development

We use the phrase "cognitive development" to refer to the development of the processes of perceiving, reasoning, imagining, and problem solving (Zimbardo, 1985) that subserve spoken language but are separate from it. This is a complex area, with more questions than answers. We don't know, for example, where to draw the line dividing language and cognition, or even if such a division makes sense.

The relationship between cognition and fluency is also complex. On the one hand, persons with cognitive deficits, especially those who have severe deficits such as those who are retarded, have a high incidence of stuttering (Van Riper, 1982). This appears to suggest that a deficit in cognitive ability increases the risk of a deficit in fluency. As Starkweather (1987) suggests, stuttering in retarded individuals may be related to their slower acquisition of speech and language. Their extended period of acquisition may make them more vulnerable to speech breakdown because of competition for limited neurological resources over a relatively long period of time. It is also possible that individuals with retardation may not have the neural plasticity to adapt when disfluencies do occur during speech and language learning.

The recent study by Yairi, Ambrose, Paden, and Throneburg (1996) provides some evidence that poorer cognitive skills even in nonretarded individuals are associated with lack of ability to recover from stuttering. Of 32 children who began to stutter, 12 continued to stutter for 36 months or more. Those with persistent stuttering scored significantly lower on a test of nonverbal abilities, i.e., the Arthur Adaptation of the Leiter International Performance Test (Arthur, 1952), compared with scores of a control group, although their scores were not below the normal mean for the test. Those who recovered did not score significantly different from the controls. Thus, some abilities associated with cognition may be related to a neural resilience allowing recovery from stuttering.

Let us consider the demands that the development of cognition may place on the development of spoken language. To the extent that cognition and language are separate, some aspects of cognitive development may compete with spoken language development for the same neuronal resources and thereby jeopardize fluency. Consider the stages of cognitive development described by the Swiss psychologist, Jean Piaget. He believed that from 14 to 18 months of age, infants go through a Sensorimotor Period, in which cognitive growth is fostered by sensory and motor activities. From 2 to 6 years, children progress through the Preoperational Period, in which they come to understand numbers,

---

[4] See Bloodstein, 1995, p. 181ff; Starkweather, 1987, p. 220ff; and Van Riper, 1982, p. 405ff, for reviews.

Age	LANGUAGE	FINE MOTOR	GROSS MOTOR	SELF-HELP	SOCIAL
5-0 yr.	Tells meaning of familiar words	Prints first name (four letters)	Swings on swing, pumping by self	Goes to the toilet without help	Shows leadership among children
4-6	Reads a few letters (five+)	Draws a person showing at least three parts—head, eyes, nose, mouth, etc.	Skips or makes running "broad jumps"	Usually looks both ways before crossing street	Follows simple rules in board games or card games
4-0 yr.	Follows a series of three simple instructions	Draws recognizable pictures	Hops around on one foot without support	Buttons one or more buttons	Protective toward younger children
	Understands concepts — size, number, shape			Dresses and undresses without help, except for tying shoelaces	
3-6	Counts five or more objects when asked "how many?" Identifies four colors correctly	Cuts across paper with small scissors Draws or copies a complete circle	Hops on one foot without support	Washes face without help	Plays cooperatively, with minimum conflict and supervision
	Combines sentences with the words "and," "or," or "but"		Rides around on a tricycle, using pedals	Toilet trained	Gives directions to other children
3-0 yr.	Understands four prepositions—in, on, under, beside	Cuts with small scissors	Walks up and down stairs—one foot per step	Dresses self with help	Plays a role in "pretend" games—mom-dad, teacher, space pilot
2-6	Talks clearly, is understandable most of the time	Draws or copies vertical lines	Stands on one foot without support	Washes and dries hands	Plays with other children—cars, dolls, building
	Talks in two- to three-word phrases or sentences	Scribbles with circular motion	Climbs on play equipment—ladders, slides	Opens door by turning knob	"Helps" with simple household tasks

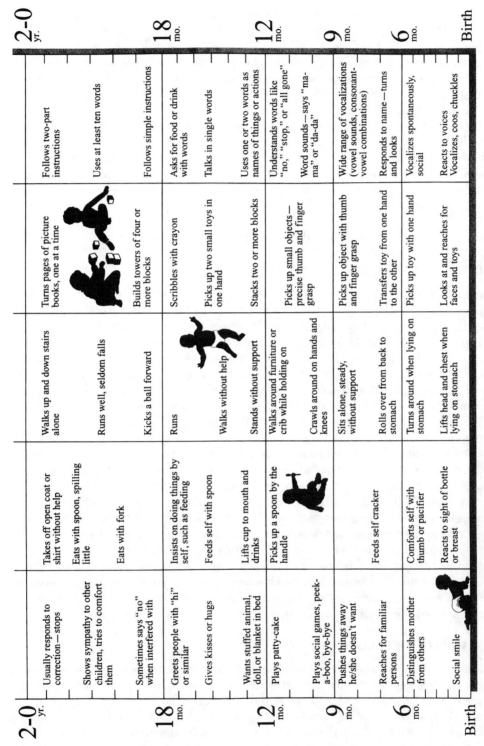

Figure 3.2. Child development in the first 5 years. (Courtesy of Harold Ireton, Ph.D.)

to classify, and to reason. During this span, children are occupied with developing higher level cognitive abilities at the expense of such sensorimotor processes as the expression of language with newly emerging motor speech skills.

Lindsay (1989) points out that during this period of cognitive development, a child goes through many transitional periods in which new cognitive learning must be assimilated and accommodated with current knowledge. These transitions are times when the child's linguistic and cognitive systems are temporarily unstable, before new concepts are mastered. As a consequence, speech and language production during this period of adjustment may be vulnerable to disfluencies.

Our understanding of the relationship between fluency and cognition is tenuous, but we have some idea of the questions that need to be asked. We need research on the extent and type of cognitive deficits in retarded individuals and the stuttering they manifest. We also need research on the potential disparity between cognitive development and motor speech development in children of normal intelligence before and after the emergence of stuttering.

Social and Emotional Development

INTERFERENCE WITH SPEECH BY EMOTION

In early childhood, a child's immature nervous system may permit "cross-talk" or interference between the limbic system—structures and pathways involved in the regulation and expression of emotion—and structures and pathways used for speech and language. This may be even more likely for children predisposed to stutter, whose slower maturing speech and language functions may not be optimally localized and closer to centers of emotion, as discussed in Chapter 2. Thus, when such children are emotionally aroused, fluency may suffer because neural signals for properly timed and sequenced muscle contractions may be interfered with in some way. We see evidence of this when we ask parents when their child first began to stutter. Parents frequently tell us they first noticed stuttering at a time when their child was highly excited about something.

Excitement is also mentioned in the literature as a common stimulus for disfluency. Starkweather (1987) noted that "all children speak more disfluently during periods of excitement." Dorothy Davis (1940), who conducted one of the first studies of normal disfluency, reported that of the 10 situations in which children showed repetitions in their speech, "excitement over own activity" was the situation in which children most frequently repeated sounds and words. Johnson and associates (1959) asked parents of children identified as stutterers to describe the situation in which they first observed their child's stuttering. The conditions most often reported to be associated with the first appearance of stuttering were when the child was in a hurry to tell something or was in a state of excitement. Thus, we see that both stuttering and normal disfluency seem to occur most often or noticeably during states of transitory emotional arousal.

STAGES OF DEVELOPMENT

Some stages of development may provide more social and emotional stress than others. For example, the processes of separation and individuation are known to be periods of stress. After a child passes his second birthday, he strives harder for autonomy, creating the conflicts of the "terrible twos." Parents gradually relinquish control and, at the same time, help their child learn the limits to his freedom. In some cases, the change from a dependent infant to an independent preschooler may be too rapid for a parent or a child. If the child is pushed toward independence faster than he wants, he may feel frustrated and insecure because his mother seems less nurturing. A mother may become alarmed if she isn't ready for the child's quest for independence and respond by restraining him. The child may conform but feel angry and frustrated. Yet, he cannot easily express those feelings to someone he depends on so much. The result may be disfluency in those interactions in which such ambivalence creates an emotional conflict that affects motor control of speech (Lidz, 1968).

SECURITY

As a young child grows older, other members of the family play a part in social and emotional changes. On the one hand, the child's father and brothers and sisters provide a wider support system. On the other hand, the child's resentment at having to share his mother's attention may elicit feelings of anger, aggression, and guilt. If such feelings are punished or ignored, they may result in temporary disfluency, or they may make stuttering more severe.

One of the more common provocations for feelings of resentment is the birth of a sibling. We discuss the effect of a sibling's birth on fluency later in the section on environmental factors, but it is worth mentioning here, too, because a child's strong feelings often reflect his developmental level as well as the environmental event. Theodore Lidz (1968, p. 246), a developmental psychiatrist with an interest in speech and language, describes a good example:

> Psychoanalytically oriented play therapy with children also indicates that many of their forbidden wishes and ideas have relatively simple access to consciousness. A six-year-old boy who started to stammer severely after a baby sister was born was watched playing with a family of dolls. He placed a baby doll in a crib next to the parent dolls' bed and then had a boy doll come and throw the baby to the floor, beat it, and throw it into a corner. He then put the boy doll into the crib. In a subsequent session, he had the father doll pummel the mother doll's abdomen, saying, "No, no!" At this point of childhood, even though certain unacceptable ideas cannot be talked about, they are still not definitely repressed.

Although we feel, as does Lidz, that stuttering may be triggered by the birth of a sibling, our belief about the underlying cause is not so freudian. Many threats to feelings of security create emotional stress and may disrupt the speech of children who are predisposed to stutter. As is evident in the section on treatment, we have found that therapy strategies that increase the child's sense of security and help him learn to speak more fluently will usually suffice.

SELF-CONSCIOUSNESS AND SENSITIVITY

The development of self-consciousness, which begins during the child's second year, may be another source of social and emotional stress. This is the growing awareness by the child of how he is performing relative to adult expectations. Although it is not thoroughly understood, Jerome Kagan presents an interesting description of the process in his book, *The Second Year* (1981). In a relevant example, Kagan proposes that the self-corrections a child makes in his speech are evidence of this self-awareness. Taking this further, we can surmise that this increasing self-awareness, in a child who is excessively disfluent, might lead to self-corrections that only worsen the problem.

In Chapter 2, we briefly discuss clinical reports and a few studies suggesting that persons who stutter, as a group, may have an unusually sensitive temperament. Research on temperament in nonstuttering children, especially the longitudinal studies of Calkins and Fox (1994) and Kagan and Snidman (1991), indicate that the social-emotional traits of fearfulness and withdrawal that accompany a more sensitive temperament can change over the course of a child's preschool years. Some children become better able to modulate their temperamental tendencies, but others remain hostage to their temperaments. These individual adaptations may be crucial in determining which children who begin to stutter will continue to do so and which children will stop.

Before we leave this section, we want to comment on stutterers' psychological adjustment in general. Many people who have little exposure to stuttering believe that stutterers are essentially nervous people or that stuttering is a sign of neurosis. If this were true, we would have found evidence of psychological maladjustment or excessive anxiety in people who stutter, particularly when stuttering first begins in childhood. However, research on personality and adjustment in people who stutter has found no convincing evidence that they differ from nonstutterers in these ways (Bloch & Goodstein, 1971; Bloodstein, 1995; Van Riper, 1982). A few findings suggest that adults who stutter may not be as socially well adjusted as those who do not, but this can probably be attributed to the influence of stuttering on social experiences (Bloodstein, 1987).

Summarizing the effect of social and emotional development on fluency, we have suggested that many of the normal social and emotional stresses that children experience may result in disfluent speech, although our evidence is mostly anecdotal. Moreover, we suspect that children who are neurophysiologically vulnerable to stuttering may be especially prone to difficulty when social conflicts and emotions create extra "noise" in their neural circuitry for speech. Children who stutter appear to be as psychologically well adjusted as nonstutterers, despite the extreme emotional stress that stuttering itself can impose.

Speech and Language Development

Stuttering usually begins when speech and language are developing most rapidly (Van Riper, 1982; Bloodstein, 1995). Consider how much this rapid growth may affect fluent speech. In the first place, the child is having to learn to control a speech mechanism that is continuously changing size and shape because he is growing rapidly. He is also having to synchronize his speech to the rates and rhythms of parents and siblings with whom he has a growing urge to communicate. In addition, his speech motor skills must accommodate his expanding linguistic abilities.

In the single year between ages 2 and 3 years, the child's vocabulary jumps from 50 to well over 500 words; in fact, toward the end of this year he may be learning five to seven new words a day (Studdert-Kennedy, 1987). At the same time, his utterances are developing from successive single word pairs with sentence-like intonations and durations into multiword sentences (Branigan, 1979).[5] As he is expanding his sentences, the child is also overhauling his language storage system. At first, he stocked his shelves with whole words in the form of articulatory routines or gestural patterns; then he changes strategies and stores, not whole words, but segments that can be combined variously into a multitude of words (Kent, 1985; Nittrouer, Studdert-Kennedy, & McGowan, 1989; Stemberger, 1982). During these same early preschool years, the child also progressively learns active, negative, and passive constructions and present, future, and past tenses. At the same time, he increases the length and linguistic complexity of his sentences together with the rate of his utterances.[6] This multitude of tasks inevitably takes a toll on a preschooler's fluency.

---

[5] This mode of sentence development may be yet another reflection of language planning leading speech production ability.

[6] The connection between increasing length of utterance and increasing rate is discussed by many authors, including Malecot, Johnston, and Kizziar, 1972; Starkweather, 1987; and Umeda, 1975, 1977.

To imagine how this might happen, remember that the child's brain is a system with a finite amount of resources that must be parceled out to tasks he is engaged in. Moreover, tasks that use similar areas of this cerebral system may have to share neural resources. During periods of rapid language acquisition available neural resources may not be shared rapidly enough for the task of speech production. However, as more language is acquired and utterances become longer, speech rate usually increases. But in a system with finite resources, there must be a speed-accuracy trade-off; that is, if speed increases, accuracy decreases. If a child, who is already burdened with increasing complexity of language, attempts to produce his utterances more quickly before available resources can meet that demand, he may make more errors. Depending on the child, this trade-off may manifest itself as stuttering, phonological simplifications, or some other form of less mature spoken language.

Bernstein Ratner (1997) provided an excellent discussion of the particular demands that children may experience as they reorganize their language production systems during the very years when stuttering onset is most frequent. Drawing on theoretical perspectives, such as those of Bates, Dale, and Thal (1995), Bernstein Ratner proposed that children move from a lexically based to a grammatically based production system during this period. Evidence suggests that this change is promoted by (or at least accompanied by) the "double whammy" of a spurt in vocabulary growth and an increased mastery of grammatical rules. Thus, as neural resources are devoted to acquiring and organizing new language learning, speech production capabilities may also be burdened by increasingly complex utterances, and all this is occurring during the same time children are trying to gain mastery of their rapidly growing speech anatomy and physiology. It is no wonder that many children experience instability in their speech and language production at this time, which may appear as normal disfluency or as stuttering.

The notion that developmental spurts of spoken language may diminish fluency is not new. Peggy Dalton and W. J. Hardcastle (1977), for example, commented that "it is tempting to see the ever-increasing demands on linguistic competence and articulatory proficiency as a major factor in the onset of some disfluency." Joseph Sheehan (1975) put it this way: "The age of onset of stuttering is consistently related to certain stages in the developmental sequence. Most notably, the 'period of resonance,' or high readiness in language learning, noted by Lenneberg . . . is also the period during which stuttering develops and flourishes." Andrews and associates (1983) pointed to the demand placed on speech by rapidly developing language by saying, "stuttering [has] a maximal frequency of onset at a time when an explosive growth in language ability outstrips a still-immature speech-motor apparatus."

The reduction in fluency during the rapid development of spoken language may result in another similarity between normal disfluency and early stuttering. Bloodstein (1995) has noted that there is considerable evidence of a connection between language development and stuttering and that part of this evidence is the tendency for many children—both stutterers and nonstutterers—to become more disfluent during certain stages of intense language development. Evidence of increased stuttering as children attempt to use more complex structures can be found in observational studies by Gaines, Runyan, and Meyers (1991), Logan and Conture (1995), and Brundage and Bernstein Ratner (1989).

In addition, experimental studies show that both stutterers (Bernstein Ratner & Sih, 1987; Stocker & Usprich, 1976) and nonstutterers (Gordon, Luper, & Peterson, 1986; Haynes & Hood, 1978; Pearl & Bernthal, 1980) show increased disfluencies as language complexity is increased. Unfortunately, there is little longitudinal research that directly bears on the question of how and when emerging language is associated with normal disfluency.

One of the few descriptive studies was the analysis of disfluencies in four nonstuttering children by Norma Colburn using data originally gathered by Lois Bloom for her work on normal language development. The published reports of this analysis (Colburn & Mysak, 1982a,b) suggested that normal disfluencies appeared not when these children first learned a new language construction, but as they began to master it and started to use it regularly. Suggested explanations for this result include the possibility that the child has incompletely automatized the use of the construction and allocates fewer resources than are necessary for production (Kent & Perkins, 1984) and the idea that, having mastered a construction, the child produced it at an increased rate, thereby straining capacity (Starkweather, 1987).

A single-case approach was used to explore the relationship between syntax acquisition and normal disfluencies in a study by Frank Wijnen (1990). Weekly speech samples were obtained from a boy from ages 2 years 4 months to 2 years 11 months. The number of repetitions, revisions, and incomplete phrases were assessed in relation to the length and complexity of utterances. It was reported that although disfluencies were randomly distributed at first, they eventually clustered on function words and sentence-initial words and then declined. Although speech rate was not measured and increased rate might have accounted for some of the increased disfluencies, the disfluencies were not highly correlated with the lengths of the child's utterances. Instead, Wijnen concluded that the decline in the child's disfluencies was associated with his development of a routine type of sentence (pronoun + verb + some other word) and that learning this routine involved so much processing capacity that speech production was short-changed. This preliminary study needs to be followed up with many more cases to test the hypothesis that the process of learning to make sentence production more automatic through routinization of several sentence types is related to normal disfluency. With a larger sample size, multiple regression analyses could be used to determine which of many possible factors best predict instances of disfluency.

There is some indication that children who have difficulty mastering speech and language during this period of development are at high risk for persistent stuttering. The study of factors that predict recovery from stuttering that was cited earlier (Yairi, Ambrose, Paden, & Throneburg, 1996) noted that poorer performance on tests of phonology and language skills were predictive of continued stuttering for 36 months or more after stuttering onset. The acquisition of spoken language may strain neural resources in many children, precipitating disfluencies. For those who have extra difficulty acquiring speech or language, the continued demand on these neural resources may hamper their efforts to compensate or reorganize speech production processes to enable fluency, and thus lead to persistent stuttering.

Earlier we suggested that the increased incidence of stuttering among children who are retarded may be explained by the fact that their acquisition of speech and language is delayed, or more to the point, their learning period is longer than normal. These children may be trying to acquire language from infancy to adulthood, increasing the risk period for developing stuttering. Our own clinical experience supports this and suggests more specifically that competition for neuronal resources may explain why fluency suffers when spoken language is learned. A mother of a child with Down syndrome told us that her son's stuttering increased dramatically in frequency and severity when he made great gains in vocabulary and syntax. This suggests that some aspect of acquiring language may make a child more vulnerable to stuttering. In individuals with more limited central capacities, the strain placed on resources by language learning may be particularly great.

As with other demands on a child's resources, rapid speech and language development may or may not affect a particular child's fluency. Whether these particular demands will precipitate stuttering and when that will occur is likely to depend, in part, on other developmental demands the child is facing, the child's resources to respond to these demands, and the support the child receives from his environment.

ENVIRONMENTAL FACTORS

Some children may show initial signs of stuttering in response to developmental pressures alone, but most who become stutterers probably are affected by environmental pressures also. These are factors outside the child. Typically, they are attitudes, behaviors, or events that occur in their homes. An example may be the child's family's anxiety about or nonaccepting responses to disfluency. Or, families may affect children's fluency by unknowingly placing pressure on them to speak at a level beyond their developmental capacity. For example, children who are at an early stage of speech development may encounter a listener's impatience when they are speaking slowly and haltingly. Responding to the listener's impatience, they may begin to stutter because they try to speak at a rate beyond their capacity. Or, the psychological stress caused by a listener's impatience may disrupt their smooth motor coordination.

When we described the effects of developmental factors on a child's speech, we used the analogy of a computer that is overloaded by too many simultaneous tasks. We can use the computer analogy for environmental factors, too. However, we now ask you to imagine that a computer is being used for programs that exceed its speed or memory capacities, is subjected to periodic power surges, or given commands it is not programmed to process. Imagine that this, in turn, may create fluency breakdowns in the vulnerable child. These environmental pressures also worsen the symptoms of stuttering, as seen in Chapter 5.

We begin this section on environmental factors by reviewing research on the most important factor in the family environment, the parents of children who stutter.

Parents

In the 1930s and 1940s at the University of Iowa, Wendell Johnson developed the "diagnosogenic" theory of stuttering. This theory, which is described more fully in a later section, suggests that a child's parents erroneously diagnose normal disfluencies as stuttering. Their reaction then causes the child to struggle and avoid these normal interruptions in speech in a way that becomes real stuttering. Johnson's diagnosogenic theory generated a great deal of research on parents of stutterers. Were they different from the parents of nonstutterers? Were they unusually critical? Did they have unreasonably high standards of speech?

One of the first studies of parents of stutterers was conducted by John Moncur (1952). Moncur interviewed the mothers of both stuttering and nonstuttering children about their parenting practices. He found that mothers of stuttering children tended to be more critical, more protective, and more domineering toward their children than mothers of nonstuttering children. Not long afterward, Frederick Darley, a student of Wendell Johnson at the University of Iowa, investigated the attitudes of stutterers' parents in more detail. Using interview techniques based on the famous sex studies of Alfred Kinsey, Darley (1955) questioned the parents of 50 stutterers and 50 nonstutterers. Although there was a great deal of overlap in the attitudes of these two groups, the parents of children who stuttered showed significantly higher standards and expectations, particularly with regard to speech. They believed in early intervention with nonfluencies; they had greater sensitivity to speech deviations; their overall drive and need for domination was greater.

Darley's study was expanded by Wendell Johnson and his research associates (1959) to the parents of 150 stuttering and 150 nonstuttering children. Again, there was much overlap between parents of stutterers and parents of nonstutterers, but again, parents of children who stutter were found to be more perfectionistic and to have higher standards of behavior than the other parents. These studies by Moncur, Darley, Johnson, and others are largely responsible for the widespread belief that parents are a key factor in the onset of stuttering. Parents could transmit a culture's "competitive pressure for achievement or conformity," which may be the environmental factor most likely to be linked with stuttering (Bloodstein, 1987).

We should emphasize that there are many conflicting findings in the literature and that parents of stutterers, if they do differ from parents of nonstutterers, differ only slightly. Because these studies have not used additional control groups of parents of children who with other disorders, we can't dismiss the possibility that, rather than causing stuttering, these differences may be the result of stuttering. Perhaps any parent of a child with a disorder would appear to have high standards for him. We note, also, that these are group differences; many parents of stuttering children are more accepting and less competitive than many parents of nonstuttering children.

Even if parents of children who stutter do have high standards and a degree of perfectionism, this factor would not by itself produce stuttering. After all, a stutterer's brothers and sisters may thrive under this influence. And as we have suggested before, most children of demanding parents do not become stutterers. But for a child who is vulnerable—constitutionally predisposed to stutter—it may be just the straw that broke the camel's back. One can imagine a child feeling self-conscious in a family that strives for perfection, especially in speech. Such a child could become so concerned about minor disfluencies that he tries too hard to be perfectly fluent and begins to labor and struggle when his speech is disfluent. Some children who become stutterers may not be highly vulnerable and have only slight constitutional predispositions, but may encounter overwhelming environmental pressures. For example, a child with few evident disfluencies may gradually develop stuttering under relentless pressure to perform at higher levels socially, academically, or athletically.

Let us digress for a moment from the Iowa studies that found competitive pressure to be common in the homes of stutterers. Different results were found in England. Gavin Andrews and Mary Ann Harris (1964), whose work is described in Chapter 2, collected and analyzed data from an ongoing study of families in Newcastle, England. Combining medical records and home visits, Andrews and Harris compared the parents of stutterers with the parents of nonstutterers. They found that both groups of parents, most of whom were mothers, were generally similar in personality but differed in some key traits. The parents of stutterers were lower in intelligence, had poorer school records when they were younger, had poorer work histories, and provided poorer housing for their children. There was no evidence that these parents criticized or pressured their children. This finding is a far cry from the evidence of excessively high standards in the stutterers' homes in Iowa.

Why are these results so different from those of the Iowa studies? There may be many reasons, but two come easily to mind. The first is that stuttering may emerge in children under many types of stress. In industrial England, the greatest stress may have come from social and economic disadvantages, but in Iowa, the greatest stress may have been the high standards of upwardly mobile parents. A second reason for these differences may be a difference in researchers' expectations and biases of two decades ago. Americans tend to believe that all men are created equal. American researchers, especially those in the heartland of the United States, would be predisposed to look for influences, not in heredity, but in stutterers' environments. On the other hand, many Britons believe that inheritance plays a major role in determining life outcomes, and researchers in Britain would be more likely to look for causes of stuttering in the parents' intelligence and social class.

The hypothesis that lower class homes can provide stress on stutterers was not new in Great Britain. John Morgenstern (1956), who investigated stuttering in Scottish children, found that stuttering was most prevalent in lower class homes (with skilled manual weekly wage earners) than those in the Iowa studies. This, however, was a stratum that in Scotland was upwardly mobile and may have expressed ambitions through high speech standards for their children. Here, we have a combination of forces, if Morgenstern's hypothesis is correct. The stress of lower class homes lies not in their deprivation, but in the cultural pressure to perform well to rise above humble beginnings.

More recent studies of parents of children who stutter present mixed results. Some reported that they are more rejecting or anxious than are parents of children who do not stutter (Flugel, 1979; Zenner, Ritterman, Bowen, & Gronhovd, 1978), but others have found only small or no differences between the two groups of parents (Goodstein, 1956; Goodstein & Dahlstrom, 1956). In his thorough review of the home environments of children who stutter, Yairi (1997b) concluded that the mix of diverse findings boil down to the likelihood that children who stutter grow up in unfavorable environments. But Yairi noted that, although many studies suggest that parents of children who stutter may be somewhat anxious, overprotective, socially withdrawn, and negatively evaluative of their children, there is no evidence that these parental tendencies cause stuttering. Yairi went on to point out that since risk for stuttering is often inherited, the parents of these children may themselves stutter or have stuttered or had contact with other family members who stuttered. Thus, their negative traits may be a result of their own experiences with this disability.

Our own view is in accord with Yairi's, but we would put this fine point on it: at least some of the children with persistent stuttering may have a vulnerable temperament (Oyler & Ramig, 1995), which may be inherited. Their parents, the genetic source of this temperament, may be those anxious, overprotective mothers or fathers described in the literature on stutterers' parents. This child, then, is in double jeopardy for persistent stuttering because of his own temperament and because one or both parents are overly concerned about his stuttering because of their temperament. On the other hand, some parents may have an ameliorating effect on a child's vulnerable temperament. With a parent's help, it is possible for a child who begins to stutter and who is emotionally reactive to recover from stuttering. In their discussion of the influence of the environment on biological predispositions in nonstuttering children, Calkins and Fox (1994, p. 209) said that "the child's interactions with a parent provide the context for learning skills and strategies for managing emotional reactivity."

Again we see that influences on stuttering are numerous and complex, coming both from the child and from the environment. Some may precipitate disfluencies, and others may interact to make remission more difficult. Still others may provide the kinds of support that make remission possible.

Speech and Language Environment

Because a preschool child is so heavily influenced by the speech and language around him, especially that of his parents, the speech and language used by others may be an important source of pressure on the stuttering child. As the child tries to imitate adult models of speech and language, to use longer words and longer sentences, to try less familiar words, and to pack more meaning into his utterances, he will be more likely to stutter. Van Riper (1973. p. 381) thought that the child may be vulnerable to this pressure when he is most rapidly developing language: "Stuttering usually begins at the very time that great advances in sentence construction occur, and it seems tenable that, when the speech models provided by the parents or siblings of the child are too difficult for him to follow, some faltering will ensue."

Two writers have moved beyond clinical speculation to develop informal theories about the influence of adult models on a child's fluency. Crystal (1987) proposed an "interactive" view of many speech and language disorders, which suggested that demands at one level of language production (e.g., syntax) may deplete resources for other levels (e.g., prosody or phonology), resulting in breakdown. His supporting data nicely illustrate how stuttering, in particular, may be exacerbated by a child's use of advanced language. He recorded evidence that the more complex the syntax and semantics a child used, the more he stuttered. Starkweather (1987), describing a demands and capacities view of stuttering, commented that "the production of speech and the formulation of language place a simultaneous demand on the young person. If the demands in either of these two dimensions are excessive, performance in the other dimension may be reduced." These two views imply that stuttering may increase when an individual uses longer words, less frequently occurring words, more information-bearing words, and longer sentences. Stuttering may also increase when the individual is uttering a more linguistically complex sentence.[7]

What do we know about the speech and language of the parents of stutterers?[8] Unfortunately, very little. One study focused directly on speech of parents. Susan Meyers and Frances Freeman (1985a,b) compared the speech of mothers of stutterers with the speech of mothers of nonstutterers. They found that mothers of stutterers spoke more rapidly than did mothers of nonstutterers.[9] This may be critical, since a mother's high speech rate has the potential to make a child try to speak faster than his optimal speed (e.g., Jaffe & Anderson, 1979). The possibility that a rapid speech rate may lead to stuttering is supported by Johnson and Rosen's (1937) finding that adult stutterers were more likely to stutter when they spoke more rapidly than normal. Children who stutter may be even more vulnerable than adults who stutter to fluency breakdowns during rapid speech, by virtue of the fact that children's natural rate of speech is slower and their temporal coordination less (e.g., Kent, 1981).

Several studies subsequent to those of Meyers and Freeman (1985a,b) have failed to find speech rate differences between parents of children who stutter and parents of children who don't stutter. Kelly and Conture (1992) found no differences in the speaking rates of mothers of these two groups of children; Kelly (1994) found no differences in the speaking rate of fathers of the two groups; Yaruss and Conture (1995) found no difference in articulatory rate (the rate at which each phrase is spoken, as opposed to speaking

---

[7] The interested reader should consult pp. 175–176 of Starkweather's *Fluency and Stuttering* (1987) for more discussion of these phenomena and for references to this research.

[8] Kasprisin-Burelli, Egolf, and Shames (1972) studied the parent-child interactions between parents of stuttering children and between parents of nonstuttering children. They found that parents of stutterers tended to make a much higher proportion of negative statements in their conversations than did parents of nonstutterers. Although these findings do not tell us about models of speech, per se, they suggest that stuttering children may be under more negative emotional pressure in talking with their parents.

[9] In this study, mothers of children who stutter spoke faster than mothers of nonstuttering children, whether they were talking to their own children or to the nonstuttering children. But mothers of nonstuttering children spoke faster to children who stuttered than they did to nonstuttering children. Thus, it may be the case that stuttering itself will influence a mother to increase here speech rate.

rate, which includes pauses between phrases) between mothers of stuttering children and mothers of nonstuttering children.

There are several possibilities why the earlier studies found differences between parents' speaking rate and later ones didn't. Zebrowski (1995), in her fine review of conversational patterns in families of children who stutter, discussed this disparity between earlier and later studies. She suggested that differences in measurement techniques and the fact that Meyers and Freeman (1985a,b) had a larger number of severe stutterers in their sample may account for the differences in the studies. We think it is possible also that parents of children just beginning to stutter are becoming increasingly aware of the importance of speaking slowly because of publicity aimed at stuttering prevention. These parents may try to speak more slowly than usual under the scrutiny of clinical researchers, thus adding to the likelihood that more recent studies may not show differences in the speaking rates of parents of stutterers and nonstutterers.

Another suspected stressor in parents' conversations, in addition to rapid speech rates, is the frequency with which parents interrupt their children. One of Meyers and Freeman's reports (1985a) presented some unexpected evidence about interruptions. Both mothers of stutterers and mothers of nonstutterers interrupted most frequently when the children were disfluent. It seems possible that such parental interruptions, some of which may have been elicited by the child's disfluencies, may, in turn, elicit changes in the child's speech. Some children might increase tension and rate and thereby develop the struggled behaviors of stuttering. Others might suppress disfluencies to avoid interruptions and eventually be "taught" by their parents not to be disfluent.

In a more recent study, Kelly and Conture (1992) found no significant differences in interruptions between mothers of stuttering children and mothers of nonstuttering children. However, a closer inspection of their data revealed a correlation between the duration of "simultalk" (one person talking at the same time that another is talking) of the mothers of children who stutter and the children's severity of stuttering. Thus, mothers of more severe stutterers did more simultalk when their children were talking than did mothers of children who stuttered less severely. In a later study of fathers, Kelly (1994) found no difference in interruptions between fathers of children who stutter and fathers of children who don't stutter. Moreover, for these fathers, the correlation between simultalk and severity of stuttering was not significant.

Besides the modicum of research cited above, there is a wealth of clinical material suggesting that the speech and language environment of a child is an important influence on his fluency. In *The Treatment of Stuttering* (pp. 380–383), for example, Van Riper cites nine references in which clinicians point to parental speech models as a major source of stress on a child's fluency. This stress includes not only the parents' speech and language, but also the conditions under which the child tries to speak. Advice for parents of stutterers, given by clinicians with experience treating young stutterers (e.g., Ainsworth & Fraser, 1989; Starkweather, Gottwald, & Halfond, 1990; and Van Riper, 1973), often includes observing and, when appropriate, changing the speech and language environment in the home. In their publications, clinicians have noted that the speech and language stresses listed in Table 3.1 are likely to increase stuttering.

These stressful conditions appear to pressure many children with average speech abilities to the point that they become mildly disfluent. But what about the child who is also experiencing difficulty with fine motor coordination for speech or who is delayed in language? This child may be especially vulnerable to speech and language stresses in the home. Fluency may break down as he struggles to produce spoken language at a rate and complexity far beyond his reach. He may also be vulnerable because he is frequently misunderstood. For example, a child who misarticulates several sounds or is notably delayed

Table 3.1. Speech and Language Stresses

Stressful Adult Speech Models	
Rapid speech rate	Complex syntax
Polysyllabic vocabulary	Use of two languages in home

Stressful Speaking Situations for Child	
Competition for speaking	Hurried when speaking
Frequent interruptions	Frequent questions
Demand for display speech	Excited when speaking
Loss of listener attention	Many things to say

in language may develop a conviction that talking is hard and he is an inadequate speaker. Bloodstein (1995) cited several accounts of the appearance of stuttering in children with delayed language development or articulation problems; their parents' models of speech and language and their attempts to improve the child's speech appear to have contributed to the child's stuttering.

Research by Merits-Patterson and Reed (1981) may also be relevant. They found that children receiving language therapy had more stuttering-type disfluencies (part-word repetitions, word repetitions, prolongations, and fixations) than did children with either language delay or normal speech who were not receiving treatment. Although their findings are weakened by the fact that the disfluencies of the two groups of language-delayed children may have differed, this study suggests that the communicative pressure created by treatment may result in an increase in stuttering-type disfluencies. It may not be stretching the point too far to suggest that language-delayed children in a home environment of fast and complex language may be experiencing pressure somewhat similar to those in treatment.

Researchers and clinicians do not feel, however, that language treatment should be avoided for children who stutter. On the contrary, as long as the clinician is sufficiently aware of the effect of language pressure, therapy can provide a critical boost to improve children's overall communication skills and thereby indirectly improve their fluency.

Life Events

Certain events in life can deliver a blow to a child's stability and security. When this happens, stuttering may suddenly appear out of nowhere, or previously easy repetitions may be transformed into hard, struggled blocks. To have someone close to you die, to be hospitalized for an operation, or to have parents divorce is difficult for any of us, but it is especially difficult for children. Obviously, many children go through such events and adapt to them without major problems. But children who are vulnerable to stuttering often show the effects of these events in their speech. Kagan (1994a) noted that even some children who begin life with a relaxed temperament may become shy and fearful under the onslaught of stressful events. This may well set the stage for stuttering if other constitutional factors predispose the child for it.

There is little research on the relationship of difficult life events to stuttering, but many authors have observed the connection. Starkweather (1987), for example, wrote, "All children speak more disfluently during periods of tension—when moving or changing schools, when their parents divorce, or after the death of a family member." This increased disfluency could easily result in the onset of stuttering or increased stuttering in those children who are most vulnerable. Johnson and associates (1959) noted that among

16 situations in which parents first noticed their child's stuttering were these: (*a*) child's physical environment changed (e.g., moving to new house), (*b*) child became ill, (*c*) child realized his mother was pregnant, (*d*) a new baby arrived. Van Riper (1982), in discussing the onset of stuttering, acknowledged that various studies have found no differences in the amount of emotional conflict in the homes of children who developed stuttering versus those who didn't. "Nevertheless," said Van Riper, "we have studied individual cases in which stuttering did seem [to be] triggered by such conflicts, and it is difficult for us to ignore these experiences."

Our own clinical experience is similar. For example, in the past several years during which we've evaluated about 20 children who stutter, we've encountered four children in four different families who began to stutter when their parents were in the early stages of divorce. However, this turmoil was not the only factor in their stuttering. Three of the children had relatives who stuttered, and the father of the fourth child was a clutterer. Moreover, all four were preschoolers and were likely experiencing various growth and development pressures. But for all of them, their parents' divorce appeared to us to be the factor that pushed them from normal speech to stuttering.

In another case of a life event precipitating stuttering, a 9-year-old girl with normal fluency began to stutter when her classroom teacher had an emotional breakdown. The teacher's outbursts of anger and crying, interspersed with high demands for rapid performance on frequent examinations, apparently created extreme stress for this student. Under this stress she developed tight blocks, with physical tension at the level of the larynx and abdomen, a pattern described by Van Riper (1982) as "Track III" stuttering. Even though we were convinced, through extensive interviews of the family, that the child had no prior stuttering, we noted several factors predisposing for stuttering. First, the girl's younger sister had significant learning disabilities, including auditory processing problems. Second, the girl's mother described herself and the daughter who stutters as shy and emotionally reactive. These two factors—family history of learning disability and presence of vulnerable temperament—may have provided a fertile matrix for the sudden germination of stuttering when a stressful life event occurred.

In a few cases, traumatic life events appear to precipitate stuttering in children (and adults) who appear to have no predisposition to stuttering. These unusual onsets are discussed when we explore "psychogenic stuttering" in a later chapter. These individuals often stutter in unusual ways, which differ from the "garden variety" stuttering seen in those who begin to stuttering when a stressful life event interacts with various predisposing conditions. The list in Table 3.2 contains some of the life events that we have found to be stressful to children's fluency.

Table 3.2. Stressful Life Events That May Increase a Child's Disfluency

1. The child's family moves to a new house, a new neighborhood, or a new city.
2. The child's parents separate or divorce.
3. A family member dies.
4. A family member is hospitalized.
5. The child is hospitalized.
6. A parent loses his or her job.
7. A baby is born or another child is adopted.
8. An additional person comes to live in the house.
9. One or both parents go away frequently or for a long period of time.
10. Holidays or visits occur, which cause a change in routine, excitement, or anxiety.

THEORIES ABOUT DEVELOPMENTAL
AND ENVIRONMENTAL FACTORS

The three views presented in this section represent three different conceptualizations of how developmental or environmental stresses or both may contribute to stuttering. One view (diagnosogenic) takes normal disfluency as a starting point and assumes that stuttering develops when parents mistakenly diagnose it as "stuttering." The other two views look more broadly at circumstances from which stuttering might arise. One of these views (communicative failure and anticipatory struggle) assumes that some form of communication difficulty precipitates stuttering; the other view (capacities and demands) presumes that almost any developmental or environmental pressure may precipitate it. As you read this section, keep in mind that these three views differ not only in their concept of the roles of development and environment but also in their specificity. The first (diagnosogenic) proposes particular elements that create stuttering; the last (capacities and demands) presents general principles by which many different variables may interact to produce stuttering. The specificity of the middle view (Communicative Failure) lies somewhere between the others.

Diagnosogenic Theory

In the 1930s, Wendell Johnson and other researchers at the University of Iowa began studying the onset of stuttering in children. As Johnson examined the speech of young stutterers and nonstutterers, he noticed a similarity. The most common disfluencies for both groups were repetitions. As Johnson contemplated this evidence, he was struck by the possibility that all of these children may have had the same disfluencies to begin with but that those who were stutterers developed more serious disfluencies by overreacting to their repetitions. Why? Their parents or other listeners may have mislabeled their repetitions as stuttering. In so doing, they may have made the children so self-conscious that they tried hard to speak without any disfluencies. This effort to avoid disfluencies may have become, with the help of further negative listener reactions, what we generally regard as stuttering (Johnson et al., 1942).

Johnson's hypothesis, which came to be called the diagnosogenic theory (meaning that the disorder begins with its diagnosis, or in this case, misdiagnosis) was the most widely accepted explanation of stuttering throughout the 1940s and 1950s. It was a strong indictment of environmental factors in the onset of the disorder. It placed the blame solely on the negative reactions of parents and other listeners and ignored the role that constitutional predispositions for stuttering may play.

Johnson and his associates continued gathering data on the disfluencies of stuttering children and their nonstuttering peers to further support the diagnosogenic theory. The results of several studies were summarized in a landmark book, *The Onset of Stuttering* (Johnson & associates, 1959). Table 3.3, taken from this book, gives an overview of the similarities and differences in the disfluencies reported by stutterers' and nonstutterers' parents.

It is immediately evident that certain types of disfluencies were reported far more commonly for stuttering than nonstuttering children. Syllable repetitions, sound prolongations, and complete blocks were recalled to have occurred much more frequently at stuttering onset. Phrase repetitions, pauses, and interjections were reported more frequently in the nonstuttering control group. What does this mean? Other authors have interpreted these findings as evidence that the two groups of children were different at the

**Table 3.3. Percentage of Parents of Stutterers and Nonstutterers
Who Reported Child Was Performing Each Speech Behavior
When They First Thought Child Was Stuttering**

| | Repetition | | | Other Nonfluency | | | |
Group	Syllable	Word	Phrase	Sound Prolonga-tion	Silent Intervals	Interjec-tions	Complete Blocks
Control (Nonstutterers)							
Fathers	4	59	23	3	36	30	0
Mothers	10	41	24	4	41	21	0
Experimental (Stutterers)							
Fathers	57	48	8	15	7	8	3
Mothers	59	50	8	12	3	9	3

From Johnson, W., and Associates. (1959). The Onset of Stuttering. Minneapolis: University of Minnesota Press. Copyright © 1959 by the University of Minnesota. © 1987 Edna Johnson. Reprinted by permission of the University of Minnesota Press.

onset of stuttering.[10] Johnson, on the other hand, emphasized the similarity of the data. He pointed out that both groups of children were reported to show at least some of each type of disfluency. The same disfluency types that some parents considered normal in their children were reported by other parents as the earliest signs of stuttering in their children. This left Johnson still convinced that part of the problem was parents' interpretation of their child's disfluencies, or as some often put it, "the problem was not in the child's mouth but in the parent's ear."

However, Johnson and his associates also observed that stuttering children had significantly more sound/syllable repetitions, complete blocks, and prolonged sounds. Johnson acknowledged that some of the problem might be more than parents' abnormal reactions, and his modified view (Johnson & associates, 1959, Chapter 10) saw stuttering as a result of the interaction among three factors: (*a*) the extent of the child's disfluency, (*b*) listeners' sensitivity to that disfluency, and (*c*) the child's sensitivity to his own disfluency and to listeners' reactions. This revision of the diagnosogenic theory still implicates the environment as a potent influence on the development of stuttering, but it also acknowledges the important contribution of factors within the child.

To illustrate the diagnosogenic view, we take an example from a masters' thesis that Johnson directed (Tudor, 1939). At that time, the diagnosogenic theory had not been formally proposed, but undoubtedly Johnson and others must have entertained the possibility that labeling a child as a stutterer would create more hesitancy in his speech. The thesis was an exploration of that idea. Johnson's student, Mary Tudor, screened all the children at a nearby orphanage for speech and language disorders. Selecting six who were normal speakers, she told these children that they should speak more carefully because they were making errors when they talked. She told them they had symptoms of stuttering. She also warned caregivers that these children should be watched closely for speech errors and corrected when they slipped up. After several months, Tudor went back to the orphanage and found that a number of the selected students showed stuttering-like behaviors. Although she tried to treat them, at least one was reported to continue stuttering for some time thereafter (Silverman, 1988).

---

[10]McDearmon (1968) has shown that these differences between stuttering and control children at onset to be statistically significant. He argued that the data from Johnson and associates' study suggest stutterers' typical first disfluencies (e.g., repetitions of syllables, sound prolongations) are categorically different form normals' first disfluencies (e.g., repetitions of phrases, pauses).

Tudor was remorseful about the results and regretted this experiment. Nonetheless, it reinforced Johnson's strong conviction, which he held throughout his career, that if a child is made self-conscious about his normal disfluencies, he may develop stuttering.

Communicative Failure and Anticipatory Struggle

This theory, developed by Oliver Bloodstein (1987, 1997), suggests that stuttering may develop when a child experiences frustration and failure when trying to talk. The child's original difficulty in talking need not be disfluency. Many types of communication failure may lead the child to anticipate future difficulty with speech. It is common, Bloodstein noted, to find articulation problems, language deficits, cluttering, and many other speech problems in the histories of children who begin to stutter. Table 3.4 lists some of the circumstances that Bloodstein suggests may cause some children to experience speech as difficult. If a child cannot make himself understood or is penalized for the way he talks, he may begin to tense his speech muscles and fragment his speech. These become the core behaviors of the child's stuttering. And they, in turn, form the experiences of frustration and failure in communication that the child anticipates with dread.

Other aspects of the child's "internal" and "external" environments play important parts also. The child's personality may be perfectionistic, or he may harbor a need to live up to parental expectations. His family may have high standards for speech or intolerance of any speech abnormality or may otherwise pressure the child to conform to standards beyond his reach. The presence or absence of such environmental pressures may cause some children to interpret an articulation difficulty, language problem, or disfluency as a failing, whereas others only shrug it off.

This perspective on stuttering accounts for the wide variability of disfluency among children. Most normal children experience enough temporary frustration when learning to talk to produce the mild fragmentations of speech we associate with normal disfluency. Children who stutter for just a few weeks may encounter unusual difficulty when first learning to talk but soon master the fundamentals and feel successful. Children who become chronic stutterers may repeatedly experience communication failure and grow up in an environment fraught with communicative pressure.

Here is a case that illustrates some of the environmental pressures that often surround children who begin to stutter. Susan grew up in the oil fields of Oklahoma, where her parents set themselves apart from the rest of the community by their aloof manner and precision of speech. They raised their children to feel that they were more cultured than their neighbors; in fact, Susan's father would often say, "We speak better than other people." Unfortunately, Susan was delayed in talking. When she did begin to speak, her parents couldn't understand her, so her older sister interpreted what she was saying to her parents. When Susan was 3 years old, her mother became pregnant, miscarried, and fell into a depression. Looking back as an adult, Susan remembers thinking that her mother's silence

Table 3.4. Experiences That May Make
Some Children Believe That Speaking Is Difficult

1. Normal disfluencies criticized by significant listeners
2. Delay in speech or language development
3. Speech or language disorders, including articulation problems, word finding difficulty, cerebral palsy, and voice problems
4. Difficult or traumatic experience reading aloud in school
5. Cluttering, especially if listeners frequently say "Slow down" or "What?"
6. Emotionally traumatic events during which child tries to speak

and depression reflected disapproval of her speech. Susan's unintelligible speech soon became stuttering. She escalated from repetitive stutters to tightly squeezed blocks within the course of a year. For the next 25 years she felt deeply ashamed of her stuttering.

Although we have no way of knowing for sure, Susan's critical home may have been a major factor in the onset of her stuttering. Many other children go through a period of unintelligible speech in their second and third years, but don't develop stuttering. On the other hand, her delayed speech, perhaps an inherited or congenital deficit, was also an important factor. Neither may have been sufficient, by itself, to create stuttering, but combined, these factors may have been enough to tip the balance.

Capacities and Demands

A third interactional view of stuttering onset is the "capacities and demands theory."[11] This view suggests that disfluencies, as well as real stuttering, emerge when the capacities of the child for fluency are not equal to the demands of the environment for speech performance. We briefly discuss this view in Chapter 2, in our description of the reduced capacity for internal modeling theory of stuttering. Andrews and associates (1983) stated that "whether one will become a stutterer depends on one's neurological capacity . . . and the demand posed by the speech act."[12] They indicated that some demands come from the rapid development of language between ages 3 and 7 years. Others may come from fast-talking parents whose speech rates may be hard for a child to keep up with. Demands for speech performance are sometimes from within the child, sometimes from outside stimuli, and sometimes from both.

Joseph Sheehan (1970; 1975) expressed an early variation of the capacities and demands view when he wrote that "a child who has begun to stutter is probably a child who has had too many demands placed on him while receiving too little support." The demands that Sheehan pinpointed are primarily those of parents who have high standards and high expectations for their child's behavior. The support Sheehan refers to can be seen as a capacity of the environment to provide love, care, and encouragement. Among the demands a child experiences, Sheehan acknowledged developmental factors, such as "differences in the rate of maturation," which result in a greater incidence of stuttering in males. Moreover, he believed that "there are persisting reasons for retaining the possibility that some kind of physiological predisposition for stuttering exists." Thus, Sheehan, who, ironically, is best known for a theory that stuttering is learned, in fact professed the view that stuttering is precipitated by the demands of the environment interacting with the limitations of the child's rate of development and his predisposition to stutter.

Starkweather (1987) has added considerable detail to the concept of capacities and demands as an explanation of stuttering onset. The normal child's capacities, he points out, include the potential for rapid movement of speech structures in well-planned and well-coordinated sequences, with the rhythms of his language. Demands on the child include those of his internal environment, such as increasingly complex thoughts to be expressed, which require increasingly sophisticated use of phonology, syntax, semantics, and pragmatic skills to express them. The external environment often places its demands on the child's fluency through parents' interactions. They may ask questions rapidly, interrupt

---

[11]This is sometimes referred to as "demands and capacities," but we prefer "capacities and demands" because it seems more logical to place first those aspects that are likely to be inherent in the child prior to the appearance of demands.

[12]The reader interested in further references on the topic of capacities for information processing should seek out Neilson and Neilson (1987), as well as the references in that article.

frequently, and use complex sentences choked with big words. They may show impatience with the child's normal disfluencies. They may make the child feel that he meets their expectations only when he's performing at high levels. These kinds of interactions can stress any child, but they are likely to push a slow-developing child beyond his capacity for fluency.

Because a child's capacity develops in spurts and because environmental demands fluctuate, stuttering may wax and wane in rapid cycles. A child may be highly fluent for a day or a week when he has mastered new speech and language skills and external demands are low. But his stuttering may suddenly flare up if his capacities become strained by the emergence of more advanced syntax or if the demands of the external environment suddenly increase when his fast-talking, interrupting big-city cousins arrive for the Fourth of July holiday weekend.

The capacities and demands view provides a way to account for not only the day-to-day variability of stuttering within an individual, but also the great differences between one individual who stutters and another. As Adams (1990) pointed out, some children may grow up in an environment with normal levels of demand but have limited capacities in speech production. Others may have normal capacities for speech production but grow up with excessive demands for rapid, fluent speech.

Treatment based on this model would begin with a careful evaluation of the capacities and demands within the child and in his environment. Therapy would then be designed to enhance capacities, decrease demands, and provide support for the child and his family while these changes are taking place. Starkweather and his colleagues have used this approach to formulate a sensible and reportedly effective program of stuttering prevention (Gottwald & Starkweather, 1984, 1985; Starkweather & Gottwald, 1990; Starkweather, Gottwald, & Halfond, 1990;). Figure 3.3 illustrates the ratios of capacities and demands in a child predisposed to stuttering. In one view, the demands are greater than the child's capacities and stuttering appears. In the second, the demands are lessened and, although capacities stay the same, stuttering is diminished.

To illustrate the capacities and demands view, we take a case from our own experience. Gina was a bright, happy 7-year-old. Her mother had been a severe stutterer as a child, but through treatment and her own perseverance, she had largely recovered. When Gina began the second grade, she had no history of stuttering nor any problem with school. Some time before Christmas that year, however, when her class was learning to read, Gina began to dislike school, and her mother soon discovered that she was having problems academically. After some testing, it was discovered that she had a learning disability; it had been hidden before, but once reading was required it became obvious. As Gina struggled throughout the rest of the second grade to cope with her reading problem, she began to stutter. Over the course of the next 2 years, she stuttered in a noticeable way but did not receive therapy. She was, however, given extra help for her reading disability. By the fourth grade, Gina was making headway with reading, and her stuttering had diminished to an inconsequential level without treatment.

Although there are many ways to interpret Gina's onset of stuttering and her recovery, a capacities and demands view would see it this way: Gina was predisposed to stuttering, but it lay dormant until she was faced with the challenge of reading. Reading, at least when first learned, involves highly conscious control of linguistic processes, in contrast to the more automatic linguistic processing in listening and speaking. Consequently, learning to read puts a large demand on the pool of available resources for speech and language processing. This demand may result in reduced capacity (fewer available resources) for speech production, which, for a vulnerable child, may result in disfluency. In this case, Gina did not seem to develop a long-lasting fear of speaking as a result of her

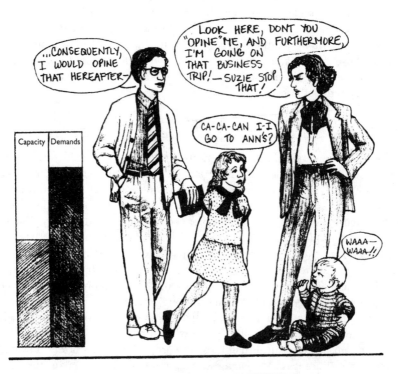

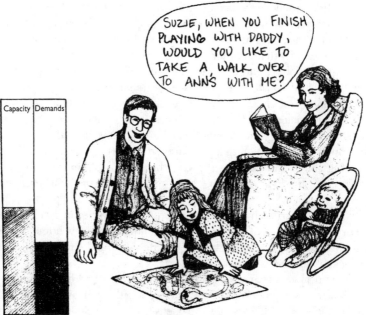

Figure 3.3. Two different ratios of capacities and demands and their hypothesized effect on fluency.

stuttering. Thus, when she overcame her initial reading difficulty and reading became more automatic (demanding fewer resources), her available capacity for speech processes increased, and she "outgrew" her stuttering.

Once again, the reader is reminded that the capacities and demands view is a metaphor for describing relationships that appear again and again but are not well understood.[13] As such, its major function is to help the student of stuttering organize complex interrelationships of variables into a set of principles that may guide treatment and suggest research hypotheses.

SUMMARY

Stuttering usually emerges during the period of children's most rapid growth in physical, cognitive, social-emotional, and linguistic domains. Researchers have speculated that this rapid development depletes neural resources needed for fluency and results in both normal disfluency and stuttering. Clear evidence in support of this speculation is lacking, but indirect evidence exists for competition between language and fluency. For example, studies have shown that both stuttering and normal disfluency are greater when children produce utterances with greater linguistic demands. Other studies support this notion of competition for resources by demonstrating that a risk factor for persistent stuttering is delay in language development. Such a delay would presumably increase the competition neural resources because of the child's prolonged struggle to develop language.

Stresses in the environment are also thought to influence the onset and development of stuttering. Studies of parents of children who stutter have often indicated that they may be more anxious or critical than those children who don't stutter. However, some studies show no differences between these two groups of parents, making this yet another area in which the evidence is not clear-cut. Stress from the child's speech and language environment has been suggested as another precipitator of stuttering. In searching for evidence of such stress, researchers have uncovered some evidence that mothers of stutterers talk more rapidly than mothers of nonstutterers, although other studies have disputed this. A more robust finding is that mothers of stutterers interrupt their children more than mothers of nonstutterers. These researchers also found that mothers of nonstutterers also interrupt children who stutter more frequently than children who don't stutter, making it unclear whether the mothers' interruption precipitate stuttering, the children's stuttering precipitate the mothers' interruptions, or both.

Some support for the notion that pressures from the environment may be associated with stuttering comes from studies showing that language therapy—a controlled environment with pressure to improve language—may generate disfluencies in nonstuttering children.

A different type of stress hypothesized to precipitate stuttering is a life event, such as the death or hospitalization of a family member, moving to a new home, or the birth of a sibling. Evidence for a connection between a life event and stuttering is limited to repeated clinical observations and parent reports.

Three theoretical views were presented linking stuttering with developmental and environmental factors. Wendell Johnson's diagnosogenic theory hypothesizes that stuttering emerges when a normal child becomes hypersensitive to his disfluencies because of listener reactions and tries too hard to avoid disfluencies. Oliver Bloodstein's communicative fail-

---

[13]In an insightful article entitled "Resources—A Theoretical Stone Soup?" David Navon (1984) casts doubt upon the legitimacy of his own capacities and demands theory in information processing. He suggests "capacities" or "resources" is a useful metaphor rather than a verifiable theory.

ure and anticipatory struggle view also proposes that "trying too hard" can lead to stuttering, but this notion indicates that many different experiences with communicative difficulty—including critical listener reactions, frustration about any speech or language problem, or the stress of corrective therapy—can cause the child to develop the anticipatory struggle behaviors of stuttering. The capacities and demands view is a loose conceptualization of stuttering as the product of a child's natural capacity for fluency being pushed beyond its limits by demands coming from the child himself or from his environment.

As we noted at the beginning of this chapter, the importance of developmental and environmental factors is less well established by research than constitutional factors. Developmental and environmental factors are probably very different in different children and fluctuate greatly in each child. Investigations that use group designs to investigate one factor at a time may not be ideal. However, clinical observation has often reported the apparent effect of these factors on stuttering onset, and efforts to lessen their stress has frequently resulted in increased fluency if not total recovery. Thus, we have a strong suspicion that they are important influences. In the next chapter, we speculate on how these factors interact with a child's constitutional makeup to create the signs and symptoms of stuttering.

STUDY QUESTIONS

1. The effect of a child's development on fluency has been likened to the effect of multiple tasks for a computer. Explain this analogy.
2. It has been said that children usually do not learn to walk and talk at the same time. What does this suggest about how motor development might affect fluency?
3. There is a high incidence of stuttering among retarded individuals. What might this suggest about the relationship between cognition and fluency?
4. What aspects of social and emotional development might threaten fluency?
5. What evidence is there that emotional arousal might increase fluency?
6. What is the possible connection between atypical hemispheric localization and the effect of emotion on fluency?
7. Why would speech and language development be likely to put greater pressure on fluency than would physical or cognitive development?
8. What aspects of parents' behavior might put pressure on a child who is disfluent?
9. Identify several characteristics of parents' speech that may create a difficult model for a disfluent child to emulate.
10. Name several life events that have been suggested to increase a child's disfluency.
11. What is the central hypothesis of the diagnosogenic view?
12. The communicative failure and anticipatory struggle view proposes that an experiencing communication failure may cause a child to anticipate difficulty speaking and begin to stutter as a result. What characteristic of the child may be another important factor?
13. How would the capacities and demands view account for the fact that some children don't begin to stutter until they are in elementary school?
14. Johnson and associates' (1959) revised view of stuttering suggested that it is a result of interaction among these three factors: (*a*) the extent of the child's disfluency, (*b*) the listener's sensitivity to that disfluency, and (*c*) the child's sensitivity to his own disfluency and to the listener's reaction. Relate these factors to constitutional, developmental, and environmental factors in stuttering.

SUGGESTED READINGS

Andrews, G., & Harris, M. (1964). *The syndrome of stuttering.* London: W. Heinemann Medical Books.

These authors present data from longitudinal studies of a thousand families in New-castle, England. The interpretation of results presents evidence that both genetic and environmental influences are at work to create stuttering. This book gives an early version of the view that stuttering is due to a lack of capacity for some aspect of speech and language processing.

Bernstein Ratner, N. (1997). Stuttering: A psycholinguistic perspective. In R. Curlee & G. Siegel (Eds.), *Nature and treatment of stuttering: New directions,* 2nd ed. Boston: Allyn & Bacon.

This is an insightful review of the many connections between language to stuttering. The author's background allows her to use linguistic theories and evidence from child language studies to discuss how language influences the loci of stuttering in speech, how parent-child interactions may affect stuttering, how language development may be important in stuttering onset, and the role of feedback on speech, language, and stuttering development.

Bloodstein, O. (1995). Inferences and conclusions. In *A handbook on stuttering.* San Diego: Singular Publishing Group, Inc.

This chapter presents the communicative failure and anticipatory struggle view of stuttering onset. Bloodstein musters the evidence he has summarized in earlier chapters of this handbook to argue convincingly that stuttering develops from an interaction between the child and his environment.

Crystal, D. (1987). Towards a "bucket" theory of language disability: Taking account of interaction between linguistic levels. *Clinical Linguistics and Phonetics, 1,* 7–22.

A theoretical discussion of interaction among levels of speech and language, with an illustrative case of a child whose stuttering increases when language demands are greater. The article makes a clear argument for the influence of speech and language development on stuttering.

Johnson, W., & Associates. (1959). *The onset of stuttering.* Minneapolis: University of Minnesota Press.

This book presents extensive data on parents' perceptions of the onset of their child's stuttering compared with other parents' perceptions of their child's normal disfluency. Johnson eloquently lays out his view of stuttering as the product of an interaction between the child's disfluency, his sensitivity, and the listener's reactions.

Kagan, J., Reznick, J.S., & Snidman, N. (1987). The physiology and psychology of behavioral inhibition in children. *Child Development, 58,* 1459–1473.

This article discusses the findings of Kagan and his colleagues that behaviorally inhibited children show high levels of laryngeal tension. Neurophysiological mechanisms are also discussed, as well as possible genetic and environmental contributions. Recommended for those interested in the hypothesis that behavioral inhibition may be a component in some stuttering.

4

An Integrated View of Stuttering

ETIOLOGICAL FACTORS
IN STUTTERING

In the previous chapters we depicted constitutional, developmental, and environmental influences on stuttering and described some of the theoretical speculations that have been made in these areas. We now present our own speculations, which integrate previous theoretical views and new information from other fields into a comprehensive understanding of stuttering that may guide your endeavors in therapy.

ch Findings and Clinical Observations About Stuttering

ve on the etiology of stuttering must try to account for established research findings as well as common clinical observations about stuttering. We begin by summarizing this material.

Stuttering occurs in all cultures of the world, but its prevalence and incidence are limited. It typically appears in children 2 to 5 years old, after they have been speaking fluently for a time. It often runs in families and may be transmitted genetically, although there are many cases of stuttering in which there is no family history of the disorder.

The earliest signs of stuttering are most often repetitions of single syllables, although prolongations and blocks may also occur very early in some children. It appears slightly more frequently in boys than girls, and this disproportionate ratio grows larger with age, probably as a result of more frequent recovery among girls. Recovery in both genders often occurs during childhood, with almost 80% of children who stutter becoming fluent by their teens.

Despite individual differences, the development of stuttering follows a specific course: after the early repetitions and prolongations (and some blocks), those who don't recover by about age 4 years typically increase the frequency and duration of their stutters, develop secondary behaviors, and acquire negative feelings and attitudes about their stuttering. Persistent stuttering in older children, adolescents, and adults occurs most frequently as part-word repetitions, prolongations, or blocks at the beginnings of sentences. Individuals who continue to stutter into adulthood have a lot in common with each other. Most can anticipate which words they will stutter on, are consistent in their loci of stuttering, and become more fluent if they read a passage several times over. A number of conditions, increase fluency for most people who stutter; for example, talking slowly and speaking in time to a rhythm.

As a group, people who stutter differ in specific ways from people who don't. Stutterers score slightly lower on intelligence quotient (IQ) tests, perform slightly poorer in school, and may be slightly more at risk for language and articulation disorders. Stutterers have slower reaction times, are poorer at tasks of central auditory processing, and have slower movements of their articulators even when they are apparently fluent. In addition, there is some evidence that those who stutter may be more likely than nonstutterers to process speech and language in the right hemisphere or bilaterally.

Clinical observations suggest that children are likely to begin to stutter or get worse during periods of cognitive, linguistic, and physical growth. Stresses of social-emotional development may exacerbate stuttering. There is some evidence, mostly anecdotal, that stresses in the environment are associated with the onset and aggravation of stuttering. Examples of such stresses include threats to the child's emotional security or family expectations for rapid and complex speech.

These are some of the findings that must be explained. Explanation is made more complicated by the fact that people who stutter are a heterogeneous group. Many stutterers are within the normal range in terms of intelligence, language, articulation, and sensory-motor coordination. Moreover, no one who stutters does so all the time; the disorder waxes and wanes under such influences as fatigue, health, and self-confidence. Thus, we are not looking for gross neurological lesions producing widespread disfunction, but subtle differences in neurological functioning that vary from moment to moment and day to day. With these caveats in mind, we now describe our view of the etiology of stuttering.

Atypical Organization of Neural Activity
for Speech and Language Processing

Studies of sensory-motor coordination, central auditory processing, and hemispheric dominance support the hypothesis that stutterers' speech and language processing is not as left-hemisphere dominant, nor as efficient as nonstutterers' processing. These clues, plus evidence that a predisposition to stutter is genetically transmitted or is associated with perinatal brain damage and that stuttering typically emerges in early childhood, point toward differences in the neurophysiology of speech and language as a likely constitutional basis of stuttering.

NEURAL DEVELOPMENT

The evolution of neural networks for language and learning begins soon after conception with the proliferation, migration, and differentiation of neural cells, a process guided by genetic predisposition and affected by such external events such as experience, injury, and disease (Chase, 1996). As neural cells continue to proliferate and differentiate, millions of synapses are formed, and pathways of communication emerge as clusters of cells send information back and forth in response to stimulation. Functional neural circuits organize themselves to perform various tasks, and, after birth, as the infant interacts with the outside world, groups of circuits bind together forming "maps" to process information and produce motor responses (Edelman, 1992).

Environmental interactions with the genetic blueprint shape the evolution of these functional neural circuits, which, in some cases, are not well organized and are therefore vulnerable to disruption. Because brain development continues at a rapid pace throughout early childhood, normal developmental processes enable some dysfunctional circuits to reorganize and establish efficient neural functions. Other inefficiently organized circuits, however, may require special training or experience if their reorganization is ever to take place.

As children grow, the connections among groups of cells all over the brain become more firmly established; those that are activated most frequently are strengthened, those that are activated less frequently are weakened and some may die (Edelman, 1992).

ATYPICAL NEURAL ORGANIZATION

Exactly what neural misorganizations predispose a person to stuttering are not known. We suspect, however, that there is not just one single answer, but many different possibilities. Every individual's functional neurocircuitries—the patterns of neural activity he has developed to accomplish tasks—develop in unique ways, only loosely guided by genetic codes that are always affected by environmental influences. This appears to lead to many individual differences in neurological functioning, even among nonstutterers, and may account for the wide variety of signs and symptoms in those who stutter.

Evidence from studies of hemispheric activation in people who stutter, cited in Chapter 2, indicate less left hemisphere processing of speech and language in stutterers than in nonstutterers. We hypothesize that because of genetic design or perinatal interference with neural development, some stutterers' earliest patterns of neural activation for speech and language tend to use more right than left hemisphere pathways. But other persons who stutter may establish patterns of neuronal activity for speech and language in damaged left hemisphere structures that result in less than efficient functioning. Certainly, many other unique patterns of activity will develop in response to early damage or anomalies in the speech and language areas of the brain.

The individual differences that arise when atypical neural activity patterns for speech and language develop may be likened to the many individual routes to a city that cars may take when traffic is detoured by an accident on a main highway. All the cars are detoured, and they all take many different circuitous paths and will arrive in the city at many different times. No wonder there are so many differences among people who stutter.

INFLUENCES ON NEURAL PROCESSING

Individual differences in the atypically organized patterns of neural activity may explain why people who stutter perform differently from each other on a variety of tasks, but not why stuttering is so variable. Why does an individual's stuttering vary so much from situation to situation and from day to day?

One explanation may be that speech and language processing in stutterers is vulnerable to interference from competing processes that also vary from day to day and situation to situation. Interference by emotions such as anxiety, excitement, and fear may occur if the brain functions in such a way that resources used for *one* function diminish the available resources for *another* process going on at the same time. Kinsbourne and Hicks' (1978) model of interference in neural processing suggests that this kind of interference between two simultaneous tasks is greatest when the tasks are carried out in similar areas of the brain; thus, two right hemisphere tasks carried out at the same time will interfere with each other more than two simultaneous tasks in opposite hemispheres. The possibility that stutterers' neural circuitry is atypically or anomalously organized may mean that the pathways of neural activity for speech production traverse areas that also serve nonspeech emotional, cognitive, and motor functions; thus, the speech production circuitry of stutterers may be vulnerable to the day-to-day and situation-to-situation variability of these other processes.

Another possible source of the variability of stuttering is that the layout of stutterers' speech-processing circuitry allows a variety of different pathways to be used at different times and while performing different communication activities, thus adding to the overall variability of stuttering.

The anomalous localization of some brain activity patterns may be not only susceptible to interference from competing activities but also slower and less efficient. To the extent that right hemisphere areas are substituted for left hemisphere areas, the rapid processing of brief speech segments may be affected because, as described in Chapter 2, right hemisphere processing is typically used for tasks with longer temporal units such as those of music. When right hemisphere areas are used for processing spoken language, either the speaker must slow down or temporal discoordination of the sequential motor behaviors of speech may result. Slow processing of speech and language might also result from an atypical bilateral distribution of speech and language centers in right and left hemispheres. If speech and language areas that are normally in the same hemisphere develop in opposite hemispheres, the coordination of activities may be less efficient and require more time, more resources, or more stimulation (such as a metronome beat) to work synchronously.

To summarize our speculation up to this point, because of genetic predisposition or brain injury, individuals who stutter do not have the well-organized and efficient functional neural networks for speech and language processing that typical nonstutterers have. Instead, some or all of the stutterers' neural functioning for speech may be localized in the right hemisphere, or it may be inefficiently organized in the left hemisphere. The wide variability among stutterers as a group may result from many possible patterns of misorganized activity; on the other hand, the wide variability of fluency within an individual stutterer may result from fluctuating interference of speech processing by competing emotional, cognitive, and motor activities. We also speculated that some of the situation-to-situation variability may arise from the option to use different neural circuitry (some less efficient; some more efficient) for different speaking tasks.

Atypical neural patterns for speech production may be only one etiological factor in stuttering; we now turn to a second possible factor.

Temperament

The hypothesis that individuals who stutter have an inefficiently organized pattern of neural activity for speech may explain the disfluencies of children at the onset of stuttering. However, it fails to provide a convincing explanation as to why some children begin to stutter with mild, repetitive stuttering but develop persistent stuttering that is characterized by increased physical tension and many learned reactions. Nor does it explain why some stuttering begins suddenly, with the tense blocks we are more used to seeing in more advanced stuttering. We believe that many cases of persistent stuttering may involve a second factor that interacts with the vulnerable neural pathways being used for speech and language.

KAGAN'S STUDIES OF INHIBITED CHILDREN

Jerome Kagan's research on behavioral and neurophysiological correlates of inhibited or sensitive temperament furnishes us with a hypothesis that may explain at least some persistent stuttering. Even though Kagan's work is focused on children who do not stutter, it is relevant to stuttering because of the evidence, presented earlier, that some stutterers may have an inherently sensitive temperament.[1] Kagan, Reznick, and Snidman (1987) postulated that some children inherit a temperament that makes them more reactive to unfamiliar, threatening, or challenging situations. This sensitivity is biologically based: these children have lower thresholds of reactivity in the part of the brain that mediates emotion and behavior—the limbic system, particularly neural circuits of the amygdala and hypothalamus. Kagan and his colleagues' experiments show that more sensitive children manifest their reactivity by generating higher levels of physical tension, particularly in laryngeal muscles, when they are speaking in unfamiliar or threatening situations.

If children who inherit or acquire vulnerable neural speech circuits are also born with a more sensitive temperament, they may be especially reactive to their early disfluencies (or other speech difficulties). Such reactivity of the limbic system may increase physical tension in speech musculature. This added physical tension may compound a child's initial disfluencies or disruptions in speech, making them more severe and more likely to be experienced as distressing to both the child and his listeners.

---

[1] It is interesting to note that Calkins and Fox (1994) have shown that temperamentally sensitive children show proportionately more right than left hemisphere activity during tasks designed to elicit emotion. Thus, if some children have speech production networks atypically functioning largely in the right hemisphere and they are also temperamentally more sensitive, they may be particularly vulnerable to disruption of speech during situations that elicit emotion. It is also possible that these two tendencies may be related; whatever inherited or acquired predispositions made localization of some neural pathways for speech in the right hemisphere more likely may have also created a tendency for emotions to produce greater right hemisphere activity.

KINSBOURNE'S VIEW ON LATERALIZATION OF EMOTION

Marcel Kinsbourne's research (Kinsbourne, 1989; Kinsbourne & Bemporad, 1984) on emotions in normal and brain-damaged individuals provides further, although indirect, support for the speculation that emotional arousal may lead to tense stuttering repetitions, prolongations, and blocks. Kinsbourne's studies of emotional regulation in neuropathology, psychopathology, and normal functioning led him to propose that emotional regulation is lateralized, with the right hemisphere having a proclivity to regulate emotions that accompany avoidance, withdrawal, and arrest of ongoing behavior, and the left hemisphere having a proclivity to regulate emotions that are associated with approach, exploration, and release of ongoing behavior. This speculation, combined with Calkins and Fox's (1994) finding that temperamentally sensitive children are right hemisphere-dominant for emotion, supports the perspective that children with this temperament have a proclivity to inhibit ongoing motor behavior, including speech, by means of arrest, withdrawal, and avoidance. This triad of inhibitory tendencies may be the neurophysiological basis for tense blocks, escape, and avoidance behaviors.

GRAY'S BEHAVIORAL INHIBITION SYSTEM

Another line of research also supports the hypothesis that increased tension is part of a biologically based response in humans. Kagan's work on sensitive children has been based in part on a model of an individual's response to stress developed by Jeffrey Gray (1987), an experimental psychologist who studies the central nervous system's responses to stress. Gray hypothesizes that the neurophysiological states for the emotions of frustration and fear are very similar, with fear being further along on a continuum of arousal. When frustration or fear are elicited, an individual's response is governed by what Gray calls a behavioral inhibition system, which increases arousal, attention to environmental stimuli, and inhibitory responses. Gray proposes that the inhibitory responses may take three forms: freezing (muscular contractions that produce tense and silent immobility), flight, or avoidance. These three behaviors are analogous to the core, escape, and avoidance behaviors that often develop in stuttering.

Thus we see that the research and theorizing of both Gray and Kinsbourne suggest biologically based responses that may underlie the development—and in some cases, the onset—of stuttering. For most children who stutter, these responses (inhibition/freezing, withdrawal/flight, and avoidance) may develop only after disfluencies emerge as a product of the atypical organization of neural processing for speech and language. These children may be predisposed to the emotions of fear and frustration when they experience the uncontrollable initial disfluencies and their initial disfluencies become transformed (by inhibition/freezing, withdrawal/flight, and avoidance) into tense repetitions, prolongations, blocks, and escape and avoidance behaviors. For other children, the emotions of fear and frustration may occur without prior disfluencies, but in response to social situations; their initial disfluencies may be characterized by tension, escape, and avoidance.

TEMPERAMENT AND SUSCEPTIBILITY TO CONDITIONING

The perspective on emotional reactivity and physiological tension responses gives rise to another hypothesis: that many children who react to early disfluencies with tension because of a sensitive temperament may also be more susceptible to fear conditioning than are other children. This hypothesis is based on the fact that the amygdala, whose reactivity results in increased tension according to Kagan and others, is known to play a major role in fear conditioning (LeDoux, 1997; LeDoux, Cicchetti, Xagoraris, & Romanski,

1990). According to LeDoux, neural circuitry of the amygdala mediates rapid, noncon-scious responses to threatening stimuli and stores memories of these stimuli, which make classical (pavlovian) conditioning much more likely.

We discuss the role of conditioning in stuttering later in this chapter, but the point we wish to emphasize here is that converging evidence from different lines of research points to the possibility of a biological predisposition in some stutterers to react to stress during speech by increasing the physical tension of their speech musculature; these same chil-dren may also be highly vulnerable to conditioning tension responses to more and more speaking situations.

TWO PREDISPOSITIONS FOR STUTTERING

As said earlier, not all stuttering begins as easy, effortless repetitions. Some stuttering be-gins with tense blocks; these may occur when a child's emotional reactivity contributes more to his predisposition to stutter than do anomalous neural activity patterns for speech and language. By contrast, some children are highly disfluent, with relatively tension-free repetitions; they may never develop tense stutters or escape or avoidance behaviors; for them, the anomalous neural activity patterns for speech and language behaviors may be their only predisposition for stuttering. Likewise, what is a predisposition among children may be an acquired anomaly for some adults.

In cases of late-onset stuttering following brain damage, neural activity for speech and language may be disrupted by disease, stroke, or injury and subsequently reorganized in an inefficient manner, giving rise to the repetitions common in this type of onset.

The two major biological predispositions for stuttering just described may both be in-herited in cases in which stuttering appears and persists. They may be two factors in the polygenic multifactorial model of genetic transmission of stuttering proposed by Kidd (1984). One gene might carry the information leading to the organization of inefficient neural pathways for speech and language (leading to mild disfluencies), and another gene might transmit a sensitive temperament with a reactive limbic system (which would ex-acerbate speech breakdowns). If either or both of these biological predispositions are present, the onset of stuttering and its characteristics would be influenced by a child's de-velopment and environment, which we consider next.

Interaction With Developmental Factors

In this section, we describe possible interactions between the two etiological factors just discussed (atypically organized neural processing and sensitive temperament) and the child's development. We suggested in an earlier chapter that a child's development—in physical, cognitive, emotional, and linguistic domains—may increase the risk for stutter-ing, especially because demands on resources are great during growth spurts. We now wish to emphasize that these developmental changes are, to some extent, related to changes in the two constitutional factors just reviewed.

Let us begin with a child who, through genetic inheritance or early trauma, begins to acquire speech with inefficient speech and language pathways. The functional plas-ticity in the child's brain attempts to reorganize and repair circuitry to more efficiently process speech as the child strives to communicate, but the exponential growth in the child's speech and language at this time may compete for resources, straining the child's capacity to handle both demands at the same time. Imagine yourself as a stu-dent who has let part of the semester slip by without studying. After you bomb the first two exams of semester, you resolve to change your study habits and catch up, but at the same time your professors pile on more work than before. You, like the child, may or may not be able to adapt to increasing demands at the same time you are spending energy to reorganize.

There will also be many individual differences in ability to adapt. For example, girls are known to be more likely to recover from early stuttering, which may be related to their inherently greater organizational plasticity because of their more widely distributed neural activation patterns for language (Shaywitz et al., 1995). Their bilateral neural activation patterns may allow more flexibility in dealing with biological predisposition for an atypical functional organization of speech and language. Some males may also be genetically endowed with more flexibility than average for reorganizing circuitry and thus may recover more readily than others.

Now let us consider the effect of development on a child's constitutional bias for inhibited temperament. This child may be particularly sensitive to the difficulties and mistakes that occur in response to his emerging speech and language skills. For example, the difficulties encountered by a child with delayed speech motor development might elicit increased tension in the speech muscles of a temperamentally sensitive child, transforming "normal" disfluencies or articulation errors into stuttering.

What might be the effect of a constitutional bias for an inhibited temperament in a child who had essentially normal neural organization for speech and language? On the basis of our clinical experience, we hypothesize that some children fitting this description might be hesitant to speak and may be referred for a stuttering evaluation, but would not manifest the typical signs of stuttering. Their hesitancies may be in the form of long pauses, phrase repetitions, or both, when their right hemisphere proclivity toward avoidance, withdrawal, and arrest of ongoing behavior manifests itself during the act of speaking. Such hesitancies may diminish with time as myelinization of subcortical connections between the hemispheres progresses and the left hemisphere has an increasingly modulating effect on right hemisphere-modulated emotions.

Interaction With Environmental Factors

We now consider the influence of the environment on anomalous speech and language neural networks and on constitutional bias toward inhibited temperament.

As the child's developing central nervous system adapts to his inherited or acquired differences in the neural substrates for speech and language, the environment plays a role through various listeners' responses to the child's emerging speech and language skills. Obviously, a child's family will have the most opportunity to provide acceptance and support. The familiar accommodations that they can provide, like a slower speech rate and fewer interruptions, may foster neurological adaptations, just as the use of slow speech transitions is reported to assist learning disabled children (Travis, 1996). In contrast, increasing the speech and language pressures in a child's environment will likely inhibit successful adaptation.

The work of Calkins (1994), Kagan and Snidman (1991), and others suggests that families can have a strong influence on temperament. As Calkins and Fox (1994) expressed it, "the child's interactions with a parent provide the context for learning skills and strategies for managing emotional reactivity." In addition, environmental factors we have called "life events" can influence the development of temperament. As noted earlier, Kagan (1994b) suggests that certain life events can cause a child who was not particularly reactive to become more reactive and inhibited.

Implications for Treatment

The conditions that we have just been describing may be malleable by a supportive environment and specific therapy approaches. By judicious control of speech and language processing demands, the environment may support the child's adaptive neuroplasticity, enabling him to improve the efficiency of his neural networks for speech and language. Families may also help a child to develop a less inhibited temperament by encouraging positive, assertive behaviors. Therapy, too, can help a child respond to disfluencies with few inhibitory responses. Active, positive treatment sessions often lead to improvements in a child's confidence. Training in fluency skills can provide a child with many satisfying speaking experiences, thereby reducing fear of talking. Development of a slower speaking style and the use of proprioception may help a child make the best of an inefficient speech production system. Confronting feared words and situations, reducing tension in stuttering, and improving eye contact during speech may shift a child's characteristic emotional valence from "avoidance" (right hemisphere) to "approach" (left hemisphere). In the chapters on treatment of stuttering, we expand on this theme and suggest a variety of other ways to help individuals overcome or compensate for factors that predispose them to stuttering.

Accounting for the Evidence

Let us now turn to the research findings and clinical observations that this view of stuttering must account for. The fact that stuttering is universal would not be unexpected, because it depends not so much on culture as on basic biological variations of the human brain. Many other disorders, such as dyslexia and specific language impairment, as well as variations in personality, such as sensitive temperament, are associated with anomalous activity in the central nervous system and are also universal. The fact that its prevalence and incidence are relatively low may arise from the fact that chronic stuttering usually results from a combination of at least two biological predispositions, and their co-occurrence does not happen frequently.

EVIDENCE ABOUT STUTTERING AT ONSET

Why does stuttering usually begin only after fluency at the one- and two-word stage has been achieved? Our view is that stuttering emerges first from disruptions caused by inefficient neural networks for speech and language processing. Perhaps the task of coordinating all the phonetic, phonological, syntactic, and semantic components of a complex utterance is too much for inefficient circuitry under stress. Just as in normal disfluency, the neural processing circuitry of children who stutter may be adequate to handle the light traffic of one- and two-word utterances. But once children begin to reorganize their language functions from a lexical basis to a grammatical-rules basis and try out complicated syntax, their inefficient neural organization breaks down.

Why doesn't a child's sensitive temperament affect speech before the multiple repetitions and prolongations of early stuttering emerge? It may, in a few cases. There are children who begin to stutter with tense blocks, that do not appear to follow a period of repetitions and prolongations. For most children who stutter, however, tension responses, as well as escape and avoidance reactions, are elicited only by the frustration and fear provoked by early stuttering.

How do we explain both genetic transmission of stuttering and the fact that evidence of genetic transmission is lacking in some cases? Genetic transmission of stuttering in

many cases may be through the two factors we have just described: anomalous neural organization for speech and sensitive temperament.

In some cases of childhood stuttering, genetic transmission may be in doubt because
no other family members seem to be affected. We think this may occur because persistent stuttering may require both predisposing factors. Some family members may inherit
one factor and some the other factor, but unless both factors are inherited by the same
individual, persistent stuttering may not develop. Another reason for the absence of stuttering in other family members may be that the predisposing factors were the result not
of genetic inheritance, but of environmental factors affecting fetal development and thus
creating the neural substrate for stuttering.

How does our view of stuttering explain its most common signs: repetitions, prolongations, and blocks? The immediate causes of the core behaviors of stuttering are not entirely clear in our view. All of them reflect an inability to move forward in speech, but the
effortless sound and syllable repetitions of many stutterers at onset seem somewhat different from later tension-filled repetitions, prolongations, and blocks. The sound and syllable repetitions of early stuttering more closely resemble the disfluencies resulting from
nervous system damage or "neurogenic stuttering" (Rosenbek, 1984). Thus, these early
signs of childhood stuttering—less tense repetitions and prolongations—may well arise
from breakdown in the function of inefficient neural circuits, perhaps from causes similar to neurogenic stuttering. Repetitions may occur simply because there is a lag in the
readiness of the next part of a word or sentence, although the drive to continue speaking
is strong. Signs of stuttering with tension that emerge later in many stutterers than effortless repetitions may stem from the frustration and fear elicited by a child's difficulty
in speaking. In cases in which the earliest signs of stuttering are characterized by tension
and blocking (Van Riper, 1982), an emotional response may be primary. As Van Riper
(1982) has suggested, these may be children whose onset is very sudden, usually after an
emotionally difficult period or traumatic emotional stress.

Any view of stuttering must explain its more common appearance in boys than girls.
We suspect that the reason more boys stutter than girls is that the genetic blueprints for
neural organization of speech and language is different and perhaps more flexible in females (Shaywitz et al., 1995). Neuroplasticity of the human brain is greatest in the first
few years of life and probably is much less after puberty. It is this neuroplasticity that permits reorganization of neural pathways and, in many cases, recovery. An important additional predictor of recovery, we believe, is an uninhibited temperament. We have met
several siblings of stutterers who have gone blithely through a period of stuttering but
were so unconcerned that tension and struggle never occurred, and they recovered.

Evidence About Stuttering as It Develops

Does our view account for the development of stuttering? The course of development of
stuttering seems to us to be determined in part by the biological responses of the child
to fear and frustration and to autonomic conditioning, to which a child prone to chronic
stuttering may be particularly sensitive. We provide details on development of stuttering
in Chapter 5.

How do we account for stimuli that reduce stuttering? Conditions that temporarily ame-
liorate stuttering, such as singing or speaking in a rhythm, probably improve fluency by giving more time or an external organizing stimulus to the speech and language process. Other
conditions, such as speaking when alone or when relaxed, often reduce stuttering but do
not necessarily eliminate it; these stimuli may calm a person, thereby diminishing the reactivity of limbic circuits. Some conditions, such as speaking more slowly, probably do both.

How about group differences in performance between stutterers and nonstutterers? As intimated earlier in this chapter, it seems to us that the wide range of stutterers' group performances on IQ tests, school achievement tests, and tests of sensory-motor ability may be affected by the wide range of delays and deviations in the neural substrates for these abilities that have led to their inefficient processing of speech and language. Among groups of individuals who stutter, there are likely to be some whose neural organization for sensory-motor processing is deviant enough to depress the group mean. In highly selected groups of stutterers, however, such as all males with no medical, neurological, or psychiatric diagnoses and complete right-body dominance (Ingham et al., 1996), the chance of finding significant differences between this group and a group of nonstutterers is decreased. In this regard, it is interesting that two independent studies have shown that children whose stuttering is their only disorder show no speech reaction time differences from nonstutterers, whereas children having stuttering and other language or articulation disorders show poorer reaction time scores (Cullinan & Springer, 1980; Maske-Cash & Curlee, 1995). Perhaps the coexistence of poorer sensory-motor integration performance and speech and language disorders reflect additional anomalies in neural organization and function in this subgroup of stuttering children. In other words, we propose that children who stutter have at least some degree of inefficient organization of neural circuitry for speech and language production; those children who show stuttering and poorer sensory-motor skills or other speech and language disorders may simply have greater anomalies in their functional neural circuitry, affect fluency, articulation, language, or other sensory-motor tasks.

Other characteristics of stuttering that we said must be explained by any view of stuttering, such as the influence of developmental and environmental factors, are explicitly addressed in earlier parts of this chapter. Some characteristics, findings, and observations are explained better than others. Those that aren't accounted for satisfactorily are important, however. They are a reality and the hard facts that should mold and shape any theoretical view until it is more fully explanatory.

We now turn to descriptions of the learning processes that affect stuttering after it has begun.

LEARNING FACTORS IN STUTTERING

Overview of Learning

Most of the ways in which stuttering interferes with the daily lives of those who stutter are the result of learning rather than hereditary or perinatal impairments. If clinicians understand how these interfering behaviors are learned, they can help clients change them. There are several types of learning, but we concentrate on classical conditioning and instrumental conditioning because they probably contribute most to the development of stuttering.

In his account of learning processes in stuttering, Starkweather (1997) clarifies these sometimes confusing concepts by pointing out several similarities and differences between them. Both classical and instrumental conditioning rely on *contingencies*. That is, events occurring in sequence—one thing following another. They are called *stimulus contingencies* if two stimuli occur in succession time after time and the second stimulus evokes a response. For example, if a bell is rung and then food is given, these are stimulus contingencies that can form the basis of classical conditioning. In contrast, they are called *response contingencies* if a response is immediately followed by a stimulus that influences future occurrences of that response. For example, if you push a button for an elevator and the elevator soon comes to your floor, this is a response contingency (the response of pushing a button was followed by the stimulus of the elevator arriving), which forms the basis for instrumental conditioning.

A combination of classical and instrumental conditioning often occurs in the real world, because when instrumental conditioning occurs (when a response is followed by a stimulus), other stimuli are usually present. And those stimuli become associated with the conditioning stimulus that follows the response. Let's say that you live in a small town and work in a large city. When you are in the small town where you live, you smile at people and they smile back. But in the city where you work, your smiles are seldom, if ever, returned. The stimuli of the small town become associated with the stimuli of people smiling back and the stimuli of the city become associated with the stimuli of people not returning your smile.

Now, let's relate this to stuttering. If a stutterer's attempt to speak slowly is rewarded by the stimulus of praise in the clinic room, but not at home, the stutterer will be much more likely to speak slowly in the clinic room than at home.

Let us now turn to the details of each type of conditioning to get a better understanding of how stuttering may be affected by learning.

Classical Conditioning

The famous Russian physiologist Ivan Pavlov offered the first scientific description of classical conditioning. Pavlov was studying the reflexive secretion of fluids in dogs' mouths and stomachs when they were fed. After several days, Pavlov found that the dogs were starting to drool when he walked into his laboratory in the morning, thereby delaying his experiments with food-elicited salivation. As he pondered the problem and began to examine the dogs' anticipatory drooling, he realized that the dogs were associating his presence with being fed and that this association produced premature salivation. Would they make the same association to anything that occurred just before they were fed? Pavlov tried a tuning fork. He sounded the fork several times just before a dog was fed and looked for the response. Initially, no response was forthcoming; the dog salivated only when food was presented. But Pavlov persisted, again and again sounding the tuning fork just before feeding the dog. After many such pairings, Pavlov found that the dog began to respond to the tuning fork just as it had when Pavlov walked through the door. The dog now salivated in response to the sound of the tuning fork, although food was nowhere in sight.

Pavlov's observation provided the first insight into classical conditioning. Since then, classical conditioning has been studied extensively, and scientists have been able to describe how it takes place. Figure 4.1 depicts the "paradigm" (a model or diagram of how a process takes place) for classical conditioning.

The first stage of this process is the presentation of an unconditioned stimulus (UCS), which elicits an unconditioned response (UCR). These are often reflexive or "hardwired" responses, such as flinching to a loud noise. For Pavlov's dog, the UCS was the food and the UCR was salivation. The second stage is the repeated presentation of a neutral stimulus just before the UCS. Pavlov sounded the tuning fork immediately before he fed the dog. The last stage happens when the presentation of the neutral stimulus begins to elicit the response before presentation of the UCS. After learning has occurred, the formerly neutral stimulus is called the conditioned stimulus (CS), and the response the CS now elicits, formerly the UCR, is now called the conditioned response (CR).

Note that for conditioning to take place, the pairing of the neutral stimulus and the UCS must take place in that order repeatedly. Moreover, this pairing of the CS and the

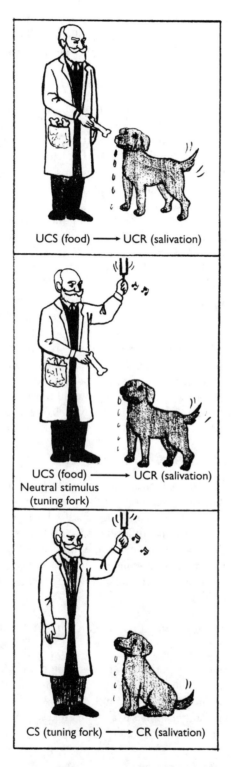

Figure 4.1. Classical conditioning paradigm. Dog salivates naturally when given food. Food is paired frequently with sound of tuning fork. Tuning fork without food then elicits salivation.

UCS must continue to occur intermittently; otherwise, the CR will cease to occur—a process called *extinction*. If Pavlov didn't occasionally feed the dog after ringing of the tuning fork, the tuning fork would cease to elicit the salivation response.

CLASSICAL CONDITIONING AND STUTTERING

First, let us examine the role that classical conditioning may play in the early stages of stuttering. An excellent theoretical account of classical conditioning and the onset of stuttering was provided by Eugene Brutten and Donald Shoemaker, a speech pathologist and a psychologist at the University of Southern Illinois (Brutten & Shoemaker, 1967).[2] These authors suggested that the earliest stuttering symptoms (repetitions and prolongations) result from the cognitive and motor disorganization that occurs in response to a child's learned anxiety in speaking situations.

Although our account owes much to Brutten and Shoemaker's pioneering work, we believe classical conditioning is seldom responsible for the earliest signs of stuttering. Instead, we believe, along with Starkweather (1987, p. 372), that "it seems likely that physiological sources play more of a role in stuttering onset, whereas conditioning processes play more of a role in stuttering development." And we agree with a very similar assessment by Van Riper (1982) that "the real contribution of classical conditioning theory as it is applied to stuttering lies in its ability to explain the development of the disorder."

Our view is that most borderline stutterers' excessive repetitions and prolongations are a result of interactions among constitutional, developmental, and environmental factors. We believe their excessive repetitions and prolongations create considerable frustration, which triggers reflexive responses of increased muscle tension and rate of repetitions. These reactions to frustration form the UCRs, which are classically conditioned to speech.

INDIVIDUAL DIFFERENCES IN CONDITIONING

We have suggested that borderline stuttering develops into beginning stuttering because of a child's reaction to the frustration created by excess repetitions and prolongations. This reaction increases muscle tension and speech rate during disfluencies. But we also believe that there are many individual differences in this response, as we described earlier in a section called "Temperament and Susceptibility to Conditioning." There, we pointed out that the process of conditioning is mediated by such brain structures as the amygdala, which is more reactive in sensitive children, making them more susceptible to fear and frustration conditioning.

EXAMPLE OF CLASSICAL CONDITIONING AND STUTTERING

We now turn to our view of the role of classical conditioning in childhood stuttering. For ease of explanation, we refer to hypothesized increases in muscle tension and speech rate during disfluencies under conditions of frustration and fear as "the tension response." The paradigm for this conditioning is shown in Figure 4.2.

To illustrate how this paradigm applies to an individual stutterer, we use a young client from our clinic, a beginning stutterer we call Richard.

---

[2] Brutten and Shoemaker provide a "two-factor" theory of learning to account for stuttering. Instrumental conditioning is the second factor. It shapes the pattern of stuttering when tension, escape behaviors, and avoidances are reinforced. We discuss the role of instrumental conditioning in the next section.

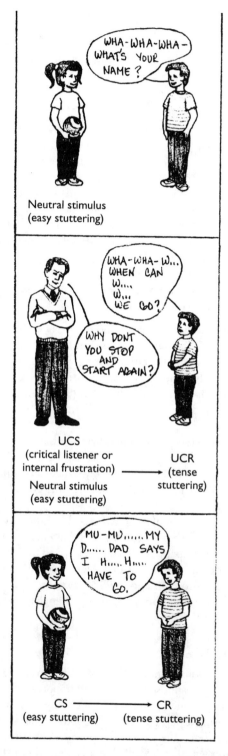

Figure 4.2. Example of classical conditioning of tension in a beginning stutterer. The repeated pairing of easy stuttering with a critical listener or internal frustration, which elicits tension, makes the easy stuttering a conditioned stimulus for tension. Consequently, tense stuttering occurs in more and more situations.

Previously Neutral Stimulus

The neutral stimulus (NS) is a child's borderline stuttering, relatively free of tension and hurry. In our example, Richard's disfluencies consisted of frequent instances of part-word repetitions, which were perceived as neither tense nor hurried.

Pairing the Neutral Stimulus with the UCS

As stuttering develops, a child's relaxed disfluencies (NS), which have not bothered him previously, become paired with an event (UCS) that elicits the tension response (UCR). This event might be a parent's frown during the child's repetitive disfluency, the child's own concern of being unable to communicate quickly, or both.

At about age 4 years, Richard became more disfluent than ever, possibly in response to having a new baby in the family and moving into a new house. His parents tried to help him by suggesting that he stop and try again when he was caught up in a particularly long and frustrating stutter. But whenever he was corrected or appeared frustrated, his repetitive stuttering became more tense and hurried.

Formerly Neutral Stimulus (Now the CS) Can Now Elicit the Formerly Unconditioned Response (Now the CR)

In this third stage of classical conditioning, the formerly neutral stimulus, now the CS (a disfluency), elicits the CR (tension response) in the absence of threatening experience. Richard appeared to show this conditioning when his increased muscle tension and speech rate during disfluencies increased in situations in which he had previously stuttered without tension or hurry, such as talking to playmates. Richard's stuttering gradually became more and more widespread, through processes to be discussed shortly.

Such rapid learning and widespread generalization that we sometimes see in stuttering children seems to parallel the "prepared classical conditioning" of animals that are rapidly and deeply conditioned to such potentially dangerous stimuli as snakes (Mineka, 1985). Children who are especially sensitive may rapidly condition to such threatening stimuli as a critical parent.

We should add that our treatment taught Richard a slower style of speaking that was free of disfluencies and therefore free from the CS that elicited the tension response. In fact, slow speech may be incompatible with tense, hurried disfluencies, perhaps because it makes linguistic-motor coordination easier, which eliminates primary disfluencies and also disarms the nervous system's rapid "flight" response. Richard now speaks more slowly only when stress threatens to bring out his disfluencies. As his system matures, this may be needed less frequently.

SPREAD OF CONDITIONING

Conditioning is an active and continuing process. Whenever the child is disfluent (CS) and experiences the tension response (CR) (a conditioned stimulus elicits a conditioned response), a host of other stimuli are present incidentally. When the child stutters, he is talking to someone, uttering a particular word or sound, speaking in a particular room, talking about a particular topic. Because of the power of classical conditioning, the pairing of these other stimuli with the CS (disfluency) gives them the potency to elicit the CR. They become CS. Thus, as conditioning takes place again and again, the stimulus becomes a complex of many things, including words and sounds, listeners, and physical surroundings or situations. This chaining of stimuli is called "higher-order conditioning."[3] Figure 4.3 illustrates the process.

It is important to note that to maintain the effects of the CS, a UCS must occur periodically. Stuttering must occasionally provoke frustration for it to also continue to elicit the tension response.

The spread of conditioning to other CS results in changes in stuttering as well. Initially, a child might emit several repetitive disfluencies, or a long prolongation, before the tension response appears. Soon, however, muscle tension occurs earlier and earlier in stutters. When other CS, such as words, elicit the tension response, the easy repetitive disfluencies may not occur at all. Instead, a child will increase muscle tension on the very first sound he tries to utter, resulting in the "fixed articulatory postures" that are a sign of beginning stuttering.

As a child's stuttering frequency increases as a result of the spread of conditioning to more and more stimuli, the duration of the child's stuttering may also increase. This may be explained by the fact that the tension response soon becomes a stimulus that elicits more tension. After all, the tension response makes it harder to utter a word, and the experience of "squeezing hard" without being able to speak for a second or two elicits frustration, leading to another tension response.

In Richard's case, his slow speech treatment included a carefully constructed hierarchy of the people and situations in which he was previously disfluent. By associating fluent speech with these situations, we were able to counteract previous conditioning and prevent these stimuli from triggering disfluency, frustration, and the tension response. This is a form of counterconditioning, a major element in treating the affective reactions in those with beginning, intermediate, and advanced stuttering. Counterconditioning should be part of well-constructed fluency shaping programs for beginning stutterers and is the essence of the desensitization phase of stuttering modification for intermediate and advanced stutterers.

CONDITIONING AS PATTERNS OF CONNECTIVITY

This description of the spread of conditioning may seem confusing. For years, clinicians and researchers have been trying to figure out why, for example, a child stutters at home but not at school, or stutters more severely during the summer than the winter. They were also baffled by the breadth of individual differences among stutterers. Why do some stutterers have a great deal of stuttering on the telephone, whereas others have little or none? Why do some stutterers stutter more with women and others with men?

Some recent cognitive models of how we learn and store knowledge may provide appropriate descriptions of this process (Rumelhart, McClelland, & the PDP Research Group, 1986). In these models, learning is viewed as the storing of patterns of connections in memory. Because nothing is learned in isolation, the stimuli associated with what is learned are also stored as part of the pattern that encodes the event. When events are experienced again and again with similar stimuli, the patterns of connectivity are strengthened. Undoubtedly, when such events are associated with strong emotions, the patterns learned are particularly strong. Applying this model to spoken language, utterances are learned and stored in patterns that reflect all of their past uses in all their emotional and cognitive contexts.

---

[3] Higher-order conditioning and related aspects of learned behavior are described with clarity and detail in Zimbardo's *Psychology and Life* (1985).

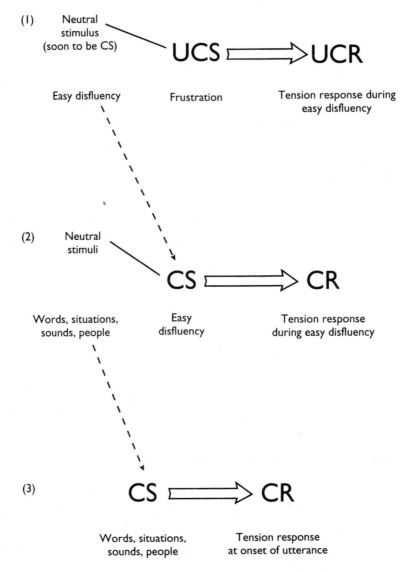

Figure 4.3. Spread of conditioning. (1) Easy disfluency repeatedly elicits the tension response, producing tense stuttering. (2) Easy disfluency, which occurs with various words, situations, sounds, and people, is then a conditioned stimulus that elicits the tension response and tense stuttering. (3) Words, situations, sounds, and people become the conditioned stimuli, which elicit the tension response at the onset of an utterance, producing fixed articulatory postures (or blocks) when the child begins an utterance.

The application to stuttering is this: A child stutters in a variety of places, on various words, with various listeners. Memories of these experiences form interconnected patterns that encode much of the context in which stuttering occurred. As stuttering develops, certain connections are strengthened more than others because they occur more frequently or with stronger emotion. In the ongoing process of evaluation, clinicians should try to discover which stimuli have the strongest connections for triggering stuttering. In treatment, clinicians—behaviorist or cognitivist—should try to strengthen connections associated with fluency and weaken those associated with stuttering.

CLASSICAL CONDITIONING AND THE ONSET OF STUTTERING

In the preceding sections, we suggested that classical conditioning may come into play only after a child has developed the first signs of stuttering—an excess of normal-sounding disfluencies. There may be a subgroup of children for whom classical conditioning is a major element in the onset of the disorder. They may have experienced other difficulties in communication, which, like disfluency, have been conditioned to frustration, fear, and increased tension. Articulation disorders, cluttering, or a traumatic experience reading aloud are examples of such difficulties. Such communicative frustrations may, like disfluencies, have become associated with caustic or critical remarks by listeners or with the child's own sense of inadequacy. This may have resulted in high levels of emotion, triggering increased tension in speech, as we described in the previous section on temperament. Bloodstein's (1987) view of stuttering as the result of the belief that communication is difficult and of anticipatory struggle in response to such beliefs is largely responsible for our thinking in this regard. Our only addition to his view is that the intervening variable of the fight, flight, or freeze response, elicited by communicative failure and causing increases in tension, can create beginning stuttering without the preceding stage of borderline stuttering.

Instrumental Conditioning

Instrumental conditioning (also called operant conditioning) is a fact of daily life. It can create in us such quirks as pushing an elevator button over and over when the elevator is already on its way. It is a major force in the development of stuttering and an important therapy tool that every clinician should understand.

Instrumental conditioning has been used for centuries to train animals and discipline children. Its influence on our daily lives and its therapeutic potential weren't well understood, however, until the American psychologist B.F. Skinner published his famous book, *The Behavior of Organisms* in 1938. Building on the work of his predecessors, such as E.L. Thorndike, Skinner set up a laboratory to study the behavior of pigeons and other animals in great detail. He found that to teach a new behavior, we must reward behaviors that are successively closer and closer to the behavior we want.

Instrumental conditioning occurs when, for example, a behavior is followed immediately by a reward. This is *positive reinforcement,* and it causes the behavior to increase. Instrumental conditioning also includes *punishment,* when a behavior is followed by negative consequences. Punishment decreases the frequency of a behavior. A third kind of instrumental conditioning occurs when, for example, a behavior reduces negative stimulation. This is *escape conditioning,* which is sometimes called *negative reinforcement.* It makes a bad situation better, so the behavior occurs more often.

As Skinner explained, many human behaviors are *shaped* by instrumental conditioning. Your parents may have taught you to tie your shoes by first praising your awkward attempts to make an overhand knot, then praising gradually better and better versions of the completed bow. Think how much more effective this was than if they waited until you had tied your shoes perfectly before giving you any praise. Shaping can work in negative ways, too. Simple stuttering behaviors can be shaped into more and more bizarre and complicated patterns when struggle behaviors (such as eye blinks and head nods) are rewarded by the release of the stuttered word. Shaping can be a powerful therapy tool when used by clinicians to decrease the frequency and severity of stuttering and to replace stuttering with fluent speech.

Skinner and other psychologists showed that there are several important variables that must be kept in mind when instrumental conditioning is used to shape behavior. First, the strength of the reward or punishment is important. Big rewards are more effective than small ones, but punishment must be given in moderation. Second, timing is everything: rewards or punishments are most effective when they follow the behavior immediately. This is why behaviors that occur just before a stuttered word is finally released (such as squeezing, nodding, and blinking) are so well learned. Third, the frequency of rewards or punishments is a key to learning. To teach someone a new behavior, begin with frequent reinforcements after a fixed number of correct responses (called a "fixed-ratio schedule"), then switch to less frequent reinforcements after varying numbers of correct responses (called a "variable-ratio schedule"). In this way, the person is motivated to learn a new behavior quickly and to continue it without having to be rewarded for every correct response. The power of a variable-ratio schedule explains why some stuttering behaviors are so persistent; they are not rewarded with release of the stuttered word every time, just enough to continue them.

Three other principles of instrumental conditioning are mentioned briefly here and discussed in more detail when we talk about stuttering therapy (Chapter 8). *Extinction* is a process through which a learned response can be unlearned. If a reward no longer follows an instrumentally conditioned behavior, the behavior gradually disappears; however, behaviors that have been learned with a variable-ratio schedule are much more resistant to extinction. *Spontaneous Recovery*[4] occurs when a conditioned behavior is extinguished but returns spontaneously when the extinction procedures are stopped for a while. If therapy continues to work on extinguishing behaviors, spontaneous recovery is less likely.

Stimulus Generalization takes place when a behavior learned in one situation occurs in a situation that is similar but not identical with the original one. A child may develop severe stuttering behaviors when talking to an angry man, and these then generalize to all men. Therapeutically, you may teach a child to use a fluency technique when talking to you in the therapy room, and she may be able to generalize it when talking to you in the classroom.

EXAMPLE OF INSTRUMENTAL CONDITIONING AND STUTTERING

Instrumental conditioning can work rapidly in a young stutterer to establish and proliferate eye blinks, head nods, and other escape behaviors. Our young friend Richard, whose stuttering escalated from easy repetitions to tense and rapid ones, also began to show increasing secondary behaviors. They were attempts to escape from his core repetitive stutters. In his efforts to end long repetitions, he tried squeezing the muscles of his vocal cords, causing his pitch to increase. This trick seemed to help for a while, but after several days, it worked only intermittently. He then discovered that if he blinked his eyes in addition to squeezing the muscles of his larynx, the word seemed to come out sooner. Sometimes this worked, sometimes it didn't; however, both pitch rises and eye blinks became a regular part of his stuttering pattern.

As a result, not only did Richard's stuttering pattern grow more complex, but the times and places when he stuttered became more widespread. At first, Richard stuttered only when he was excited, tired, or afraid. Then he began stuttering many times throughout the day for several days at a time. Gradually, his stuttering started to be a regular feature of his speech whenever he talked.

---

[4] This use of "spontaneous recovery" is not to be confused with "spontaneous remission," when a child stops stuttering without treatment.

Let's look at how instrumental conditioning may have been at work here. The first time Richard squeezed his laryngeal muscles in an effort to stop a repetition, he was negatively reinforced by the terrific relief from the discomfort of stuttering when he said the word. Unfortunately for Richard, the reinforcement schedule started out as a 100% fixed ratio, because every time he squeezed his laryngeal muscles during a stutter, he was negatively reinforced by the release of the word. But soon, for reasons we don't understand, squeezing his muscles wasn't always followed by a release of the word; but sometimes it was. Richard was now on a "variable ratio" schedule of negative reinforcement for squeezing his laryngeal muscles to release himself from a stutter.

With such a powerful conditioning history, Richard's habit of squeezing his laryngeal muscles to push words out became resistant to change. On top of that behavior, Richard soon learned to blink his eyes as well, because of a similar schedule of fixed-ratio and then variable-ratio reinforcement. As time passed and Richard's stuttering became more widespread, these escape patterns proliferated and even began to occur earlier in the string of his repetitions. Stimulus generalization was responsible for the spread of both the classically conditioned (increases in tension and tempo) and the instrumentally conditioned (escape behaviors) parts of Richard's stuttering.

Without therapy, Richard might have gone on to add more and more maladaptive behaviors to his stuttering pattern. Fortunately, we were able to use a therapy program with plenty of positive reinforcement to help Richard unlearn his old stuttering patterns and learn more fluent speech. Stimulus generalization played an important role in treatment, too. The therapy setting (e.g., the treatment room) and the stimuli associated with it (e.g., parents, peers, and others) became discriminative stimuli and reinforcers for change and could be used to stimulate and reward the changes Richard learned as he worked on his stuttering.

Avoidance Conditioning

The word and situation avoidances seen in intermediate stuttering arise from the combined effects of instrumental and classical conditioning. These two learning mechanisms join forces to produce behaviors that are so well learned that they are hard to unlearn. This may be one of the reasons that stutterers often relapse after therapy.

To understand avoidance conditioning in stutterers, it may helpful to see how animals can be conditioned this way. One of the best examples comes from the work of two early experimenters in avoidance conditioning, Richard Solomon and L.C. Wynne (1953). These experimenters first trained dogs to escape an electric shock by placing them in a box divided by a low barrier and administering a shock until they learned to jump over the barrier to safety. Once the dogs learned to escape the shock promptly, the experimenters then gave a warning signal before the shock began. After only a few trials in which the warning signal preceded the shock, the dogs learned to jump over the barrier at the warning signal before the shock. This was avoidance learning.

The analogous behavior in stutterers is this: a stutterer first learns to escape from a stutter by, for example, saying another word when he is blocked, as in "I went to New Y-Y-Y . . . the Big Apple." After many pairings of anticipating a particular word and stuttering on it, he learns to use his escape behavior (e.g., substituting "The Big Apple" for "New York") before he stutters on "New York," and the stutter is avoided. Figure 4.4 depicts the transformation of an escape behavior into avoidance behavior.

Word avoidances often become less and less effective, but they continue to be used despite their intermittent success. The fact that they work sometimes (a variable ratio schedule of reinforcement) makes them all the more resistant to modification. Stutterers

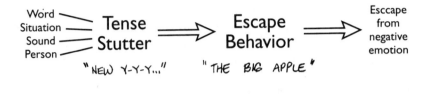

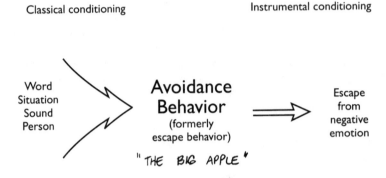

Figure 4.4. Creation of an avoidance response from an escape behavior. At first, in the presence of various words, situations, sounds, and people, a tense stutter is followed by an escape behavior, which terminates a negative emotion. Then, the words, situations, sounds, and people elicit the avoidance response (formerly the escape behavior). This is rewarded by the successful avoidance of stuttering and its negative emotion.

have a strong urge to use an avoidance device if there is a chance they might stutter. Treatment must deal with this tendency of word avoidances to be used when stuttering is expected.

The intermediate stutterer has learned to fear and avoid situations as well as words. This phenomenon is well known in the animal conditioning literature (Bouton & Bolles, 1985; Mineka, 1985). An experimental psychologist would say that when a stimulus has been conditioned to elicit a response in a particular context, the context becomes part of the stimulus that elicits the response. Other similar contexts can, by associative learning, become eliciting contexts. Thus, after stuttering badly in a classroom at school, that classroom and similar classrooms are likely to become feared situations for the stutterer, and he will do his best to avoid talking in them. If he has terrible blocks on the telephone, he begins to fear talking on the telephone and eventually avoids using it. This contextual learning, as we shall see, is an important consideration in the treatment of someone with advanced stuttering.

Experimental treatment with animals has taught us much about deconditioning avoidance learning in stutterers. Our primary method is to bring stutterers into contact with feared situations or events but at reduced levels of arousal than were experienced before. For many individuals who stutter, this often consists of teaching them ways of speaking that produce fluency and then gradually teaching them to use more and more words and sounds that were previously feared in more and more situations that were feared. Some individuals also fear stuttering itself. For them, treatment consists of teaching them to decrease their fear during stuttering, which decreases tension and rate and provides them an opportunity to change their stuttering behavior toward fluency.

STUDY QUESTIONS

1. What do brain imaging studies show about stutterers' structures and functions?
2. What might be sources of heterogeneity in stutterers as a group?
3. What are the differences between right and left hemisphere emotions, as Kinsbourne sees them?
4. How might a sensitive temperament affect speech? What is the evidence for this?
5. What are the two biological predispositions for stuttering that the author proposes?
6. In what ways might developmental factors affect each of the biological predispositions for stuttering?
7. In what ways might the environment affect these predispositions?
8. Describe two different elements of treatment that may affect these predispositions.
9. Describe why an escape behavior is used by a stutterer. Give examples.
10. How does instrumental conditioning work to increase the frequency of escape behaviors?
11. Give an example of a stutterer's (a) word avoidance, (b) situation avoidance.
12. How does classical conditioning work to generalize stuttering from a specific word or situation to many other words and situations?

SUGGESTED READINGS

Gray, Jeffrey A. (1987). *The psychology of fear and stress,* 2nd ed. New York: Cambridge University Press.

Gray's experimental work and his theoretical model of a behavioral inhibition system are clearly described here. Some of the book—those parts dealing with the effects of pharmacological agents on the brain—is for specialized readers. Much of it, however, is a readable exposition on the biological basis of learning, stress, and fear. Because this is the second edition of a popular book, we hope a new edition will be available soon.

Kagan, J., Reznick, J.S., & Snidman, N. (1987). The physiology and psychology of behavioral inhibition in children. *Child Development, 58,* 1459–1473.

This article discusses the findings of Kagan and his colleagues that behaviorally inhibited children show high levels of laryngeal tension. Neurophysiological mechanisms are also discussed, as well as possible genetic and environmental contributions. Recommended for those interested in the hypothesis that behavioral inhibition may be a component in some stuttering.

Kinsbourne, M., & Bemporad, B. (1984). Lateralization of emotion: A model and the evidence. In N.A. Fox & R.J. Davidson (Eds.), *The psychobiology of affective development.* Hillsdale, NJ: Lawrence Erlbaum Associates.

Normal Disfluency and the Development of Stuttering

In this chapter, we describe the characteristics of normal disfluency and explain how it differs from stuttering. Then we describe the development of stuttering, from its first appearance to its most advanced stages.

To highlight the important changes that often take place in stuttering over time and to clarify key elements necessary for treatment at each stage, we propose a hierarchy of five developmental/treatment levels. The first level is normal disfluency; the next four levels reflect the changes in key features that occur as stuttering progresses. In this chapter, we share our understanding of the reasons for these changes; in later chapters, we describe how to use this understanding in evaluation and treatment.

The five levels are shown in Table 5.1, along with the age ranges typically associated with them. Within each level, we have divided the characteristics of stuttering into four subcategories. The first three—*core behaviors, secondary behaviors,* and *feelings and attitudes*—are described in Chapter 1. The fourth, *underlying processes,* is introduced in this chapter to explain why the symptoms change from level to level. The explanations are hypotheses,

Table 5.1. Developmental/Treatment Levels of Stuttering

Developmental/Treatment Level	Typical Age Range
Normal disfluency	1.5–6 years, although a small amount of normal disfluency continues in mature speech
Borderline stuttering	1.5–6 years
Beginning stuttering	2–8 years
Intermediate stuttering	6–13 years
Advanced stuttering	14 years and above

based on evidence from animal and human studies of learned behavior about how stuttering behaviors become more severe and complex. This subcategory should help you understand the nature of the symptoms, as well as the treatment procedures in Section II.

These five developmental/treatment levels should become your guide for diagnosing and treating stutterers. Your client's core and secondary behaviors, along with feelings and attitudes, will indicate a developmental level and help you plan treatment. Note that our levels are based somewhat on age. We find that the appropriate treatment for an individual who stutters is determined both by how far stuttering has advanced and how old the person is. For example, an 8-year-old may have signs of advanced stuttering, but the stuttering treatment we propose for the advanced level would be inappropriate for this child because it demands considerable self-therapy. We discuss these sorts of choices in Section II.

These developmental/treatment levels do not precisely characterize all people who stutter. Many won't fit neatly into any of the levels we've constructed. Some behaviors in the same individual will suggest one level; other behaviors, another level. Generally, most stuttering behaviors can be placed reasonably well within only one level. Moreover, even though all of a person's behaviors may not reflect a single level of stuttering, treatment need not be a problem; when some aspects of a person's stuttering seem to be more advanced than others, strategies can be borrowed from other levels to treat them.

Another qualification of the hierarchy of levels of stuttering presented here is the implication that all individuals who stutter pass through each stage in sequence. This is generally true, but there are exceptions. A child may show only normal disfluencies one day and beginning or intermediate stuttering on another day. He may stop, miraculously, a week later, or he may continue stuttering unless treated. One 3-year-old boy we knew changed overnight from borderline to severe beginning stuttering after a change in his allergy medication. When it was changed back to the original prescription, he became a borderline stutterer again and then recovered completely. There are many unsolved mysteries in stuttering.

Van Riper (1982) also described a subgroup of stutterers who show a relatively sudden onset with severe symptoms. He suggested that many of these children begin to stutter after a traumatic incident and stutter with a great deal of tension, even at onset. In these cases, however, an overlay of learned behaviors soon places them in one of the levels to be described. Despite their unusual onsets, many of these clients respond well to our treatment procedures, especially if therapy begins soon after the onset of stuttering.

With these limitations in mind, we begin our description of the levels of stuttering development. We start with a behavior that is really not stuttering at all, but part of normal speech.

NORMAL DISFLUENCY

Children vary a great deal in how easily they learn to talk. Some children pass their milestones of speech and language development with relatively few disfluencies. Others

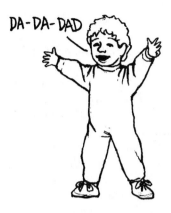

Figure 5.1. Child who may be normally disfluent.

stumble along, repeating, interjecting, and revising, as they try to master new forms of speech and language, on their way to adult competence. Most children are somewhere between the extremes of exceptional fluency and excessive disfluency, such as the 2-year-old shown in Figure 5.1.

Children also swing back and forth in the degree of their disfluency. Some days they are more fluent and other days less fluent. The swings in disfluency may be associated with language development, motor learning, or other developmental or environmental influences mentioned in the preceding chapter. In the following sections, we discuss factors that may influence disfluency, as well as specific behaviors that we categorize as normal disfluency and the reactions some children may have to them. We also highlight aspects of normal disfluency that distinguish it from early stuttering, because one of our aims in this chapter is to prepare you to make this differential diagnosis.

Core Behaviors

Normal disfluencies have been cataloged by several authors, and there is general agreement among them as to what constitutes disfluency.[1] Table 5.2 lists eight commonly used categories of disfluency.

Some of the major distinguishing features of normal disfluency—features that differentiate normal disfluency from stuttering—are the amount of disfluency, the number of

Table 5.2. Categories of Normal Disfluencies

Type of Normal Disfluency	Example
Part-word repetition	"mi-milk"
Single-syllable word repetition	"I . . . I want that."
Multisyllabic word repetition	"Lassie . . . Lassie is a good dog."
Phrase repetition	"I want a . . . I want a ice-ceem comb."
Interjection	"He went to the . . . uh . . . circus."
Revision-incomplete phrase	"I lost my . . . Where's Mommy going?"
Prolongation	"I'm Tiiiiiiiimmy Thompson."
Tense Pause	"Can I have some more (lips together; no sound coming out) milk?"

---

[1] Here are several studies that discuss categories of nonfluencies: Williams, Silverman, & Kools (1968), Colburn & Mysak (1982a,b), Yairi (1982), Yairi (1983), Bloodstein (1987), and Yairi (1997a).

units of repetitions and interjections, and the type of disfluency, especially in relation to the age of the child.

Let's discuss the amount of disfluency. This is often measured as the number of disfluencies per 100 words, rather that "percent disfluencies." Percent disfluencies implies that the disfluencies are associated with the production of particular words. For example, if you said that a child had a disfluency frequency of 10% words disfluent, it would be assumed that 10% of the words spoken were spoken disfluently. However, many disfluencies, such as revisions, interjections, or phrase repetitions, are associated with several words or occur between words. For example, a child may say "Mommy, can you . . . can you . . . um . . . can you buy me dat?" In this case, we say that the child spoke six words (Mommy can you buy me dat) and had two disfluencies (a phrase repetition and an interjection). Hence, we calculate the number of disfluencies that occur when the child speaks 100 words. More details on counting disfluencies are given in Chapter 7.

Although many researchers have measured disfluencies per number of words spoken, a good argument can be made for measuring disfluencies per number of *syllables* spoken. Andrews and Ingham (1971) first recommended the practice of assessing frequency of stuttering in relation to syllables spoken. Following their logic, Yairi (1997a) noted that as children get older, they are more likely to use multisyllable words, and it is possible to have disfluencies on more than one syllable in a word, as in "di-dinosa-sa-saur." Thus, in several important studies, Yairi has assessed disfluencies in children as number per 100 syllables (Hubbard & Yairi, 1988; Yairi & Lewis, 1984; Yairi & Ambrose, 1996).

When the frequency of all of the child's disfluencies is measured, we need to know how many of them are normal. Some of the earliest research on disfluency was conducted by Wendell Johnson at the University of Iowa. He assembled a team of researchers in the 1950s to examine the evidence for his "diagnosogenic" theory of stuttering. As indicated in Chapter 3, Johnson hypothesized that at the time the child is first "diagnosed" a stutterer by his parents, the child's disfluencies are no different from those of nonstuttering children. One of the research team's projects was to record children identified by their parents as stutterers and compare the amount of disfluency in their speech with that of nonstuttering children (Johnson & associates, 1959). One part of this study compared 68 male stuttering children with 68 male nonstuttering children. The results showed that, although there was some overlap, the stutterers had more than twice the amount of disfluency than did the nonstutterers (an average of 18 disfluencies per 100 words compared with 7 disfluencies per 100 words).[2]

Other researchers who have examined disfluencies in nonstuttering children put the amount of their disfluencies at about this level (DeJoy & Gregory, 1985; Hubbard & Yairi, 1988; Wexler & Mysak, 1982; Yairi, 1981; Yairi & Ambrose, 1996; Yairi & Lewis, 1984; Zebrowski, 1991). Bringing all these studies together, we can estimate that the average, normally disfluent preschool child has about seven disfluencies for every 100 words spoken. If measured in terms of syllables, it would be closer to six disfluencies per 100 syllables. This figure may be a little high throughout the preschool period (Yairi, 1997a), but many children go through a period of increased disfluency at age 2 or 3 years that will reach this level.

---

[2] Wendell Johnson's original interpretation was that the two groups were essentially the same because there was so much overlap in both amount and type of disfluency. Other researchers have reinterpreted the data to suggest that these are two different groups. Johnson's diagnosogenic hypothesis would not be jeopardized by this reinterpretation, however, since he believed that the child's reaction being labeled by the parents as a stutterer caused the child to engage in behavior that would differ from normal disfluency.

The range in frequency of normal disfluency is important to note also, especially if frequency of disfluency is used to make a clinical decision. Johnson and associates (1959) and Yairi (1981) found that, although many nonstuttering children have only one or two disfluencies per 100 words, at least one child in their samples had slightly more than 25 disfluencies per 100 words. Thus, frequency of disfluencies is not, by itself, a definitive clinical measure.

Another distinguishing characteristic of normal disfluency is the number of units that occur in each instance of repetition or interjection. Yairi's (1981) data suggest that typically normal repetitions consist of only one extra unit: a child might say "That my-my ball." Interjections are likely to be just a single unit, as in "I want some . . . uh . . . juice." Instances of multiple repetitions were occasionally observed in these children, but this was the exception. The rule was one and sometimes two units per repetition or interjection. This agrees with Johnson and associates' (1959) findings that the average nonstuttering child has one- or two-unit repetitions.

Another major characteristic of normal disfluency is the type of disfluency that is most common. Johnson and associates (1959) found that interjections, revisions, and word repetitions were the most common disfluency types among his 68 nonstuttering males, who ranged in age from 2½ to 8 years of age. Yairi (1981) found, in his 33 2-year-old normal subjects that there were two clusters of common disfluency types. One cluster involved repetitions of speech segments of one syllable or less (one-syllable words or parts of words were repeated). The second cluster consisted of interjections and revisions.

The most common disfluency type seems to change as a child grows older. In a follow-up of his earlier study, Yairi (1982) found that children between 2 and 3½ years showed an increase in revisions and phrase repetitions, but a decrease in part-word repetitions and interjections. Yairi suggested that his data indicate that as a nonstuttering child matures, part-word repetitions decline, even if other disfluency types increase. Moreover, the increase of part-word repetitions as a child is observed longitudinally is a sign that may warrant concern.

Although the research is far from complete, we can summarize normal disfluency types as follows: revisions are a common disfluency type in normal children and may continue to account for a major portion of their disfluency as they grow older. Interjections are also common, but usually decline after age 3 years. Repetitions may also be a frequent type of disfluency, especially single-syllable word repetitions with fewer than two extra units around age 2 to 3 years. Repetitions are more likely to involve longer segments (e.g., phrases) as the child grows older.

Table 5.3 summarizes the major characteristics of normal disfluency.

Secondary Behaviors

A normally disfluent child generally has no secondary behaviors. He has not developed any reactions, such as escape or avoidance behaviors, to his disfluencies. Although research suggests that some normal children occasionally display "tense pauses," this tension does not appear to be a reaction to the experience of disfluency. If a child shows what

---

Table 5.3. Characteristics of Normal Disfluency in the Average Nonstuttering Child

1. No more than 10 disfluencies per 100 words.
2. Typically one-unit repetitions, occasionally two.
3. Most common disfluency types are interjections, revisions, and word repetitions. As children mature past age 3, they will show a decline in part-word repetitions.

appears to be normal disfluencies, such as single-word repetitions, yet consistently displays such reactions as pauses or interjections of "uh" immediately before or during disfluencies, he should be carefully evaluated as a possible stutterer.

Feelings and Attitudes

The normally disfluent child rarely notices his disfluencies, even though they may be apparent to others. Just as a child may stumble when walking but regain his balance and keep walking without complaint, a normal child who repeats or interjects or revises usually continues talking after a disfluency without evidence of frustration or embarrassment.

Underlying Processes

Let us first review the behaviors we are trying to account for. Normal disfluency occurs throughout childhood and adulthood. It may begin earlier than 18 months of age[3] and peaks between ages 2 and 3½ years. It slowly diminishes thereafter, but also changes in form. Some types of disfluency, such as repetitions, decrease after age 3½, but other types, such as revisions, may increase. Episodic increases and decreases are also common throughout childhood.

What causes these changes in disfluency? Why are there ups and downs and changes in form? Like most natural phenomena, multiple forces probably have an impact on fluency at any one moment, but some may be more predominant at certain times. In Chapter 3, we talked about developmental and environmental influences on stuttering and normal disfluency, and we will review these influences as we discuss studies of normally disfluent children.

The development of language is certainly likely to be one major influence on fluency. As our earlier review showed, children tend to be most disfluent at the beginning of syntactic units (Bernstein, 1981; Silverman, 1974) and when the length and complexity of their utterances increase (DeJoy & Gregory, 1973; Gordon, Luper, & Peterson, 1986; Pearl & Bernthal, 1980). These findings suggest that disfluency is greatest when a child is busy planning a long or complex language structure but must, at the same time, begin to produce it, putting a heavy load on cerebral resources. It seems likely that producing newly learned language structures would be hardest of all, resulting in more frequent disfluencies on most recently acquired forms.

However, evidence gathered on four children between 2 and 4 years old suggests that normal disfluency may be greatest on structures that have been learned, but perhaps not fully automatized, thus requiring more resources than are allocated to their production (Colburn & Mysak, 1982a,b).

Pragmatics may influence disfluency, too. Studies by Dorothy Davis (1940) and Susan Meyers and Frances Freeman (1985a,b) indicate that children's disfluency increases under certain pragmatic conditions, such as when interrupting, when directing another's activity, or when asked to change their own activity. Mastering such pragmatic skills, especially those involving more complex social interactions, creates yet another challenge for

---

[3] Harris Winitz (1961) studied the vocalizations of infants during the first two years of life and found that repetitions were common throughout that period. It is not clear whether the repetitions in nonmeaningful speech are the result of the same processes that create repetitions in meaningful speech. Winitz reported that the frequency of repetitions peaked at 12 months. Curlee (personal communication, 1996) has surmised that this peak may result from the emergence of one-word utterances, potentially reflecting a different mechanism for repetitions from that underlying repeated vocalizations.

a developing child. The pressures of language acquisition, interacting with other factors, can be seen as competition for cerebral resources, which leaves fewer available resources for fluent speech production.

Another likely influence on disfluency, in addition to language, is speech motor control. Between the ages of 2 and 5 years, most children begin to reach almost all the segmental and supersegmental targets of their native tongue, as well as to increase their speech rate to produce longer and longer utterances. These maturational changes must keep the average child fairly busy, although it may not be obvious. He is continually scanning his parents' and older siblings' speech, acquiring information about talking. He is also continuously modifying his own productions to make them more and more like the speech he hears. This age, from 2 to 5 years, also encompasses intensive refinement of nonspeech motor skills. Children are mastering a myriad of other motor tasks at the same time they are acquiring the ability to speak in rapid, complex, fluent sequences. However, it is probable that motor tasks that use substantially different neural networks than speech are not as likely to interfere with fluency.

In general, the view of stuttering described earlier, suggesting that a breakdown may occur when cerebral resources are reassigned from a motor control system to be used elsewhere, may fit the nonstuttering child as well as the child who stutterers (Andrews et al., 1983; Starkweather, 1987). Some of the upswings and downswings in disfluency may occur when a normal child is occupied with language, speech production, and motor control for other things besides speech fluency.

Besides the continuing demands of normal development, there are also episodic stresses in a child's environment that may temporarily increase normal disfluency. An experiment by Harris Hill (1954) demonstrated that conditioned fear could bring about disfluency in normal adults' speech. Therefore, it is easy to imagine that there are many psychological stresses in a child's life that would also bring about disfluency. Clinically, we have observed many situations that seem to increase normal disfluency. Among them are stress from a move from one home to another, parents' separation or divorce, the birth of a sibling, and other events that decrease a child's security.

We have also seen increases in normal disfluency during periods of excitement, such as holidays, vacations, and visits by relatives. Disfluency especially increases when excitement combines with competition to be heard, such as at dinner table conversations during which everyone often talks at once or after school when several children are competing to tell Mom what happened during the day. As we speculated in Chapter 4, emotions may have an especially strong influence on fluency in children. This happens after interactions between right and left hemispheres develop during the child's first 2 years (Fox & Davidson, 1984) and overflow activity from emotional arousal in the right hemisphere may affect vulnerable, immature language production networks in the left.

Summary

Between the ages of 2 and 5 years, many children pass through periods of disfluency. Repetitions, interjections, revisions, prolongations, and pauses are commonly heard during this period. When the average child is between 2 and 3½, disfluencies reach 7 per 100 words spoken and may be even more frequent in some children. Repetitions are probably most common in younger children, whereas revisions are more common in older children. Despite the fact that children's disfluencies may occasionally attract some adult attention, normally disfluent children seem generally unaware of them in their own speech and, consequently, don't react to them or use secondary behaviors to escape or avoid them.

Some factors thought to contribute to increases in normal disfluencies include the demands of language acquisition, lagging speech-motor control, interpersonal stress associated with growing up in a typical family, and threats to security from such disruptions as relocation, family breakup, or hospitalization. Disfluencies may also increase under the daily pressures of competition and excitement while speaking.

BORDERLINE STUTTERING

Borderline stuttering has all the characteristics of normal disfluency (Fig. 5.2); however, there are more disfluencies, and they often differ from normal ones in several ways. Diagnosis of borderline stuttering is sometimes difficult because a child may drift back and forth between normal disfluency and borderline stuttering over a period of weeks or months. Some children with borderline stuttering gradually lose their stuttering symptoms and grow up without a trace of stuttering. Others develop more stuttering symptoms and progress through levels of beginning, intermediate, and advanced stuttering.

In describing the behaviors of borderline stuttering, we begin to define our view of how stuttering differs from normal disfluency. The distinction between stuttering and normal disfluency has been of great interest to theorists for many years. Some theorists (e.g., Wendell Johnson et al., 1942; 1955) suggest, as noted previously, that a stuttering child developed symptoms only after his parents mislabeled his normal disfluencies as stuttering. That is, this child's first "stuttering" symptoms were really the disfluencies of normal speech.

An opposing view maintains that there are objective differences between the speech of the normal child and the speech of a child first suspected of stuttering by his parents or another lay person. We hold the latter view, believing that, when parents first become concerned, most children who stutter are disfluent in ways that differ from peers. Although the disfluency pattern, considered as a whole, may be different, there are still many overlaps with normal disfluency. Moreover, as previously stated, these children often go back and forth between stuttering and normal disfluency over a period of months. For this reason, we use the term "borderline" to indicate that the children are neither entirely normally disfluent, nor definitely stuttering.

Core Behaviors

There is no single behavior that distinguishes borderline stuttering from normal disfluency. However, many researchers and clinicians have suggested a few guidelines. *Fre-*

Figure 5.2. Child who may be a borderline stutterer.

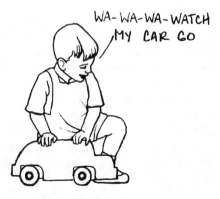

quency of disfluencies is one important aspect to consider. As we indicated in our description of normal disfluencies, nonstuttering children between the ages of 2 and 5 years may go through periods of increased disfluency. Even so, their average level of disfluency averages about 7 per 100 words. Thus, if children have many more disfluencies per 100 words (e.g., more than 10), we may consider them borderline.

Another feature that can help identify children who may have borderline stuttering rather than normal disfluency is *the proportion of certain types of disfluencies*. The study we cited earlier by Johnson (Johnson & associates, 1959) suggested that, compared with nonstuttering children, stuttering children had significantly more sound and syllable repetitions, word repetitions, phrase repetitions, broken words (phonation or airflow is stopped within a word), and prolonged sounds. There were no significant differences between the groups in their number of interjections, revisions, and incomplete phrases.

More information on types of disfluencies was provided by Young (1984), who surveyed a large number of studies that assessed which types of disfluencies were identified as stuttering and which were not. His summary impression was that repetitions of parts of words and, to a lesser extent, prolongations are the disfluency types that are likely to be classified as stuttering. Bloodstein (1987) and Conture (1982; 1990) generally concur with other writers, suggesting that "within-word" disfluencies (i.e., part-word repetitions, single-syllable word repetitions, prolongations including blocks) and broken words are the types of disfluencies most likely to be heard in stuttering children.

Yairi and colleagues (Yairi & Ambrose, 1996; Yairi, 1997a,b) propose that children who stutter can be distinguished from normally disfluent children using a grouping of "stuttering-like" disfluencies. He includes in this grouping short-segment repetitions (part-word and monosyllabic word repetitions), tense pauses, and a category introduced by Williams, Silverman, and Kools (1968) called "dysrhythmic phonations" (any within-word distortion such as a prolongation or a break in phonation that is not included in another category). Yairi (1997a,b) notes that when many previous studies of stuttering and nonstuttering children are reanalyzed using this grouping, the proportion of stuttering-like disfluencies in nonstuttering children is always less than 50% of the total number of disfluencies.

In summary, we can say that one measure that will help us distinguish the child with borderline stuttering from the normally disfluent child is a higher proportion of part-word and monosyllabic whole-word repetitions and prolongations, compared with multisyllabic word and phrase repetitions. In the next section, we see that children with the types of tension in their disfluencies that have been labeled blocks, broken words, and dysrhythmic phonations are beginning rather than borderline stutterers.

The *number of times a word or sound is repeated* in a part-word or monosyllable word repetitive disfluency appears to be another distinction between children who stutter and their normally disfluent peers. In Yairi's (1981) sample of 33 nonstuttering children, repetitions typically involved only one or two extra units of repetition (one extra unit would be li-like this). Other studies comparing stuttering and nonstuttering children (Ambrose & Yairi, 1995; Johnson & associates, 1959; Yairi & Lewis, 1984; Zebrowski, 1991) have found that the repetitive disfluencies of nonstuttering children average 1.13 extra units and that of stuttering children, 1.51. Thus, the frequent appearance of repetitions in which there is more than one extra unit is a warning sign of borderline stuttering.

We have said that borderline stuttering consists primarily of effortless repetitions and occasional prolongations. However, as Van Riper (1971; 1982) noted, these young children are often highly variable in their stuttering. Although they usually show the core behaviors of borderline stuttering, they may have brief periods of normal fluency and days when they show signs of more advanced stuttering.

Secondary Behaviors

The borderline stutterer has few if any secondary behaviors. The degree of tension may sometimes seem to be slightly greater than normal, but repetitions and prolongations generally look and sound relaxed. The child does not use accessory movements before, during, or after his stutters. In fact, there is usually nothing in his behavior to indicate that he is aware of his stutters.

Feelings and Attitudes

Because the child with borderline stuttering seems to have little awareness of his stutters, he does not show concern or embarrassment. When he repeats a sound or a syllable, even five or six times, he usually goes on talking as though nothing has happened. One exception is that, once in a while, a child with borderline stutter might appear surprised or frustrated when he is repeating a syllable several times and is unable to finish a word. Then he may stop and comment, "Mommy, I can't say that word." But, in general, the borderline stutterer shows no evidence that he has more problems than anyone else.

Table 5.4 summarizes the major characteristics of the borderline stutterer.

Underlying Processes

We hypothesize that the symptoms of borderline stuttering are the result of the constitutional and environmental factors described in Chapters 2, 3, and 4. The constitutional factors associated with borderline stuttering—differences in cerebral organization—often first show their effects as an excess of normal disfluencies.[4] As previously stated, environmental and developmental pressures may be great between the ages of 2 and 3½, and during this period borderline stuttering typically emerges. The converging demands of expressive language and motor speech development ordinarily peak between ages 2 and 4 years, "when an explosive growth in language ability outstrips a still-immature speech motor apparatus" (Andrews et al., 1983). This age is also filled with psychosocial conflicts, as a child copes with security needs as an infant and longs to grow more independent as a toddler. The child can be ready to explore, but also fearful. A new brother or sister may be born, triggering the child's insecurity with the threat of being replaced. An older sibling may turn belligerent toward him because of the older child's own need to express aggression as a prelude to puberty. Just as these stresses wax and wane in strength during preschool years, so does stuttering.

After age 4½ or 5 years, developmental stresses taper off for most children. Some of the parent-child conflicts are resolved, and children may feel more integrated within

Table 5.4. Characteristics of Borderline Stutterer

1. More than 10 disfluencies per 100 words
2. Often more than 2 units in repetition
3. More repetitions and prolongations than revisions or incomplete phrases
4. Disfluencies loose and relaxed
5. Rare reaction of child to his disfluencies

---

[4] Constitutional, developmental, and environmental factors sometimes precipitate stuttering that is far more involved than an excess of normal disfluencies at onset. We deal with this in the next section, on beginning stuttering.

themselves and within their families. Articulation and language skills, although still not at adult levels, have been mastered sufficiently for most children to say what's on their mind and to be understood. They have also mastered other motor skills, such as walking and running, as well as riding a tricycle or a bike with training wheels. They may have adjusted to a new, younger sibling as well and made at least temporary peace with an older one.

By now, the capacities of a great many children who may have had a modest predisposition to stutter can easily meet most environmental demands. Therefore, many children who were borderline stutterers will have acquired normal fluency skills by the time they are 4½ or 5 years old. Others may still have many disfluencies at this age, but will eventually outgrow them, perhaps because they are not frustrated by them and do not respond with tension or by rushing. They are functioning well in general, feel accepted, and can use their resources to compensate for whatever difficulty in speaking remains.

Some children do not outgrow borderline stuttering. They may continue to stutter and their symptoms may worsen. These may be children who have a substantial predisposition to stutter, which cannot be offset by a "good enough" environment (Winnicott, 1971). Their ability to produce speech and language at the rate and level of complexity used by parents and peers may be insufficient. Their continuing efforts to meet adult speech and language targets may result in excess disfluency that does not diminish as they pass their third and fourth birthdays. Their frustration tolerance for the multiple repetitions that many 2-and 3-year-olds experience may be low. Rather than shrugging it off, they may begin struggling to produce flawless speech, thereby making it worse. Still other children may continue to stutter because environmental and developmental stresses do not diminish. Their insecurity may continue from sibling rivalry, breakup of their family, or a parent's death. They may have language or articulation problems, as well as stuttering, which limit their communication abilities throughout their preschool years. Deficits in processes underlying speech and language development, plus the frustration of being unable to communicate easily, may be devastating to fluency. This may lead to the increased tension of beginning stuttering. A child in this situation is unlikely to outgrow stuttering unless parents and professionals provide extensive support.

Summary

Children with borderline stuttering usually have a greater amount of disfluency than do normal children—more than 7 nonfluencies per 100 words. They are also likely to repeat units more than once in many of their part-word and single-syllable word repetitions and to have many more part-word and single-syllable word repetitions and prolongations than multisyllable word and phrase repetitions, revisions, and interjections. At the same time, their disfluencies, like those of nonstuttering children, are usually loose and relaxed-appearing. Also, like nonstuttering children, children with borderline stuttering show little or no awareness of their speaking difficulty. Only rarely do they express frustration about it.

Among the underlying processes behind borderline stuttering are probably some of the speech and language-processing anomalies described in the earlier chapter on constitutional origins of stuttering. These deficits in resources may interact with demands from speech and language development, the pressure from higher rates of speech, more complex language, competitive speaking situations, and other attributes of a normal home. In addition, some of the psychosocial conflicts described earlier, which increase normal disfluency, are likely to be active in creating borderline stuttering.

BEGINNING STUTTERING

When stuttering persists, the child who has been a borderline stutterer often begins to tense and speed up repetitions, as the child in Figure 5.3 appears to be doing. At first, the child may do this only occasionally, when excited or stressed. Then, gradually tension and hurry may become a regular part of stuttering. The child's borderline stuttering is now becoming beginning stuttering. The child is stuttering more often and is less tolerant of it. He is impatient with his stuttering and consequently begins to use a variety of escape behaviors. For example, he may stop long repetitions by using a quick blink of his eyes or a sudden nod of his head. These signs, and his stuttering in general, may still come and go, as in the borderline stutterer. In the beginning stutterer, however, periods of increased stuttering may last for several months, whereas the periods of fluency may last only a day or so.

As these signs occur consistently, tension increases, and struggle is more evident. Instrumental and classical conditioning processes increase the frequency of struggle behaviors, complicate the pattern of stuttering, and spread the symptoms to many more situations.

It should be noted that some children evidence beginning stutterer at onset, without passing through a stage of borderline stuttering. Van Riper (1971; 1982) described several different profiles of stuttering with tense blockages at onset. Many of the children he depicted as more severe at onset were relatively older (4, 5, or 6 years old) when their stuttering first appeared. Onset seemed to be related to one of two factors: delayed language development or emotional events. Yairi and Ambrose (1992b) described onsets of stuttering that were characterized by the signs we have called beginning stuttering in 28% of their sample of 87 children. Many of these children had relatively sudden onset, with normal fluency changing to beginning stuttering within 1 day or, at most, 1 week.

Core Behaviors

The core behaviors of beginning stuttering differ from those of borderline stuttering in several ways. Repetitions begin to sound rapid and irregular. The final segment of a repeated syllable, if it is a vowel, often sounds abrupt, as if suddenly cut off, or as though a neutral or schwa vowel ("uh") has been substituted for the appropriate one, as in "luh-luh-luh-like." Repetitions are also produced more rapidly, sometimes with an irregular

Figure 5.3. Child who may be a beginning stutterer.

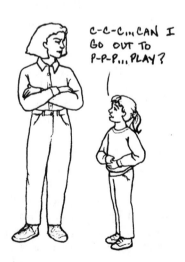

rhythm. Rather than patiently repeating a syllable as the borderline stutterer does, the beginning stutterer hurries through a repetitive stutter, as though juggling a hot potato.

As symptoms progress, the beginning stutterer increases tension throughout the speech mechanism. Stuttering is often accompanied by a rise in vocal pitch, resulting from increased tension in the larynx. Pitch rises may first appear toward the end of a string of repeated syllables, but in time appear earlier and earlier in the repetition.

The beginning stutterer sometimes prolongs sounds that would have previously been repeated. Initially, he may prolong the first sound of a syllable, but as stuttering grows more severe, he also may prolong the middle sound, and this, too, may be accompanied by an increase in pitch.

As beginning stuttering progresses, the first signs of blockages appear. These are significant landmarks that indicate that a child is stopping the flow of air or voice at one or more places (Van Riper, 1982). He may inappropriately jam his vocal folds closed or wide open, interrupting or possibly delaying the onset of phonation (Conture, 1990). Shutting off the airway is usually heard as a momentary stoppage of sound in a child's speech and is sometimes accompanied by a visual cue: the child may seem momentarily unable to move his mouth or may make groping movements as he tries to get air or voice going again. When stoppage of movement, voice, or airflow first begins, it may be so fleeting that we don't notice it unless we are listening and watching carefully. As these blocks worsen, they become so obvious that they often overshadow the repetitions and prolongations that may remain.

Secondary Behaviors

As a beginning stutterer's symptoms progress, secondary behaviors are added. They are called secondary because they appear to be responses to the muscle tension that has emerged. In addition, although hard evidence is lacking, the core behaviors of tension and speeding up seem to be "involuntary," to have begun as a reaction, that is, beyond the stutterer's ability to control. In contrast, the secondary behaviors to be described seem to have begun "voluntarily." They are, at least initially, deliberate. Among the earliest are "escape" behaviors, which are maneuvers used to stop a stutter and finish a word. Beginning stutterers often show escape behaviors after several repetitions of a syllable. They nod their head or squint their eyes just as they try to push a word out. This extra effort often seems to help—in the short run. They escape, for the moment, from the punishing repetition or prolongation. Alternately, they may insert a filler such as "uh" or "um" after a string of fruitless repetitions. The "um" seems to release the word, perhaps by relaxing the tightly squeezed larynx or by unlocking the lips. The "um" can always be said fluently, and once uttered, phonation and movement for the word often begin. The filler works like a little push you might give your sled if it were stuck in the snow as you start down a hill; the "um" gets the child going again when he is stuck in a stutter.

The beginning stutterer starts to use escape behaviors earlier and earlier in the stutter. The first appearance of these behaviors is usually after a child has repeated a sound several times and is thoroughly frustrated with it. It may sound this way: "Luh-Luh-Luh-Luh-Luh-umLet's go!" Soon, however, the child does not wait until he has tried to say the sound five times. He finds himself about to say a word, feels convinced it won't come out, then, perhaps instinctively, uses the escape behavior when he is first starting to stutter: "L-umLet's go!" Such "starters" may even appear before the first sound of the word, in this fashion: "umLet's go!" Their use, however, is more common among children with intermediate stuttering, even though they occasionally appear in the speech of a child with beginning stuttering.

Feelings and Attitudes

The child with beginning stuttering has stuttered many times. He is aware of stuttering when it happens. The feelings the beginning stutterer has just before, during, and after a stutter are often strong. Frequently, frustration is a major feeling. The child may stop in the middle of a stutter and say, "Mom, why can't I talk?" This momentary frustration grows into momentary fear when the word or sound is stuck for several seconds. He feels helpless and out of control.

Although a child with beginning stuttering is conscious that he has some "trouble" when he talks, he has not developed a belief that he is a defective speaker. His lack of a negative self-image may be attributed, as Bloodstein (1987) and Van Riper (1982) suggest, to the "episodic" nature of stuttering. Some days it's there; some days it's not. Sometimes the child feels that he has problems when he talks; other times he forgets about it.

The essential characteristics of beginning stutterers are shown in Table 5.5.

Underlying Processes

The signs and symptoms of beginning stuttering that we described can be observed by any experienced clinician. We have witnessed them in hundreds of children who stutter. But the processes underlying these behaviors are not so easy to see. In Chapter 4, we suggested that beginning stuttering may result from the interplay between constitutional and environmental factors, especially from a child's reactive temperament. We will review our hypotheses about the core behaviors of beginning stuttering, as well as the learning processes that are likely to perpetuate the core behaviors and the child's secondary reactions.

INCREASES IN MUSCLE TENSION AND TEMPO

One of the first signs of beginning stuttering is the appearance of extra muscular tension in repetitions and prolongations and increased tempo or rate in repetitive stutters (Van Riper, 1982). Why do these changes occur? Oliver Bloodstein (1987) suggests that facial tension and strained glottal attacks in the speech of young children who stutter may reflect extra muscular effort that emerges when they anticipate difficulty. Edward Conture (1990) offers a related view. He conceptualizes the increased articulatory and laryngeal muscle tension as a child's attempt to control the sound-syllable repetitions, which are so distressing to him and his parents. We, ourselves, have described this tension as the child's effort to control a frustrating and scary behavior of his own body, an attempt to stiffen the speech muscles to brace himself against the perturbations of seemingly involuntary, runaway repetitions (Guitar et al., 1988).

Table 5.5. Characteristics of Beginning Stutterers

1. Signs of muscle tension and hurry appear in stuttering. Repetitions are rapid and irregular, with abrupt terminations of each element.
2. Pitch rise may be present toward the end of a repetition or prolongation.
3. Fixed articulatory postures are sometimes evident when the child is momentarily unable to begin a word, apparently as a result of tension in speech musculature.
4. Escape behaviors are sometimes present in stutterers. These include, among other things, eye blinks, head nods, and "um's."
5. Awareness of difficulty and feelings of frustration are present, but there are no strong negative feelings about self as speaker.

The other early sign, increased rate in repetitive stutters, is cited by a number of authors as a sign that stuttering is worsening. Van Riper (1982), in describing the developmental course of the majority of children who stutter, suggests, "the tempo changes as the disorder develops. The repetitive syllables become irregular and are often spoken more rapidly than other fluent syllables." Starkweather (1987) explains this increase in speed of repetitions as the product of the pressure that children feel as they becomes more aware of the extra time it takes them to produce an utterance.

But why are these increases in tension and tempo so common in the development of stuttering, and why are they so difficult to change in therapy? In Chapter 4, we described our view that children in whom stuttering persists may be especially sensitive to certain kinds of experiences. Faced with frustration or fear, we hypothesized, they react with elements of their biologically based freezing or flight responses. The signs of beginning stuttering appear to have similarities with these reactions. The excessive muscle tension in beginning stuttering can be viewed as a way the child's limbic system causes him to freeze in the face of his frustrating or frightening repetitive disfluencies, transforming them into abrupt, tense repetitions, blocks, or prolongations.[5] Research bears out the speculation that at least some adults who stutter contract their muscles in such a way that movement and phonation are immobilized. Freeman and Ushijima's (1978) and Shapiro and DeCicco's (1982) studies indicate that stuttering is associated with abnormal muscle co-contraction of adductor and abductor muscles in the larynx. Such co-contraction would be a means of stiffening the phonatory structures and silencing vocal output. Other studies of stuttering have demonstrated co-contraction in the articulatory structures (Fibiger, 1971; Guitar et al., 1988; Platt & Basili, 1973), which would also produce immobility and silence.

Unfortunately, little research directly supports the notion that the increased rate of repetitions has its basis in the flight response. We have some tentative evidence that stutterers have more rapid productions during repetitions than do nonstutterers. An unpublished study (Allen, 1988) carried out in our clinic indicated that the durations of beginning stutterers' repeated segments and the silences between them were shorter than similar durations in the disfluencies of nonstuttering children matched for age. This finding has been confirmed in the recent work of Throneburg and Yairi (1994), who found that the silent intervals and the total durations of the repetition disfluencies were significantly shorter in stuttering children compared with control nonstuttering children. Such shortening of segments results in a faster speech rate, at least for the stuttered elements. This increased rate may derive from the "great increase in activity" seen in the flight response, although these particular data do not exclude the possibility that stuttering children were more rapid speakers to begin with.[6]

Thus, the possibility that increased muscle tension and rapid repetitions are a result of a biologically based freezing or flight response is highly speculative at this time. If these responses are part of the human's neural wiring designed for survival, this may be a potential explanation of why some children develop stuttering so rapidly and why the tension response is so difficult to change.

---

[5] As we have mentioned, some children appear to show tense blocks at the onset of their stuttering. These may be children who have a high degree of emotional sensitivity and whose very first manifestation of stuttering may be the result of fear-based responses to speaking experiences.

[6] Kloth, Janssen, Kraaimaat, & Brutten (1995) found that rapid speaking rate was a predictor of which young children with a family history of stuttering and who were fluent at the time of testing would eventually stutter. The rapid rate in these children might be related to a reactive limbic system, although there is no evidence that speech rate is related to such reactivity.

EFFECTS OF LEARNING ON STUTTERING

We are not sure whether the increases in tension and rate are voluntary or involuntary or both, but we do know that these reactions increase with persistent stuttering. This is likely to be the result of classical and instrumental conditioning. These are the forces at work when stuttering escalates from an occasional tense and hurried repetition to speech that is riddled with tense and hurried repetitions. Learning also turns occasional eye blinks or head nods during stutters into the stereotyped pattern of blinking and nodding that transforms innocuous disfluency into something so obvious that listeners gape in surprise and parents look away. Let us examine these learning processes closely, so that we can better understand those who come to us for help.

Classical conditioning, we surmise, is responsible for previously "neutral" experiences and situations eliciting tense and hurried stuttering in the child's speech. This occurs after many experiences in which the child's repetitive stutters have elicited an emotional response that has triggered an increase in tension and hurry. Classical conditioning spreads this more severe stuttering to more and more situations. In a few children, tension appears at the onset of the disorder because they experience a high degree of emotion during a speaking situation. We also hypothesized that children whose stuttering persists are highly susceptible to being conditioned because of their reactive nervous systems.

Instrumental conditioning is responsible for the increase in frequency of escape behaviors in beginning stuttering, we hypothesize, because the child is reinforced for such things as head nods or eye blinks when they are followed by a gratifying release of the word that a child may be stuttering on. Instrumental conditioning generalizes the escape behaviors to more and more situations and causes escape behaviors to occur earlier and earlier in the stutter, so that escape behaviors eventually become "starters."

Summary

The principal differences between the borderline and the beginning stutterer are these:

• The beginning stutterer shows more tension and "hurry" in his stuttering. This is often manifested in abruptly ended syllable repetitions, irregular rhythms of repetitions, evident stoppages of phonation, and momentarily fixated articulatory postures. The beginning stutterer also evidences such secondary behaviors as escape devices and starters. In addition, the beginning stutterer sees himself as someone who has trouble talking.
• We speculate that one major factor underlying beginning stuttering is a child's sensitivity to stress, which may easily result in the emotion of frustration, triggering a tension response. Classical conditioning then links this unconditioned response sensitivity to disfluency (when the child is disfluent, he feels threatened, frustrated, or afraid), leading to the rapid, tense disfluencies that begin to appear in the beginning stutterer. After repeated pairing, the disfluency itself elicits increased tension and rate. Classical conditioning also links the child's disfluency to more and more people and places. A third factor in beginning stuttering is instrumental conditioning, which increases and then maintains use of escape devices. These behaviors are negatively reinforced when the frustration of a stutter is terminated by an escape behavior and positively reinforced when the stutterer completes his communication.

INTERMEDIATE STUTTERING

The youngster with intermediate level stuttering, who is typically between the ages of 6 and 13 (Fig. 5.4), has two major characteristics that distinguish him from the child with

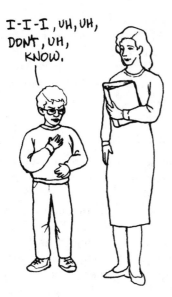

I-I-I, UH, UH,
DON'T, UH,
KNOW.

Figure 5.4. Child who may be an intermediate stutterer.

beginning stuttering. First, he is starting to *fear* stuttering, whereas the beginning stutterer is only frustrated, surprised, or annoyed by it. Second, he reacts to his fear of stuttering by *avoiding* it, something the beginning stutterer doesn't do. These new symptoms emerge gradually as a young stutterer experiences negative emotion more frequently during stuttering. For example, he blocks and feels helpless, listeners respond with discomfort or pity, and after this has happened frequently, he becomes afraid.

The fear may be attached first to the sounds and words on which he stutters most. He starts to believe that these sounds are harder for him. Then he begins to scan ahead to see whether he might have to say them. When he anticipates them, he tries to avoid them. For example, he may say, "I don't know" to questions, or he may substitute "my sister" for his sister's name when talking about her. He may start a sentence, realize a feared word is coming up, then switch the sentence around to avoid saying it, producing a maze of half-finished sentences.

The intermediate stutterer's fear of stuttering may be attached to situations as well as words. The youngster may find that he stutters more in some situations than in others. At first, he approaches these situations with dread, but later, he may go to great lengths to avoid them. Van Riper (1982) suggested that the development of these situational fears and avoidances depends on listener reactions. Interventions with key listeners in the stutterer's environment may help prevent them.

Core Behaviors

What are the intermediate stutterer's moments of stuttering like, when he doesn't avoid them? What are his core behaviors? Although he still repeats and prolongs, his most notable core behaviors are now blocks. The blocks of children with intermediate stuttering seem to grow out of the increasing tension seen initially in beginning stuttering. The child at the intermediate level usually stutters by stopping airflow, voicing, or movement (or all three), and then struggling to get his speech going again. His stutters seem to surprise him less than when he was a beginning stutterer. Instead, as evidenced by his voice and manner in certain situations, he anticipates stutters.

We have the impression that the intermediate stutterer's blocks are frequently characterized by excessive laryngeal tension, but he often blocks elsewhere as well. He may squeeze his lips together, jam his tongue against the roof of his mouth, or hold his breath. Even though he is not highly conscious of just what he's doing during a block, he has a vivid awareness that he is stuck, that he feels helpless, and that the word he wants to say won't seem to come out.

Secondary Behaviors

The blocks just described can be devastating to a child who stutters. He is frustrated not only with his inability to make a sound, but he is often faced with a surprised and uncomfortable listener as well. Even patient listeners may not know what to do. They may interrupt, look away, or fidget, leaving the stutterer then to conclude that he is doing something wrong and should try to escape or avoid these painful moments.

The escape behaviors, which a stutterer uses to free himself from his stutters, are present in the beginning stutterer, but they are far more frequent in the intermediate stutterer. They are often more complex, too. An intermediate stutterer may blink his eyes and nod his head in an effort to escape a block. Sometimes, he may do both, and if he is still unable to say the word, he may resort to yet another device, such as slapping his leg. As these patterns grow more complex, they also may become disguised to look like natural movements and are performed more rapidly.

In addition to escape behaviors, the intermediate stutterer uses both word and situation avoidances, as previously mentioned. Word avoidances develop after a child has had repeated difficulty with a particular word or sound and discovers how to take evasive action before he has to say it. For example, a young stutterer in our clinic was once asked his name by a particularly stern nun. He blocked severely on it and subsequently became fearful of saying his name, as well as other words starting with the same sound. He could usually think up synonyms for other words but found it awkward to substitute a word for his name. He then learned to get a running start on his name by beginning with "My name is . . . " whenever he was asked his name. This permitted him to avoid stuttering about half of the time. It is a subtle form of avoidance that many clinicians call a "starter." More obvious examples of avoidances are given in the following text.

Van Riper (1982) cataloged many word avoidance techniques used by stutterers. His list includes *substitutions* (substituting one word or phrase for another when stuttering is expected, as in "he's my u-u-u . . . my father's brother"), *circumlocutions* (talking all around a word or phrase when stuttering is expected, as in "well, I went to . . . yes, I really had a good time there, I saw the Empire State Building."), *postponements* (waiting for a few beats or putting in filler words before starting a word on which stuttering is expected, as in "My name is. . . . . .Bill") and *anti-expectancy devices* (using an odd manner or funny voice to avoid stuttering when it is anticipated). Like escape behaviors, these word avoidance techniques often become more rapid and more subtle with time. A clever stutterer can disguise his word avoidances to look like normal behavior. For example, he may put on a pensive expression and appear to search for a word while he postpones the attempt to say a feared sound. Experienced clinicians learn to pick up subtle cues in the rate and manner of speaking that tip them off to the use of such avoidances.

Situation fears and avoidances are also beginning to appear in the intermediate stutterer. Past stuttering in specific places or with specific people are the seeds from which situation fears grow. In school, stutterers usually have more trouble reading aloud or giving oral reports. Most stutterers (and many nonstutterers) have dreaded those classes in which the teacher calls on students by going up and down the rows. As in our earlier example, a stutterer's fear steadily mounts as a teacher goes down the row, getting closer and closer to him. Then, if he's called on, he may take a failing grade rather than give his oral report. In contrast, other situations in school, especially casual ones like gym class or lunch period, are likely to hold little fear and expectation of stuttering for him.

Situation fears quickly generate situation avoidance. The student who fears giving answers in class may try to slouch low in his seat in hopes of being overlooked. A stutterer who is afraid of making introductions will contrive to let other people handle them. As a teenager, the author coped with his fear of ordering in restaurants by ducking into the bathroom when the waitress arrived, leaving friends to order for him. Every stutterer has his own pattern of situation avoidances, which may provide an important focus for therapy in many cases.

Feelings and Attitudes

The youngster with intermediate stuttering has gone well beyond the momentary frustration and mild embarrassment observed in those with beginning stuttering. He has felt the helplessness of being caught in many blocks and runaway repetitions. The anticipation of stuttering and the subsequent listener penalty have been fulfilled many times. These experiences pile up like cars in a demolition derby to create an entanglement of fear, embarrassment, and shame that accompanies moments of stuttering. These feelings may not be pervasive or dog the stutterer all the time. But stuttering has now changed from an annoyance to a serious problem.

The intermediate stutterer shows his increasingly negative feelings about stuttering in many ways. He looks away from a listener during stutters and flushes with embarrassment afterward. He becomes stiff and uneasy at the prospect of speaking. His stuttering pattern includes an increasing number of avoidance devices, and he is beginning to evade situations in which he may stutter. These are all signs that his feelings and attitudes are becoming pervaded by fear.

Table 5.6 gives the characteristics of intermediate stutterers.

Underlying Processes

Many of the intermediate stutterer's symptoms result from the same processes that underlie those of beginning stutterers. However, there are major differences. In the intermediate stutterer, the classically conditioned tension response is more evident, conditioned frustration is becoming a more intense fear reaction, and avoidance conditioning has become a factor in shaping stuttering behaviors.

Avoidance conditioning transforms *escape* behaviors, such as the use of "um" to escape from a stuttering block, into *avoidances*, such as saying "um" before saying a word on which stuttering is expected. This learning process also leads the individual with in-

---

Table 5.6. Characteristics of Intermediate Stutterers

1. Most frequent core behaviors are blocks in which the stutterer shuts off sound or voice. He may also have repetitions and prolongations.
2. Stutterer uses escape behaviors to terminate blocks.
3. Stutterer appears to anticipate blocks, often uses avoidance behaviors prior to feared words. He also anticipates difficult situations and sometimes avoids them.
4. Fear before stuttering, embarrassment during stuttering, and shame after stuttering characterize this level, especially fear.

termediate stuttering to avoid words, to change sentences around, and to avoid speaking situations entirely. Avoidance learning generalizes from one word to another, from one situation to another.

Summary

The intermediate level of stuttering is characterized by increasingly tense blocks, repetitions, and prolongations. This increased tension results from feelings of frustration, fear, and helplessness. These feelings trigger tension responses, which interfere with fluency and, in turn, produce more frustration, fear, and feelings of helplessness. As tension mounts, this vicious cycle continues: blocks are longer and more noticeable, more listeners react with surprise and impatience, and the stutterer's fear increases in response to these reactions.

These negative feelings spur stutterers to use various devices to escape from blocks. Instrumental conditioning increases the frequency of escape behaviors. Classical conditioning generalizes the conditioned anticipation of stuttering to specific sounds, words, and situations. These anticipations give rise to both word and situation avoidance behaviors.

ADVANCED STUTTERING

The last developmental/treatment level, advanced stuttering, is characterized more by the age of the stutterer than by differences in stuttering pattern or underlying processes. The advanced level comprises older adolescents and adults (Fig. 5.5). Treatment at this level is unique because the client can take much of the responsibility for therapy, including substantial work outside the clinic.

An advanced stutterer's increased capability in therapy may compensate for another characteristic of this level, a long history of stuttering. The advanced stutterer's pattern is highly overlearned because of this history and therefore more difficult to change. The advanced stutterer's self-image is also a consideration. After many years, an adult who stutters increasingly thinks of himself as a stutterer, rather than as someone who has occasional difficulty speaking. Except for a few safe situations, in which he may be relatively fluent, most speaking situations hold some fear for him, and he shapes his life accordingly. His friends, his social activities, and his job are often influenced by his view of him-

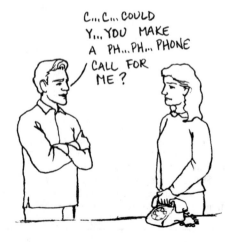

Figure 5.5. Individual who may be an advanced stutterer.

self as a stutterer. He may believe that his stuttering is as noticeable to others as having two heads, and just as unacceptable.

Core Behaviors

Core behaviors in advanced stuttering are typically blocks—stoppages of airflow or phonation or both. These behaviors may be longer and more struggled in an advanced stutterer than in the intermediate stutterer, but they are essentially the same. Because blocks are longer, tremors of lips, jaw, or tongue may be more apparent.

Some advanced stutterers' blocks are hardly evident at all. These stutterers have honed their avoidance devices to such a fine edge that core behaviors are scarcely noticeable. If stuttering does become evident, it usually devastates them. Consequently, much of their energy is spent anticipating blocks that don't occur and mustering avoidances to keep anxiety at bay. One such individual, a delightful woman named Lenore whom the author knew, said she had stuttered since childhood. Yet, she almost never had a repetition, prolongation, or block that we could see. She was highly competent at everything she did, but limited her life severely because of fear that she would stutter.

Individuals with advanced stuttering, like those at the intermediate level, have repetitions as well as blocks. These are not the easy, regular repetitions of borderline stuttering, but are more like those of beginning stuttering: tense, with a rapid, irregular tempo. They may be repetitions of syllables, li-li-li-like this, or mixed with fixed articulatory postures of tense blocks, l. . . . l. . . . .li-li-li. . . . like this. The latter look as if the speaker recoils from a momentary fixation and then gets stuck again.

Secondary Behaviors

Advanced stuttering has many of the same word and situation avoidances of intermediate stuttering, but the avoidances are likely to be more extensive. Some behaviors are more obvious than others. There may be several attempted word-avoidance devices (such as "uh . . . well . . . you see," and a gasp of air) followed by a block of long duration that is filled with unsuccessful escape attempts before, finally, a release showing great effort. Others approach feared words cautiously and use subtle mannerisms, such as appearing to think just before saying them, so that most listeners wouldn't realize they were stuttering.[7] These stutterers are usually on guard much of the time, scanning ahead with their verbal early-warning systems.

Many advanced stutterers also control their environments carefully so that they can avoid situations in which they are likely to stutter. They may feign sickness when they have to give a speech, use answering machines rather than answering the telephone, or arrange to have their spouses or children deal with store clerks.

Often, with careful questioning of these advanced stutterers who use avoidance a great deal, we can learn what occurs when avoidances don't work. Even the most skillful avoiders are sometimes caught with their defenses down and become stuck in block. Core behaviors may also be elicited by asking some stutterers to stutter openly, without using secondary behaviors. Stutterers who can do this, especially those who can do this without excessive discomfort, are more amenable to change.

---

[7] Several well-known television and radio personalities fit into this pattern, using bizarre speaking styles to avoid stuttering. The next time you see or hear someone in the media with an odd manner of speaking, consider whether he or she might be a successful avoider.

Feelings and Attitudes

The feelings and attitudes of an advanced stutterer, like his stuttering pattern, have been shaped by years of conditioning. Over and over, the stutterer has learned that much of his stuttering is unpredictable. When it is predictable, it comes when he wants it least—when he wants more than anything to be fluent. As a result, he often feels out of control. Figure 5.6 reflects one individual's depictions of his own feelings of being out of control when stuttering.

These uncomfortable internal feelings are confirmed by the stutterer's perception of how others see him. Listeners' reactions look overwhelmingly negative to him. Even

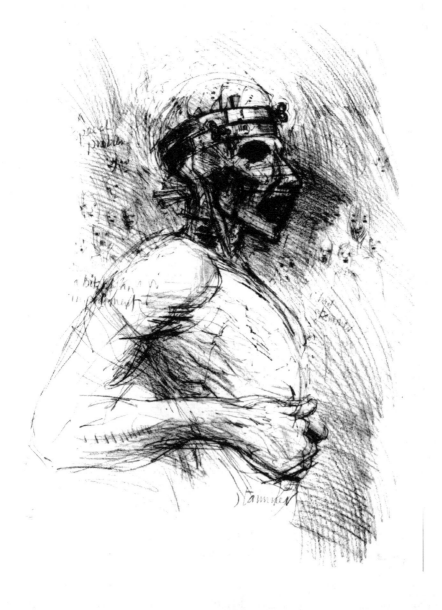

Figure 5.6. "How I feel when I stutter" by Mike Peace. (Courtesy of Dr. Trudy Stewart.)

when listeners say nothing, their faces say everything. It is as though stuttering is a rattletrap car that always stalls in heavy traffic amid honking drivers. Such experiences gradually shape an advanced stutterer's attitudes toward feelings of helplessness, frustration, anger, and hopelessness.

Of course, individual responses to stuttering vary greatly. If the person who stutters has many talents and abilities for which he is recognized and has an assertive personality, he may be less devastated by stuttering. But if he has many other problems and a highly sensitive nature, his feelings and attitudes about stuttering may be an important component of his problem.

The point is that by the time a stutterer is an adult, he has had years of experiencing stuttering, feeling frustrated and helpless, and developing techniques to minimize pain. Unless he has strong attributes to compensate, he will likely feel that stuttering is a big part of whom he presents to other people. It is a part that he hates, a part on which he blames many other troubles and a part he wants to eliminate.

On the other hand, some stutterers who have reached the advanced level have become reconciled to their handicap. If they are in their 20s or 30s or beyond, there may be some natural resistance to treatment because stuttering has become part of their identity. After years of doubt and turmoil, they've grown accustomed to themselves as stutterers. To contemplate treatment is to reject themselves, to open old wounds. Those who risk change, enter treatment, and succeed will find the risk to have been worthwhile. But those who enter treatment and fail may suffer twice, from the pain of failure as well as the loss of what had been gained before but was given up.

Table 5.7 lists the major characteristics of advanced stutterers.

Underlying Processes

In advanced stuttering, unlike in the lower levels of stuttering, the original constitutional, developmental, and environmental factors are minimally influential. The effects of home environment, developmental pressures of speech and language, and maybe even some differences in central nervous system function have been diminished by maturation and learning. However, conditioned habits that are learned in response to these early factors are stronger than ever. Their effects have been magnified by years of experience. Moreover, a stutterer's characteristic patterns of tension, escape behaviors, and word and situation avoidance have become almost automatic through years of practice. For example, he may have a string of avoidance and escape behaviors, but he only remembers that "the word got stuck."

The advanced stutterer's disorder is affected by cognitive learning as well. He has developed a self-concept as an impaired speaker, and this carries, for most, highly negative connotations. Self-concepts begin to be formed in preschool years and initially are based on a picture of what one can do, rather than what one is (Clarke-Stewart & Friedman,

Table 5.7. Characteristics of Advanced Stutterers

1. Most frequent core behaviors are longer, tense blocks, often with tremors of lips, tongue, or jaw. Individual will also probably have repetitions and prolongations.
2. Stuttering may be suppressed in some individuals through extensive avoidance behaviors.
3. Complex patterns of avoidance and escape behaviors characterize the stutterer. These may be very rapid and so well habituated that the stutterer may not be aware of what he does.
4. Emotions of fear, embarrassment, and shame are very strong. Stutterer has negative feelings about himself as a person who is helpless and inept when he stutters. This self-concept may be pervasive.

1987). More enduring traits are added as a result of social interactions in later childhood, adolescence, and beyond (Roessler & Bolton, 1978). Therefore, a stutterer's self-concept at the earliest levels of development is determined in part by his perception of how he talks. It may be a fleeting notion, not necessarily negative, that sometimes he has difficulty talking. At later levels of development, the reactions of significant listeners—parents, peer group, other adults—have a major impact. Now his self-concept may become filled with relatively enduring negative features as a result of listeners' impatience and rejection. A negative self-concept is formed not only by perceptions of listeners' reactions, it also in turn affects those perceptions.

Researchers studying the psychology of disability suggest that "one's perception of self influences one's perception of others' views of oneself, rendering social interaction more difficult" (Roessler & Bolton, 1978). Applied to an advanced stutterer, this suggests that he is likely to project his own rejection of his stuttering onto his listeners, thereby inhibiting his interactions with them. This vicious cycle can only be stopped when an outsider helps a stutterer test the reality of his perceptions.

In addition to working on cognitive aspects of the problem, therapy for the advanced stutterer also deals directly with avoidances he has learned so well. As mentioned in the discussion of intermediate stuttering, as avoidance conditioning progresses, the stutterer fears not only words and situations, but also stuttering itself. To decondition this fear and change such responses, treatment enables a stutterer to stutter with less fear by associating the clinician's approval with a calmer, more relaxed form of stuttering. Gradually, tension and hurry fade from his disfluencies, and he feels more in control. Consequently, his fear diminishes even further.

Summary

The diagnosis of advanced stuttering characterizes a developmental level and implies a particular treatment orientation. Treatment may be easier because the stutterer can assume much of the responsibility for generalization beyond the clinic. On the other hand, treatment is more challenging because the stutterer's patterns are more thoroughly learned than at earlier levels. The advanced stutterer's core behaviors often consist of long blocks with considerable tension and sometimes visible tremors. Secondary behaviors may consist of long chains of word avoidance and escape behaviors. Situation avoidance is common.

Some advanced stutterers may hide and disguise their stuttering well enough to avoid detection by many listeners, but this is at a cost of constant vigilance. Feelings of frustration and helplessness usually accumulate over the years, leading to coping behaviors and a lifestyle that may be highly constraining. Such responses create a self-concept of an inept speaker whose stuttering is unacceptable to listeners. This, in turn, affects the stutterer's perceptions of the listener's reactions.

OVERALL SUMMARY

Table 5.8 summarizes the characteristics of the five developmental/treatment levels described in this chapter. Each individual who stutters will have his own course of development, influenced by the interaction of constitutional and environmental factors. The clinician needs to use her understanding of the underlying processes to design procedures to treat each individual's core behaviors, secondary behaviors, and feelings and attitudes.

Table 5.8. Characteristics of Five Developmental/Treatment Levels

Developmental/ Treatment Level	Core Behaviors	Secondary Behaviors	Feelings and Attitudes	Underlying Processes
Normal disfluency	10 or fewer disfluencies per 100 words; one-unit repetitions; mostly repetitions, interjections, and revisions	None	Not aware, no concern	Stresses of speech/language and psychosocial development
Borderline stuttering	11 or more disfluencies per 100 words; more than 2 units in repetitions; more repetitions and prolongations than revisions or interjections	None	Generally not aware; may occasionally show momentary surprise or mild frustration	Stresses of speech/language and psychosocial development interacting with constitutional predisposition
Beginning stuttering	Rapid, irregular, and tense repetitions may have fixed articulatory posture in blocks	Escape behaviors, such as eye blinks, increases in pitch, or loudness as disfluency progresses	Aware of disfluency, may express frustration	Conditioned emotional reactions causing excess tension; instrumental conditioning resulting in escape behaviors
Intermediate stuttering	Blocks in which sound and airflow are shut off	Escape and avoidance behaviors	Fear, frustration, embarrassment, and shame	Above processes, plus avoidance conditioning
Advanced stuttering	Long tense blocks; some with tremor	Escape and avoidance behaviors	Fear, frustration, embarrassment, and shame; negative self-concept	Above processes, plus cognitive learning

STUDY QUESTIONS

1. Name the five developmental and treatment levels of stuttering and give their associated age ranges.
2. What is the difference between core behaviors and secondary behaviors?
3. Name five types of normal disfluency and give an example of each.
4. At what ages is normal disfluency likely to be most frequent?
5. Name three influences that may cause normal disfluency to increase.
6. What are three ways in which core behaviors of normal disfluency differ from those of borderline stuttering?
7. Describe the core behaviors of the beginning stutterer.
8. What causes the beginning stutterer's increase in tension in his disfluencies?
9. Describe why an escape behavior is used by a stutterer. Give examples.
10. Give an example of a stutterer's (a) word avoidance, (b) situation avoidance.
11. What is the major secondary behavior that differentiates the intermediate from the beginning stutterer?
12. Compare the feelings and attitudes of the borderline, beginning, and intermediate stutterer.
13. Why might the treatment of the advanced stutterer be different from that of the intermediate stutterer?
14. Describe the role of the listener in the development of the advanced stutterer's self-concept.

SUGGESTED READINGS

Bloodstein, O. (1995). Symptomatology. In *A handbook on stuttering*. San Diego: Singular Publishing Group, Inc.

The subsection titled, "Developmental changes in stuttering" in this chapter describe four stages similar to our levels of stuttering development. Other schemas of developmental changes are also discussed in a clear and logical style.

Gray, J.A. (1987). *The psychology of fear and stress*. Cambridge, UK: Cambridge University Press.

This is a very readable exposition of relatively recent findings about innate fears, conditioning, and brain processes involved with escape and avoidance learning. Gray also describes his concept of the "behavioral inhibition system," a model of the role of conditioning, language, the limbic system, and anxiety on behavior.

Luper, H.L., & Mulder, R.L. (1964). *Stuttering: Therapy for children*. Englewood Cliffs, NJ: Prentice-Hall.

An excellent treatment text that describes four developmental levels of stuttering similar to our own. Although out of print, this book is available at most university libraries.

Starkweather, C.W. (1983). *Speech and language: Principles and processes of behavior change*. Englewood Cliffs, NJ: Prentice-Hall.

This book describes the principles of instrumental, classical, and avoidance conditioning that underlie much of stuttering behavior. It gives a clear account of how these principles create stuttering behavior and how conditioning is used in treatment.

Van Riper, C. (1982). *The development of stuttering.* **In** *The nature of stuttering.* **Englewood Cliffs, NJ: Prentice-Hall.**

In this chapter, Van Riper describes four developmental tracks of stuttering, three of which depart substantially from our stages of stuttering development. This chapter will give the reader a good sense of individual variability in stuttering.

Assessment and Treatment of Stuttering

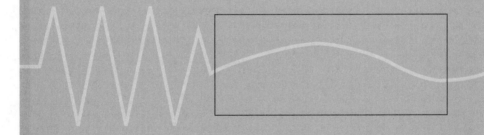

Treatment Considerations

We believe there are a number of issues the clinician needs to consider and resolve before initiating an assessment or treatment program for a person who stutters. The positions the clinician takes on these matters will guide her clinical judgment and behavior. What she believes will determine not only assessment procedures, but also long-term treatment goals and daily clinical procedures with the client.

The first issue is a clinician's beliefs about the causes and development of stuttering. Assessment strategies and therapy goals and procedures should be compatible with beliefs about the nature of stuttering.

Second, there are a number of important questions related to therapy goals that the clinician will need to consider. These include (*a*) What are the appropriate speech behaviors to target in therapy? (*b*) What are realistic fluency goals for the client? (*c*) How much attention should be given to the client's feelings and attitudes about speech? (*d*) What procedures or strategies are needed to help the client maintain his improvement? (*e*) What should be done about any concomitant speech and language problems the client has?

Finally, the clinician needs to consider the methods to be used with the client. For example, will therapy be characterized by behavior modification with its emphasis on instrumental or operant conditioning and programmed instruction principles, or will it be more loosely structured, focused on helping the client reduce struggle behaviors, while confronting his fears?

These issues are not independent of each other. The clinician's view on one influences her position on another. Nevertheless, we think it is important to discuss each of these issues separately. We outline these issues below and give our point of view. In the next eight chapters, we expand on these issues as we discuss assessment and treatment procedures.

CLINICIAN'S BELIEFS

We believe it is important for clinicians to weigh their beliefs about the nature of stuttering against the available data, then develop clinical procedures compatible with those beliefs. Our beliefs about the etiology and development of stuttering, presented in Section I, are reviewed here only in enough detail to illustrate how a clinician's theoretical view affects clinical decisions. As you may recall, we believe that predisposing physiological factors interact with developmental and environmental influences to produce or exacerbate core behaviors, which often, but not always, begin as repetitions. When the child responds to these early disfluencies with increased tension and hurry, various secondary or coping behaviors and negative feelings and attitudes are learned. Escape behaviors are learned through instrumental conditioning; speech fears are classically conditioned. Word and situation avoidances are acquired through avoidance conditioning. All of these etiological and developmental factors and their contributions to stuttering are reflected in the developmental/treatment levels described in the preceding chapter.

How does this point of view about the etiology and development of stuttering affect our clinical behavior? Let us use the treatment of school-age children who stutter to demonstrate this point. First, a child's therapy is determined by the developmental/treatment level of the child's stuttering. Therapy for each level is different. For example, we believe a second-grade beginning stutterer who is not embarrassed or afraid to talk and who is not avoiding talking should be managed differently from a fifth-grade intermediate stutterer who is beginning to develop fear and avoidance behaviors relative to his speech. Thus, knowing the child's developmental/treatment level is essential to making appropriate therapy decisions.

In discussing our developmental/treatment levels, we begin with the treatment of the advanced stutterer because stuttering modification and fluency shaping therapies are most dissimilar at this level. This will enable you to better appreciate the differences between these two major therapy approaches. Then, as we progress through treatment for intermediate, beginning, and borderline levels of stuttering, the increasing similarities of approaches will be evident. It will become clear that when stuttering behaviors are less complex and emotions play a smaller part, stuttering modification and fluency shaping approaches handle the problem in similar ways.

A second way in which our beliefs about the etiology and development of stuttering affect our clinical behavior involves our assessment procedures. Because identifying the child's developmental/treatment level is important, it is necessary that the assessment procedures provide the clinician with information essential for determining a child's treatment level. For example, for the second-grader with beginning stuttering and the fifth-grader with intermediate stuttering, it would be necessary to evaluate each child's feelings and attitudes about his speech, as well as his use of word and situation avoidances, to accurately diagnose each child's developmental/treatment level, as well as to decide which aspects of the problem to focus on first.

A third way in which our theoretical position on stuttering influences our clinical behavior is counseling the parents of these two school-age stutterers. We would discuss with each set of parents the importance of factors in the environment that could be contributing to his stuttering problem and discuss ways of modifying these factors. We would also discuss possible predisposing constitutional or physiological factors that could be contributing to their child's stuttering. It is important to let them know that they didn't cause their child's stuttering, but that they can do much to help him overcome it. These, then, are some of the ways our beliefs about the nature of stuttering influence our work with stutterers and their families. There are many others, which we discuss in subsequent chapters. We also point out how other clinicians' beliefs influence their therapies; however, the latter examples should be enough to illustrate how a clinician's views on stuttering can influence her work with clients.

SPEECH BEHAVIORS TARGETED FOR THERAPY

Which speech behaviors should be targeted for therapy? Should the clinician work directly on the client's stuttering in an effort to modify or reduce its severity, or should some other aspect of the stutterer's speech behavior be targeted, such as reducing his rate of speech? There has been considerable controversy relative to this topic for a number of years. For example, Hugo Gregory (1979) in his book, *Controversies about Stuttering Therapy,* grouped therapies for the advanced stutterer into two general approaches, the "stutter more fluently" and the "speak more fluently" approach. The "stutter more fluently" approach is based on the premise that a stutterer should first study and become familiar with his stuttering and then learn to modify it by stuttering more easily. The stutterer should also reduce his avoidance behavior. The "speak more fluently" approach involves replacing stuttering with fluent speech. To do this, various procedures are used to establish a form of controlled fluency, and then features of this initial fluency are gradually modified to obtain speech that sounds normal.

Richard Curlee and William Perkins (1984) also grouped current therapies into two approaches similar to Gregory's. They referred to the two approaches as "those that manage stuttering" and "those that manage fluency." The former group focuses on techniques to help the stutterer stutter more fluently and with less effort, whereas the latter group emphasizes teaching the stutterer how to talk more fluently. Curlee and Perkins also observed some other philosophical differences between these two approaches. Many clinicians who favor managing fluency also advocate applying behavior modification principles in their therapy. Generally, this has not been true for those clinicians who support managing stuttering. The recent revision of Curlee and Perkins' book (Curlee & Siegel, 1997) suggests, in its organization of therapy chapters, that clinicians working with adults are still divided into those who modify stuttering and those who teach a fluent speech pattern.

In an earlier publication (Guitar & Peters, 1980), we attempted to bridge the gap between these two approaches. We discussed their similarities and differences and attempted to integrate them. We referred to the two approaches as "stuttering modification therapy" and "fluency shaping therapy." We stated that, in addition to targeting different speech behaviors in therapy, these two approaches often differ in their fluency goals, attention given to feelings and attitudes, maintenance procedures, and clinical methods. In the following pages, we outline how stuttering modification therapy and fluency shaping therapy often differ on these five clinical issues and give our point of view on each.

Stuttering Modification Therapy

We described stuttering modification therapy as helping a stutterer learn to modify his moments of stuttering (Fig. 6.1). This can be done in a variety of ways. For example, the clinician can teach the client to reduce the tension and hurry in his stuttering and learn to stutter in a more relaxed, easy, and open manner. A good example of this type of therapy is Charles Van Riper's (1973) therapy for the advanced stutterer. In this therapy, Van Riper teaches the stutterer to stutter more fluently by using cancellations, pull-outs, and preparatory sets. In using these techniques, the advanced stutterer is not taught to speak normally; rather, he is taught to stutter in a more fluent, less abnormal manner. In our opinion, other proponents of stuttering modification therapy include Richard Boehmler, Edward Conture, Carl Dell, David Prins, and Joseph and Vivian Sheehan. This list is not exhaustive, but we believe these clinicians' therapies are clearly representative of stuttering modification therapy.[1] We refer to the writings of these clinicians in subsequent chapters.

Fluency Shaping Therapy

Whereas the goal of stuttering modification therapy is to modify the moments of stuttering, the goal of fluency shaping therapy is to systematically increase stutter-free speech until it replaces the moments of stuttering. This fluency is first established in the clinical setting, then is generalized to the person's daily speaking environment. Fluency shaping clinicians usually use one of two approaches or a combination of each to establish fluency in the clinic. In one approach, a basal level of fluency is established by having the stutterer produce short fluent responses, such as single words or simple phrases. These short fluent responses are reinforced, and any stuttering may be punished. The length and spontaneity of the client's responses are then systematically increased until fluent conversational speech is achieved in the clinical environment. In the second approach, the clinician helps the stutterer to establish fluency by altering his speech pattern (Fig. 6.2). For example, this may involve having him speak at a substantially slower rate; this slow, fluent pattern is then gradually modified to approximate normal-sounding speech.

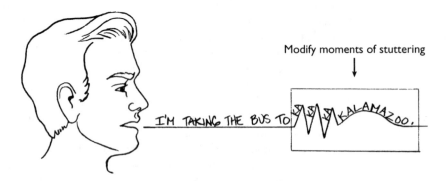

Figure 6.1. Stuttering modification therapy.

---

[1] In choosing these clinicians to illustrate stuttering modification therapy, we attempted to select those clinicians whose therapies are clear examples of this approach, just as we did in selecting clinicians to illustrate fluency shaping therapy and the integration of the two approaches. In doing so, we did not include some well-known clinicians whose therapies do not fit as well within any of the above three approaches to treatment. An example of this latter situation is Gene Brutten's two-factor behavior therapy (1970, 1975).

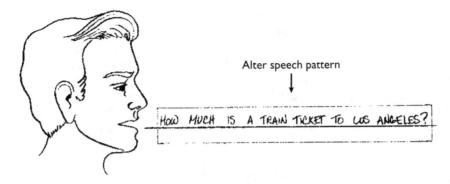

Figure 6.2. Fluency shaping therapy.

Regardless of which approach is used to establish fluency in the clinic, once it has been established, treatment focuses on generalizing fluency to the stutterer's daily speaking environment.

One writer whose therapy is representative of fluency shaping therapy is Bruce Ryan (1974). Ryan has described a number of programs for increasing or establishing fluent speech in the clinical setting. One of these is the Delayed Auditory Feedback (DAF) Program. In a DAF program, a delayed auditory feedback device helps the client to speak in a slow, prolonged, fluent manner. The delay times on the delayed auditory feedback machine are systematically reduced, which allows the client to gradually reduce his prolongation of speech sounds until his speaking rate approaches normal. He is then taken off DAF, and new fluency is gradually transferred to everyday speaking situations. In this DAF program, a person who stutters is not taught to stutter more easily; rather, fluency is first established in the therapy sessions and then transferred to the client's daily speaking environment. Other advocates of fluency shaping therapy include Martin Adams, Einer Boberg, Janis Costello Ingham, George Shames and Cheri Florance, Mark Onslow, Richard Shine, and Ronald Webster. Again, this list is not exhaustive, but we believe these clinicians' therapies are clear examples of fluency shaping therapy. In the following chapters, we refer to the therapies of these clinicians as well as our own.

Integration of Approaches

In later chapters of this book, stuttering modification and fluency shaping approaches are described in more detail for each of the developmental/treatment levels of stuttering. Many clinicians believe they need to use one approach or the other because the two approaches appear to be incompatible, even though choosing one over the other may be difficult or confusing. Fortunately, the two approaches need not be antagonistic. In fact, techniques based on one approach can be helpful to clinicians using the other approach. One of the prime goals in writing this book is to demonstrate how stuttering modification therapy and fluency shaping therapy can be integrated. Consequently, the following chapters provide many examples of ways that clinicians can combine aspects of both approaches into an integrated approach. In addition to discussing our own clinical procedures in detail, we also review the therapies of Hugo Gregory and his colleagues Diane Hill and June Campbell, C. Woodruff Starkweather, and Meryl Wall and Florence Myers. They are not the only clinicians who integrate these two approaches, but we believe they provide clear examples. For now, we outline our position on the speech behaviors that should be targeted for therapy.

We believe it can be beneficial for those with advanced stuttering to learn to stutter more easily on given moments of stuttering, as well as to learn to modify certain aspects of their overall speaking pattern, such as rate of speech, to enhance fluency. We believe these two skills are not incompatible, but in fact, can complement one another. We also believe this is true for most intermediate stutterers. For borderline and beginning stutterers, we believe that the issue of which speech behaviors to target in therapy is less critical because the differences between stuttering modification and fluency shaping therapies are less pronounced. In-depth discussions of these viewpoints are presented in the chapters on treatment.

FLUENCY GOALS

Dimensions of Fluency

What are realistic therapy goals for persons who stutter? Before responding, let's take a closer look at fluency. Starkweather (1985, 1987) suggests that speech fluency has four basic dimensions: (*a*) the continuity of speech, (*b*) the rate of speech, (*c*) the rhythm of speech, and (*d*) the effort with which speech is produced (Fig. 6.3). We examine each dimension more closely below from a clinical management point of view.

CONTINUITY

By continuity, Starkweather means the smoothness of speech versus the extent to which speech may be broken up by disfluencies. In terms of clinical management, we are interested in reducing the number of part-word and monosyllabic word repetitions, prolongations, and blocks that occur in a client's speech. Documenting therapy goals often includes assessing the frequency of stutterings remaining in a client's speech at the end of therapy. After all, most clients' complaints center on their disfluencies.

RATE

Fluency consists of more than just the absence of disfluencies; fluent speech is also rapid. Thus, we need to be concerned about clients' speech rates. This is particularly true when rate control strategies are used in therapy to eliminate or significantly reduce the number of disfluencies. For example, one technique commonly used in fluency shaping therapy teaches a person who stutters to slow speech rate by prolonging each syllable as he talks. This will reduce the number of disfluencies; but unless the stutterer is also taught

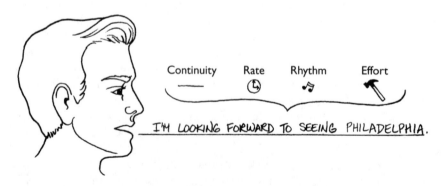

Figure 6.3. Dimensions of fluency.

how to use this technique while still approximating a normal speaking rate, our experience suggests that he will not use it in everyday speaking situations. Clients want to sound normal in this regard, too.

A few individuals who stutter speak quite rapidly before treatment and may continue to do so afterward. This may not only contribute to their disfluency but at times may make their speech difficult to understand. Therapy with these individuals may need to include work on a more normal rate of speech, slower than they are used to talking.

RHYTHM

Rhythm is a third dimension of fluency and is related to the stress patterns of speech. For a client's speech to sound normal at the end of therapy, it is important that he use normal stress patterns. He should not sound monotonous or be giving each syllable equal stress. Monotonous-sounding speech can be a by-product of fluency shaping programs that instruct clients to slow their speech by prolonging each syllable. We have also heard this quality in the speech of stutterers who have been treated in stuttering modification programs. It is important that a client's speech not sound monotonous at the end of therapy; both the stutterer and his listener will object to it. Furthermore, many stutterers will not use monotonous-sounding fluency in everyday speaking situations. They would rather stutter and be spontaneous.

EFFORT

The last dimension of fluency is effort. Starkweather observes that effort includes both physical and mental effort. We think that mental effort is more significant clinically. Normally, fluent speech is spontaneous; it does not require the constant monitoring to sound normal. The speaker pays attention to his ideas; he does not pay attention to the act of speaking. When speech is closely monitored, it is not normal. Normal speakers do not constantly monitor their speech, and stutterers do not like to constantly monitor their speech either. It requires too much effort. In our experience, people who stutter are not pleased in the long run if they have to constantly monitor their speech, whether they have been treated by stuttering modification or fluency shaping.

Speech Naturalness

A more overreaching treatment goal than the four dimensions of fluency just described is to have speech that sounds natural to both the speaker and his listeners. In recent years, clinical scientists have been concerned that treatments that produce fluency do not always result in natural-sounding speech. As Schiavetti and Metz (1997) warned, "Some stutterers may reduce their number of stutters at the expense of a speech pattern that is stutter free but not really fluent." Thus, some stuttering treatments may get rid of stuttering, but leave an individual with speech that sounds odd, unusual, or unnatural. Martin, Haroldson, and Triden (1984), one of the first investigative teams to report on this problem, found that unsophisticated listeners rated the stutter-free speech of individuals who stutter speaking under DAF as significantly more unnatural than the speech of nonstutterers. Ingham, Gow, and Costello (1985) used the same rating scale and found that the fluent speech of treated stutterers were judged to have more unnatural speech than nonstutterers. Both investigations used a nine-point, equal-appearing intervals scale to rate speakers based on judges' intuitive sense of what sounded "natural." The judges used in these and most subsequent studies showed satisfactory levels of interrater reliability and agreement, although individual rater reliability was only marginally satisfactory.

Clinically, we must be sure that clients sound as natural as possible after treatment. Otherwise, they are likely to abandon their fluency skills because of their own and their listeners' negative reactions, in favor of old, familiar stuttering patterns. Can we rate our clients' naturalness reliably? Schiavetti and Metz (1997) indicate that clinicians who have learned to become consistent raters of speech naturalness may rely on the relative values of their ratings. Thus, they can judge when one client sounds less natural than others they have treated and take appropriate steps to improve that client's naturalness before releasing him from treatment.

Effective Communication

In the early 1990s at conferences of speech-language pathologists who work with stuttering, it began to be evident that the goal of completely fluent speech was perhaps not appropriate for all people who stutter. This was particularly evident among clinicians who worked in school settings. A consensus among school clinicians in group discussions at workshops sponsored by The Stuttering Foundation of America was that many children did not achieve total fluency in the treatment setting, or if they did, they did not maintain it in the classroom or other daily situations.

The realization that many children were more fluent in the treatment setting has led clinicians to work not only on fluency skills, but also on effective communication skills that would be useful both when a person is stuttering and when he is fluent. Their goal was to help a person who stutters become able to communicate "whenever, wherever, and to whomever he or she wants" (Conture & Guitar, 1993).

Types of Fluency

Let us consider alternative fluency goals that clinicians, depending on their particular beliefs, view as successful outcomes of therapy for people who stutter. These goals are: spontaneous fluency, controlled fluency, and acceptable stuttering.

SPONTANEOUS FLUENCY

By spontaneous fluency, we are referring to the fluency of normal speakers. In terms of continuity, spontaneous fluency contains neither tension nor struggle behaviors, that is, no abnormal monosyllabic repetitions or blocks. Of course, spontaneous fluency does contain revisions, an occasional easy repetition or prolongation, and filled pauses. Its rate and rhythm are normal. With regard to the effort of speaking, spontaneous fluency is not maintained by paying attention to speech; rather, the person just talks and pays attention to his ideas.

CONTROLLED FLUENCY

Controlled fluency is similar to spontaneous fluency in terms of continuity, except that a person who stutters is monitoring and changing his manner of stuttering or speaking to maintain relatively normal-sounding speech. He may do this in a variety of ways. For example, he may use preparatory sets to modify moments of stuttering or slightly reduce speaking rate by prolonging syllables to enhance fluency. In other words, listeners, especially an experienced listener, may hear small differences in the speech of someone who stutters. The stutterer, however, will not be exhibiting noticeable moments of stuttering. It is apparent, then, that in controlled fluency, rate or rhythm or both are modified at times. On the other hand, effort is high; the stutterer must monitor his speech and modify it to maintain fluency.

ACCEPTABLE STUTTERING

The third possible outcome of therapy is acceptable stuttering. Acceptable stuttering occurs when a speaker exhibits noticeable, but not severe, disfluency and feels comfortable speaking despite it. He is not embarrassed by or fearful of his stuttering. As with controlled fluency, the individual may need to monitor his speech to maintain acceptable levels of stuttering. In this case, all four dimensions of fluency—continuity, rate, rhythm, and effort—may be adversely affected. In other cases, it is possible that a person who stutters does not need to monitor his speech to maintain acceptable stuttering. He is just talking spontaneously. In this case, effort is not significantly affected.

Stuttering Modification Therapy

We believe that advocates of stuttering modification therapy see spontaneous fluency as the ultimate goal of treatment, especially for beginning stutterers. It is less true for intermediate stutterers and much less true for advanced stutterers. If spontaneous fluency is unobtainable with the latter two groups, then most stuttering modification clinicians work for controlled fluency. If this cannot be obtained, they try for acceptable stuttering.

Fluency Shaping Therapy

Adherents of fluency shaping therapy also have spontaneous fluency as their ultimate goal for clients. If this cannot be achieved, controlled fluency becomes the goal. We believe, however, that most fluency shaping clinicians would not have acceptable stuttering as a goal for clients. It would be regarded as a failure.

Integration of Approaches

We believe that spontaneous fluency, controlled fluency, and acceptable stuttering should vary, as therapy goals, with the treatment level of a client's stuttering. Although the ultimate goal for advanced stutterers should be spontaneous fluency, most do not reach this goal on a consistent basis. They may have periods when they are spontaneously fluent. At other times, they will need to monitor their speech to use controlled fluency, or they will need to tolerate acceptable stuttering. Thus, we believe that a realistic goal for most advanced stutterers is the ability to use and be comfortable with both controlled fluency and acceptable stuttering. In other words, there will be times with friends or family when an advanced stutterer is spontaneously fluent; but at other times in more stressful situations, he will need to use controlled fluency or be willing to exhibit acceptable stuttering.

With an intermediate stutterer, that is, the child who is only beginning to avoid talking, the goal should still be spontaneous fluency. In some cases, it is more realistic to expect the outcome of therapy to be controlled fluency or, more frequently, acceptable stuttering. This is especially true as the intermediate stutterer approaches adolescence.

We try to help both intermediate and advanced stutterers accept some stuttering as a safety margin. They may be able to achieve high levels of fluency, but there is always the possibility that well-learned stuttering behaviors will reappear in times of stress. We do not want clients to be thrown for a loss by unexpected stuttering or to hold back from speaking because they feel they might stutter. In emphasizing the importance of communication over mere fluency, we are often able to help clients approach speaking situations confidently, thereby increasing the likelihood that they will succeed.

We believe, as do many others, that a realistic goal for beginning stutterers is spontaneous fluency or normal speech. Many of these children regain spontaneous fluency with a minimum of therapy. It is fortunate, both for the child and the clinician, that these young stutterers gain or regain spontaneous fluency relatively easily. Our experience suggests that it is unrealistic to expect children as young as 4 or 5 years old to carefully monitor their speech and use controlled fluency or to accept evident stuttering.

FEELINGS AND ATTITUDES

How much attention in therapy should be given to the stutterer's feelings and attitudes about his speech (Fig. 6.4)? Stuttering modification therapy and fluency shaping therapy differ substantially on this issue. This is particularly true when dealing with advanced stutterers, but less so with younger stutterers and those whose stuttering is less developed.

Stuttering Modification Therapy

Stuttering modification for an advanced stutterer places a great deal of emphasis on reducing the fear of stuttering. Much of therapy is concerned with reducing fear of stuttering and eliminating avoidance behavior associated with this fear. In addition, stuttering modification clinicians are also interested in fostering positive attitudes toward speaking. They help stutterers develop an "approach" attitude toward speaking, rather than avoidance, encouraging them to seek out speaking situations that they formerly avoided.

With younger stutterers, stuttering modification clinicians put less emphasis on modifying a child's feelings and attitudes than they do with older stutterers. As a rule, the younger the child and the less developed his stuttering, the less attention given in therapy to feelings and attitudes. This is because most stuttering modification clinicians believe that stuttering goes through stages when it persists for several years. They believe that fears, avoidances, and negative attitudes develop only after the child has been stuttering for some time and that these fears, avoidances, and negative attitudes increase in number and severity as the child matures. Thus, it makes sense to target such feelings and attitudes only when they become part of the stuttering problem.

Fluency Shaping Therapy

As a rule, most fluency shaping clinicians do not directly attempt to reduce a stutterer's fear and avoidance of words and speaking situations. This would be true for advanced

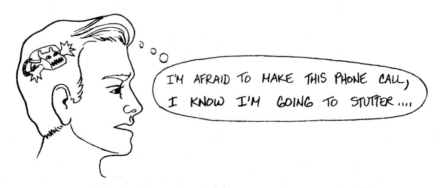

Figure 6.4. How much attention should be given to feelings and attitudes?

stutterers as well as for stutterers at lower levels. Thus, the attention given to working with the feelings and attitudes of an advanced stutterer differs substantially between fluency shaping and stuttering modification clinicians. This difference is much less pronounced in working with a borderline stutterer because neither clinician would focus directly on feelings and attitudes with very young stutterers.

Integration of Approaches

We have been strongly influenced by proponents of stuttering modification therapy on the importance of targeting feelings and attitudes in treatment. Our approach varies with the treatment level of a stuttering problem. For example, individuals with advanced stuttering exhibit chronic frustration, embarrassment, and fear associated with their stuttering. They avoid feared words and fearful speaking situations. Stuttering has become a severe handicap. Our experience has taught us that negative emotions and avoidance behaviors should receive considerable direct attention in therapy. Speech fears need to be reduced if the person who stutters is going to succeed in applying either stuttering modification techniques to reduce the severity of his stuttering or fluency shaping techniques to enhance his fluency. If a stutterer becomes too fearful in a speaking situation, the result will be excessive muscular tension in his speech mechanism. His motor control will break down, and he will not be able to alter how he produces speech.

Fears and avoidance behaviors also need to be reduced substantially if an advanced stutterer is to maintain the improvements he made during therapy. If fears and avoidances are not significantly reduced, we believe that they will become seeds for relapse, which is common among advanced stutterers.

Our approach to reducing fears and avoidances is based, in part, on principles borrowed from experimental treatments of phobias in animals, as noted in Chapter 4. In her review of animal models for behavior therapy, Mineka (1985) discussed three guidelines for successful treatment: (a) the presence of someone who is not afraid of the feared object, (b) opportunities to explore a feared object, and (c) substantial amount of time in contact with a feared object. We adapt these principles to our therapy by (a) demonstrating for the client through the use of pseudostuttering that we are not afraid of stuttering, (b) assisting and supporting the client's exploration of what he is doing when he stutters and how he feels, and (c) reinforcing the client for holding onto a stuttering block, repetition, or prolongation beyond the point when he could release it. We try to adapt these principles to each client's fears and avoidances. This is described in more detail in Chapters 9 and 11.

During treatment we try to deal with an individual's feelings by communicating our efforts to understand what those feelings are. The important element is not that we catalogue every nuance of fear and frustration, but that the client experiences our interest and ability to verbalize for him some of his fears and frustrations, which he has not been able to articulate. This ability does not develop overnight; it results from working with many clients and trying to understand what they feel when they stutter and what they think about themselves. Some clinicians feel that such sensitivity can be improved by being in psychotherapy oneself, but participating in workshops and reading about counseling and psychotherapy are also helpful. We have found the writings of Donald Winnicott and Carl Rogers to be of assistance. Some of Van Riper's writings (1973, 1975a, 1994) deal directly with the stutterer's feelings and attitudes.

Much of our approach to feelings and attitudes can be adapted to a youngster with intermediate stuttering, although he is not as affected as the advanced stutterer by years of embarrassment and fear about his speech. The intermediate stutterer does avoid some words and situations, and clinicians need to spend some time with this client, but less than with the advanced stutterer, helping the child reduce his fears and avoidances. Many intermediate stutterers benefit from a clinician's model of stuttering voluntarily without panic or avoidance. Sometimes introducing a child with intermediate stuttering to another child or adolescent who has made considerable progress in therapy is effective.

As we've noted frequently, beginning stutterers have little or no concern about their speech. They do not exhibit word or situation fears and avoidances. Accordingly, their feelings and attitudes about speech require little, if any, attention during the course of therapy. Instead, the focus of treatment is on speech behaviors, with the primary goal of increasing the child's fluency.

For children with borderline stuttering, there should be no negative feelings attached to disfluencies; however, the parents of these children may express significant concern, frustration, or guilt. If so, we need to help the parents to reduce such feelings by giving them information about stuttering, providing an understanding and supportive environment, and developing a program for them to help promote the child's fluency. We may need to work on the feelings and attitudes of parents of children with beginning and intermediate levels of stuttering as well. There are many good books and chapters to help clinicians perfect their skills in helping parents, including Luterman (1996), Curlee (1988), and Starkweather (1994).

MAINTENANCE PROCEDURES

What strategies or procedures, if any, do clinicians need to employ to help a person who stutters maintain the progress he has made during therapy? Once clients become fluent, do they automatically maintain their fluency, or do they need to work at being fluent? Stuttering differs from most other speech and language disorders in this regard. Most clients with other speech and language disorders, once they have generalized their new target behaviors to their everyday speaking environments, maintain these new behaviors with little apparent effort. This is not true with many stutterers, especially advanced stutterers, who are noted for relapsing. Beginning stutterers, on the other hand, tend to maintain fluency more readily and with much less effort.

Let's look at what stuttering modification and fluency shaping clinicians do with regard to maintenance.

Stuttering Modification Therapy

Once a child with borderline stuttering is well on his way toward normal fluency because of changes in his environment or other key modifications, the clinician's task is to continue to provide whatever support is needed. Such children often maintain normal fluency without further intervention. However, some may go through brief periods of recurrence of stuttering, often during holidays or other times of stress. Thus, clinicians should prepare the family to deal with these temporary relapses and be available for brief consultations.

Because beginning stutterers tend to regain spontaneous or normal fluency as a result of therapy, they also tend to maintain their fluency rather easily. They may have an occasional mild relapse, but it is often short-lived. At these times, most stuttering modification clinicians will bring the child back into therapy for a booster session or two, which is usually all that is needed.

With some intermediate stutterers and almost all advanced stutterers, relapse is a significant problem. Stuttering modification clinicians tend to rely on the following to combat relapse. They urge clients not to avoid words or situations. They stress the importance of keeping speech fears at minimum levels. They help clients master their stuttering modification skills more thoroughly. And they help clients assume more responsibility for their own therapy.

Fluency Shaping Therapy

The fluency shaping approach to a child with borderline stuttering is essentially the same as that used by stuttering modification clinicians. Thus, maintenance involves being available for further consultation in the unlikely event that relapse occurs. Because fluency shaping clinicians ordinarily monitor the frequency of stuttering for several months after normal fluency is achieved, they will be guided by their data to intervene earlier if stuttering returns.

Like stuttering modification clinicians, fluency shaping clinicians have few problems with beginning stutterers having relapses after they have generalized fluency to everyday speaking environments. If they do relapse, they are recycled through part of the fluency shaping program they completed earlier.

Like stuttering modification clinicians, fluency shaping clinicians find relapse to be a significant problem in their work with older stutterers. To help these clients maintain fluency, fluency shaping clinicians typically stress the importance of their clients' mastery and continuing practice of fluency enhancing skills, for example, using a slower speech rate, which they learned in their treatment program. The assumption is that, if clients thoroughly master and use these skills, they will maintain their ability to use controlled fluency. If stuttering does recur, they will be recycled through the fluency shaping program again.

Integration of Approaches

We believe that a client's developmental/treatment level should determine the procedures used to maintain his fluency. For maintaining improvement with an advanced stutterer, we rely a great deal on stuttering modification strategies. It is important for someone who stutters to keep his speech fears and avoidances at a very low level. We help him become comfortable with both controlled fluency and acceptable stuttering and encourage him to thoroughly master stuttering modification and fluency shaping techniques so that he can both modify his moments of stuttering and enhance his fluency. Finally, we help him learn to be his own clinician.

We believe that youngsters with intermediate stuttering, who are beginning to avoid talking, usually need help in maintaining improvement—whether it is spontaneous fluency, controlled fluency, or acceptable stuttering. They need to be impressed with the importance of not avoiding talking and may need continued work on desensitization of speech fears. They may also need to develop greater skill and confidence in their ability to use stuttering modification or fluency shaping techniques or both in everyday environments.

We have found that beginning stutterers generalize and maintain their fluency much more readily than do older or more developed stutterers. Thus, we believe that clinicians need only provide a setting in which a beginning stutterer can develop spontaneous fluency and then organize the conditions that will allow fluency to generalize. Maintenance usually takes care of itself. If not, a brief return to therapy may be needed.

When we work with parents of borderline stutterers, we prepare them to deal with recurrences of stuttering, which are most likely to happen during times of developmental or environmental stress.

CLINICAL APPROACH

We use clinical approach to refer to two dimensions of the therapy process: its structure and data collection. Stuttering modification therapy and fluency shaping therapy differ substantially with regard to these two aspects of therapy.

Stuttering Modification Therapy

With regard to the structure of therapy, we have observed that in stuttering modification therapy, the person who stutters and the clinician typically interact in a loosely structured manner. With adults and older children, the structure of therapy is characterized by a teaching/counseling interaction. With the younger child, the context of treatment is often in play.

In terms of the second dimension of the therapy process, stuttering modification clinicians traditionally have not put much emphasis on the collecting and reporting of objective data, for example, the frequency of stuttering before and after therapy. It is not that they are not interested in a client's progress; rather, they consider both their and the client's global descriptions and impressions of progress as more valid than rates of stuttering made in the treatment environment.

Fluency Shaping Therapy

In contrast, fluency shaping therapy is usually performed in a highly structured manner. With their roots in operant conditioning and programmed instruction, fluency shaping clinicians put a great deal of emphasis on behavioral objectives and sequencing antecedent events, responses, and consequent events in a series of steps. Specific instructions and materials are often prescribed. Specific responses from the client are targeted, and specific reactions to these responses are required from the clinician.

As might be anticipated from their theoretical orientation, fluency shaping clinicians put much emphasis on the collection and reporting of objective and reliable data. They regard such information as extremely important in documenting their client's progress.

Integration of Approaches

So what should clinicians do about these treatment issues? There are strong advocates of both approaches. With regard to the structure of therapy, we have used both approaches and now find ourselves borrowing from both. Sometimes we use one approach, but at other times we use the other. Often, our therapy is characterized by the loose application of programming principles. Each clinician, however, has to make up her own mind on this matter.

On the issue of data collection, we are less ambivalent. Our position has been strongly influenced by fluency shaping advocates. We believe it is important for clinicians to collect data routinely on clients so that she knows if therapy procedures are having their intended effect on clients' problems. This is a critical ingredient to effective therapy. In addition, with today's emphasis on accountability, record keeping has become more and more important for public school clinicians who must write an Individual Education Program (IEP) for each child.

We routinely obtain data before, during, and after treatment. At a minimum, we measure a client's frequency of stuttering and rate of speech. These data are always obtained from samples of a client's speech before and at the termination of treatment and are sometimes obtained in probes during a therapy session. Furthermore, we attempt to assess a client's speech at home and school. We also try to assess the client's feelings and attitudes toward his problem. More is said about these matters when we discuss assessment procedures in Chapter 7 and our clinical methods in the treatment chapters that follow.

TREATMENT OF CONCOMITANT SPEECH AND LANGUAGE PROBLEMS

As noted in our review of research in Chapter 2, children who stutter, or a substantial subgroup of these children, are described as delayed in their articulation and language development. Thus, most clinicians are likely to encounter a number of children who stutter and who also have concomitant speech and language problems. Until recently, little has been written about the clinical management of such compound problems. In the past 10 years, however, Bernstein Ratner (1995), Conture (1990), Gregory and Hill (1980), Starkweather (1997), Wall and Myers (1995), and others have discussed evaluating and treating these children. These clinicians suggest that children with moderate to severe concomitant problems should be treated for these other problems along with their stuttering. They recommend that care be given to regulating the demands placed on fluency when the child is learning to stretch his abilities in other areas. For children whose mild concomitant disorder does not seriously affect communication—a mild articulation problem, for example—we may leave that problem untreated for a while, and monitor it as we treat the child's stuttering. For still other children, with mild stuttering that appears as we are treating another disorder, we may only monitor the stuttering and leave it untreated unless it gets substantially worse. We continue to treat the concomitant disorder in ways that do not put undue stress on fluency.

In the chapters on therapy (Chapters 8 through 14), we describe our own and other clinicians' approaches to this issue. To illustrate the types of concomitant problems you may encounter, we briefly describe two children seen in our clinic and expand on these cases later.

CASE EXAMPLES

Bob, age 8, stutters at the intermediate level and has a substantial language problem involving short-term memory and narrative sequencing. When telling a story, he frequently inserts fillers in his speech, either because he is avoiding a moment of stuttering or because he has difficulty accessing the appropriate language, or both. Each therapy session focuses on both stuttering and language because we believe the problems may be interactive. The more difficulty Bob has in accessing language, the more he stutters; moreover, both his stuttering and language problems have kept him from participating in classes.

Adam, another child we worked with, had a moderately severe problem producing /r/ when we first began to work with him at age 6. We left his articulation problem untreated because he was extremely sensitive about his stuttering and we felt it was unwise to concern him with yet another problem. By the time he was 9, his articulation problem had disappeared, and he was making substantial progress with fluency.

We describe our decision making process for these and other children in the chapters to come.

SUMMARY

We have suggested that clinicians' beliefs on treatment issues affect not only their goals for clients, but also their daily clinical behaviors. Thus, it is important for clinicians to give serious thought to seven treatment issues.

The first issue is a clinician's beliefs about the onset and development of stuttering. We stress the fact that beliefs about the nature of stuttering influence clinical decisions. To illustrate this point, we described how our belief in developmental levels of stuttering significantly influences our clinical goals and procedures.

The second issue involves the speech behaviors targeted for therapy. With an advanced stutterer, we believe it is important to integrate aspects of both stuttering modification and fluency shaping therapy. This enables a person who stutters to learn to stutter with less struggle on given moments of stuttering, as well as to change certain aspects of his speech pattern to increase fluency. This integration is less critical with beginning stutterers because the differences between stuttering modification and fluency shaping therapies become less pronounced with young children.

The next issue is the type of fluency expected as a result of therapy. The three possible outcomes are spontaneous fluency, controlled fluency, and acceptable stuttering. We believe that the type of fluency expected varies with the client's developmental/treatment level. For the advanced stutterer, we believe that development of his capacity to use both controlled fluency and acceptable stuttering is the most realistic goal. With the intermediate stutterer, the goal should be spontaneous fluency, but controlled fluency, or especially acceptable stuttering, is the more realistic outcome to expect. Spontaneous fluency is a realistic expectation for borderline and beginning stutterers.

The fourth issue is the attention given to feelings and attitudes in therapy. Again, we believe this varies with treatment level. With the advanced stutterer, this dimension of therapy needs to receive considerable attention; with the intermediate stutterer, some attention should be focused on the client's feelings and attitudes. Beginning stutterers need little attention to be given to feelings and attitudes in therapy.

The next issue is the choice of procedures or strategies, if any, to help a client maintain his improvement. Older stutterers—that is, intermediate and advanced—require considerable help to keep avoidances and speech fears at a minimum and to master the stuttering modification and fluency shaping skills that allow them to modify their stuttering or improve their fluency, or both. Beginning stutterers seldom need help in maintaining the fluency they acquire in therapy.

The sixth issue deals with clinical approaches. Some clinicians prefer loosely structured therapy characterized by a teaching/counseling interaction. Others prefer a highly structured approach that emphasizes behavioral objectives and antecedent events, client responses, and consequent clinician events sequenced in a careful series of steps. Regardless of the approach, we encourage the use of data collection to document the effects of therapy.

The last issue involves treating concomitant speech and language problems in young stutterers. Several recently developed programs successfully address these needs, which we strongly support.

We return to these clinical issues again and again in subsequent chapters. Our goal is to impress upon the clinician the impact of one's clinical beliefs on one's clinical practice.

STUDY QUESTIONS

1. List the seven clinically relevant issues discussed in this chapter.
2. Give an example of how a clinician's beliefs about the nature of stuttering may influence her approach to therapy.
3. What speech behaviors are usually targeted for therapy in stuttering modification therapy? In fluency shaping therapy?
4. Define the following dimensions of fluency: continuity, rate, rhythm, and effort.
5. Define the following terms: spontaneous fluency, controlled fluency, and acceptable stuttering. Include all four dimensions of fluency in your definitions.
6. Should a clinician have the same fluency goals for a beginning stutterer as for an advanced stutterer? If not, why not?
7. How do the approaches of stuttering modification clinicians and fluency shaping clinicians differ with regard to targeting feelings and attitudes in treatment? How are they similar?
8. Why is it important for clinicians to be concerned about maintenance of fluency following treatment, especially with intermediate or advanced stutterers?
9. As a rule, how do stuttering modification clinicians and fluency shaping clinicians differ with regard to clinical methods?
10. Why is it important for a clinician to have a position with regard to the treatment of concomitant speech and language disorders in stutterers?

SUGGESTED READINGS

Gregory, H.H. (1979). Controversial issues: statement and review of the literature. In H.H. Gregory (Ed.), *Controversies about stuttering therapy* **(pp. 1–62). Baltimore: University Park Press.**

In this chapter, Gregory defines the "stutter more fluently" and the "speak more fluently" approaches to treatment. He also raises many excellent questions relevant to the evaluation and treatment of stuttering.

Guitar, B., & Peters, T.J. (1980). Comparison of stuttering modification and fluency shaping therapies. In B. Guitar & T.J. Peters, *Stuttering: An integration of contemporary therapies* **(pp. 13–23). Memphis: Speech Foundation of America.**

The similarities and differences, as well as the pros and cons, of stuttering modification and fluency shaping therapies are discussed.

Assessment and Diagnosis

This chapter is a bridge between our description of the nature of stuttering (Chapters 1 through 5) and our recommendations for treatment (Chapters 8 through 14). It is written to help clinicians develop an effective treatment program for their clients by (*a*) showing them how to assess the predisposing, precipitating, and learning factors currently influencing a client's stuttering and then by (*b*) describing how to use this information to select the appropriate developmental/treatment level. Figure 7.1 illustrates the components of assessment and diagnosis and the sequence in which we use them.

We describe assessment procedures for three age levels: the adolescent and adult, the elementary school child, and the preschool child. Age levels are used because we know a client's age before an evaluation but little else about him. Our sequence of age levels reflects the fact that very different procedures are used for assessing each age level.

We use the terms "assessment" and "diagnosis" to specify two different stages of our evaluation. Our initial data gathering is the assessment stage. The steps we follow to pull this information together to decide whether a client is indeed a stutterer and to specify the level of treatment appropriate for him is the diagnosis stage.

Components of Assessment and Diagnosis

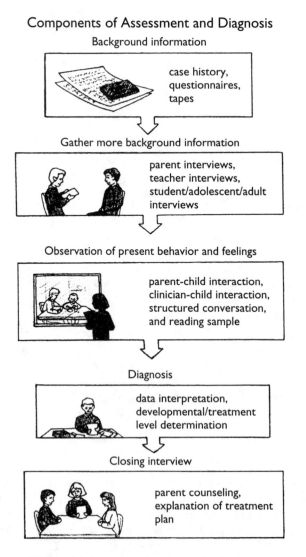

Background information

case history,
questionnaires,
tapes

Gather more background information

parent interviews,
teacher interviews,
student/adolescent/adult
interviews

Observation of present behavior and feelings

parent-child interaction,
clinician-child interaction,
structured conversation,
and reading sample

Diagnosis

data interpretation,
developmental/treatment
level determination

Closing interview

parent counseling,
explanation of treatment
plan

Figure 7.1. Sequence of assessment and diagnosis.

PRELIMINARY CONSIDERATIONS

The initial assessment session provides the clinician with an opportunity to make a significant impact. It is a time when individuals or families are motivated, ready for help, and open to change. Even the most reluctant school child, who is sent to the speech-language pathologist by teachers or parents, will have hopes of relief from frustration and fear. Thus, we begin by offering some observations and suggestions about how clinicians can be most effective at this time.

The Client's Needs

It is easy to say we must always consider a client's needs, but hard to put into practice. One reason is that we develop expectations that function as blinders. Such expectations affect perceptions of what our clients want, what caused their stuttering, what their priorities are, and many other things. Every client is different, but we have found that the more experienced we become, the more we need to resist the tendency to jump to conclusions. And a warning bell needs to go off if we find ourselves thinking, "Ah, yes, I understand this client. Just like that child I saw last year."

We must be cautious about letting referral information, past experience, and biases cloud our ability to see all aspects of the client and his problem clearly. Also, we must be wary of simple explanations and quick judgments as to which factors are critical for a client. For instance, if a child's parents tell us that they often ask the child to stop and start again when he stutters, that they both work long hours outside the home, and that dinner time is noisy and confusing, we try not to assume that pressures at home are the major problem for the child. They may be, but other things may be critical. We need to ask more questions and explore how the child responds in these and other situations before we decide where or how to begin the process of change.

Sometimes individuals' or families' requests differ from what we think they need. An individual may say that he wants "totally fluent speech," but we know this is unattainable for even the most fluent nonstutterer. Or, a family may want us to treat their 3-year-old without their having to take part in therapy, although our preferred approach for a child this age involves parent participation. We have found it best not to confront such issues in an assessment session. We make no promises but do make a concerted effort to understand what clients and families want and why. Our experience has been that after we work with a family or individual for several sessions, we build up enough trust to work together to make the changes that we mutually decide are appropriate.

In trying to meet a client's needs, we consider the person as well as the problem. The client, no matter what age, will sense quickly whether a clinician is seeing him as an individual or is only seeing his stuttering. An effective clinician is genuinely interested and empathetic; she accepts failures and backsliding as well as victories and progress. The evaluation is a clinician's first opportunity to show the client that she accepts him just as he is, without rejection or fear of his stuttering. In this atmosphere, the client can start to accept himself and his stuttering and take the first critical steps toward more fluent speech and effective communication.

Cultural Considerations

As the world becomes smaller and more people from other countries emigrate to the United States from other countries, clinicians will have more opportunities to work with clients from other cultures. Therefore, clinicians will need to develop a multicultural perspective on assessment and therapy.[1] An underlying principle of this perspective is becoming sensitive to differences in communicative style in other cultures and learning how other cultures view speech and language disorders. A number of issues are particularly relevant to stuttering. For example, some cultures do not favor eye contact in conversation; a stutterer from such a culture may look away from listeners but not necessarily because of shame or embarrassment. Moreover, in some cultures stuttering is a highly negative reflection on the family, and parents from these cultures may find it difficult to discuss the stuttering of one of their children.

Our clinic recently treated a young man from China who was referred for his accent. Only after months of treatment was he willing to talk about the greater problem, his stuttering. Until he discussed it, he thought he had successfully disguised it, even though his stuttering was obvious to the clinician.

A sensitive evaluation and treatment take into consideration not only the culture's view of stuttering but also the culture's style of verbal and nonverbal interaction. Orlando Taylor described a number of cultural differences in communication style that are relevant to an evaluation of stuttering. He pointed out that among Hispanics and Native Americans, avoidance of eye contact during speaking or listening may convey respect, not shame. Moreover, among blacks, interruptions of one speaker by another are to be expected. Persons from black and Native American cultures may not be comfortable with the personal questions often asked in an initial interview.

It may not be possible for a clinician to know all the relevant aspects of each new client's culture. But the clinician can be aware of the importance of culture in a person's response to stuttering, as well as the differences in communication styles between her culture and her clients' cultures. Such awareness can come from reading about a client's culture and, if appropriate, discussing this with the client. On some occasions, it may be beneficial to ask a client to bring a family member or friend who shares his culture to increase the clinician's understanding.

For individuals who don't speak the same language as the clinician, an interpreter is necessary. Because the interpreters in many cases are from the same culture as that of the client, the interpreter may help not only in translating, but also in providing information to the clinician to better understand important aspects of the culture. Sometimes, interpreters change the clinician's message to the client. When a message is rephrased by an interpreter to a more culturally appropriate style, therapeutic interaction will be facilitated. However, if an interpreter doesn't understand the intent of a question or statement, he or she may inadvertently convey the wrong information. A colleague who was working with non-English-speaking Haitian immigrants in Boston understood just enough French to realize that the wrong information was being given to a client by an interpreter. She rectified the situation by giving the interpreter a brief overview of what she wanted to discuss with the Haitian family and why certain elements were vital. This immediately improved the communication.

In the case of a bilingual-bicultural client, a clinician should try to ascertain the extent of stuttering in each language. As Watson and Kayser (1994) point out, it is often vital to have a friend or family member of the client to help determine which disfluencies are stuttering and which are nonfluency in the second language as well as to help identify such secondary behaviors as avoidances. In this case, the use of tape recording, if ac-

---

[1] A number of sources discuss important issues to consider in working with clients from other cultures and other social classes; these include Conrad (1996); Cooper & Cooper (1993); Culatta & Goldberg (1995); Taylor (1986); and Watson & Kayser (1994).

ceptable to the client's culture, may be helpful in a joint discussion of what stuttering behavior includes.

Similar sensitivity should be extended to different social classes within the clinician's culture. Understanding and respecting class differences in such areas as vocabulary and values are crucial. Sometimes working with people from other cultures increases our respect for class differences within our own culture. This was brought home to us in getting to know a white Australian clinician, who often worked in the aboriginal culture. This man demonstrated deep respect for the unique values of each of his aboriginal clients and those in the mainstream Australian culture as well.

The Clinician's Expertise

During an assessment, the clinician has a chance to demonstrate not only her empathy with the client's feelings but also her mastery of stuttering diagnosis and treatment. Adolescents and adults who stutter, and their family members, come with feelings of frustration, fear, and helplessness. They are looking for someone whom they can trust, someone who can successfully guide them through the often difficult process of recovery. One of the first things the clinician can do to establish trust and credibility is to show that she not only knows about stuttering, but that she is comfortable asking questions about it, duplicating it in her own speech, exploring it empathically. This provides both clients and family members with an ally, someone who is unafraid of what is so troubling to them.

As the clinician tries to understand an adult or adolescent's stuttering, she can ask him to teach her how to stutter the way he does. As she interviews the family of a preschooler, she can emulate repetitions, prolongations, and blocks as she asks about the types of stuttering the child has shown at various times and in various situations.

The clinician's statements and questions, too, convey her expertise. For example, as she interviews an older child, she can show that she knows about stuttering by making empathetic comments such as "Giving reports in front of class can sometimes be hard for kids who stutter." This allows the child to respond without feeling the direct pressure of a question, but also realize that the clinician is someone who has experience. When talking with families, she can intersperse questions with statements such as "When children keep repeating a sound that won't come out, they will sometimes make their voices rise in pitch as the repetition continues." The family can then confirm or deny whether they have noticed this in their child's speech, and, at the same time, recognize that the clinician is knowledgeable about children's stuttering. Obviously, these kinds of comments and questions are easier for experienced clinicians, but even beginning clinicians can rely on their reading, their all-too-brief practicum experiences, and their intuitions to convey their interest and understanding.

Because it has risks as well as rewards, the approach to interviewing a client or family that was just described should be used carefully. By making comments based on past experience, we may inhibit some individuals and families from telling us about experiences that differ from those offered by the clinician. It is an art to find the balance between showing an understanding and leading the witness. As your clinical judgment develops, you will learn which clients will be helped by this approach and when.

We also caution that demonstrating expertise should be secondary to understanding clients' needs. The clinician's first task is to discern what the individual or family would like from the clinician. The second task is to understand the stuttering problem. In the normal course of accomplishing these two tasks—with attentive listening, empathetic comments, and perceptive questions—the clinician's expertise will emerge naturally.

Continuing Assessment

Assessment is an ongoing process. As treatment progresses, the clinician should keep asking, "Am I using the best approach with this person? Is there something else or something different I should be doing?" She should also decide what measures of progress are important for a client and apply these measures at regular intervals. Our own approach is to assess stuttering behavior at the beginning and the end of each semester. In other settings, we often assess a client after every 10 hours of treatment. In these periodic assessments, we try (although we don't always succeed) to obtain samples of our clients' speech in a nonclinical situation, such as in the classroom or at work. We also assess our clients' stuttering when we bring them in for maintenance checkups at increasingly longer intervals after formal treatment is over.

In addition, we assess our clients' feelings and attitudes at the beginning and end of treatment, and we may assess them at other times if we are concerned about progress. If we are working on changing attitudes and feelings, change should be reflected in our measures, or we should try a different approach. Decreases in negative attitudes and feelings should be accompanied by decreases in stuttering severity, and our measures should show this. The tools for making these various assessments are described for each age level later in this chapter.

Variability of Stuttering

One of the important characteristics of stuttering that we discussed in Chapter 1 is its tremendous variability. Not only does it change as a child develops, but it differs in frequency and severity from day to day and from situation to situation within the same day. Such variability affects both children and adults, but it is most apparent with younger stutterers. Sometimes a preschool child is stuttering severely, then 3 weeks later during the evaluation will be entirely fluent.

Because of the variability of stuttering, we try to assess each individual in a variety of situations and at several points in time. We ask parents to record on tape their child's speech several times before an evaluation to obtain samples that may better reflect the range of their child's stuttering severity. We record (or at least observe) school-age children in their classrooms as well as in the therapy room. We ask adults and adolescents to record their speech in outside situations (although not all will comply) and sample not only their reading and conversation in the clinic, but also their speech on the telephone. We continue this process of multiple sampling in our assessments of the client's progress throughout the course of therapy.

ADOLESCENT AND ADULT

Preassessment

CASE HISTORY FORM

We usually send a case history form to adult clients—those over age 18 and beyond high school—several weeks before their appointment. A copy of this form is shown in Figure 7.2. Because adolescents are often seen in a school, we encourage them to fill out the form themselves but suggest that they may want to get their parents' help for parts of it.

This form requests information that would be appropriate for most speech-language disorders, so that it can be used with all adult clients referred for speech or language prob-

Note: Please complete and return this form before your appointment. Thank you.

Speech Clinic
Stuttering Case History Form — Adult & Adolescent

Date: _____

Name: _____

Address: _____ Tel: _____

_____

Date of birth: _____ Place of birth: _____

Social Security #: _____ Referring physician: _____

Sex: _____ Marital status:_____

Educational level: _____ Occupation: _____

Employed by: _____

Referred to this Center by: _____

Name of spouse/nearest relative: _____

Address: _____ Tel: _____

_____

History of Stuttering

Are there other individuals in your family background or immediate family who stutter?
_____

Give approximate age at which your stuttering was first noticed. _____

Who first noticed or mentioned your stuttering? _____

In what situation did this occur? _____
_____

Describe any situations or conditions that you associate with the onset of stuttering.
_____
_____

What were the first signs of your stuttering? (If you don't remember, you might ask
parents or siblings.) _____
_____
_____

Was the stuttering always the same or did it occur in several different ways?_____
_____

If the stuttering occurred in different ways, how were they different from one another?
_____
_____

Did the first blocks seem to be located in the tongue? Lips? Chest? Diaphragm?
Throat? (Circle your answer.)

Approximately how long did each block (on one word) seem to last? _____

Was the stuttering easy or was there force at the time when the stuttering was first
noticed? _____

Were the words that were stuttered at the beginning of sentences, or were they
scattered throughout the sentence being said? _____
_____

(continued)

Figure 7.2. Case history form for adults and adolescents.

When stuttering first began, was there any avoidance of speaking because of it? Give examples, if any._____

At the time when stuttering was first noticed, what was your reaction? (Check all that apply.)

Awareness that speech was different? ____   Indifference to it?   ____   Other? ____
Surprise?   ____   Anger or frustration? ____
Fear of stuttering again?   ____   Shame?   ____

What attempts have been made to treat the stuttering problem?_____
_____
_____

Development of Stuttering

Since the onset, have there been any changes in stuttering symptoms? (Check all that apply.)

Increase in number of repetitions per word ____
Change in amount of force used (Increased?) ____ (Decreased?) ____
Increase in amount of stuttering ____
Increase in length of block ____
Periods of no stuttering ____
More precise in speech attempts ____
Lowered voice loudness ____
Slower rate of speech ____
Change in location of force when stuttering (if force is present) ____
Looking away from listener ____
Describe any that apply _____
_____

Were there any periods (weeks/months) when the stuttering disappeared? _____
_____

Were there any periods (weeks/months) when stuttering increased? _____
_____

Can you give an explanation for these "worse" periods? _____
_____

Current Stuttering

Are there any situations that are particularly difficult? If so, please describe.
_____
_____

List any situations that never cause difficulty. _____
_____

Answer the following "yes" or "no" as they apply to your stuttering.
Do you stutter when you—

Talk to young children?   ____   Recite memorized material? ____
Say your name?   ____   Ask questions?   ____
Answer direct questions?   ____   Talk to strangers?   ____
Talk to adults, superiors at work, teachers? ____ Speak when tired?   ____
Use new words that are unfamiliar?   ____   Speak when excited?   ____
Use the telephone?   ____   Talk to family members?   ____
Read aloud?   ____   Talk to friends?   ____

Do you feel that stuttering interferes with your career? ____ Social relationships? ____
Success in school? ____ Success on the job? ____ Daily life? ____

Figure 7.2.—*continued*

Do you know any stutterers? ——— Describe your relationship with them. ————
_____
_____

Describe what your stuttering currently looks and sounds like. ————————
_____
_____
_____

Medical Development and Family History

If possible, describe your mother's health during pregnancy and/or your birth history (i.e., complications). ——————————————————————————————————
_____
_____

Describe any development problems during infancy or early childhood (i.e., late in walking, feeding problems, food allergies, late in talking). ————————————
_____
_____

Are you: Right-handed?___ Left-handed?___ Both? ___ Is there evidence of visual, artistic abilities in your family? ——————————————————————————————
_____

Were you sensitive as a child?   Would you describe yourself as sensitive now?

List any significant illnesses, injuries, and operations:

Name	Date	Fever	Complications	Treatment	Physician's Name

List all present physical disabilities.

Any chronic illnesses, allergies, or physical conditions?

Is your vision normal?   Hearing normal?

List any medications you take regularly or are taking currently.

Describe any learning or reading problems you experienced as a child or are currently experiencing.

Do any members of your family have speech or language problems or learning disabilities? If so, describe.

Social History

Hobbies
Leisure time activities

(continued)

Figure 7.2.—continued

Describe any previous therapy you have participated in to aid your fluency. When? Where? With whom? For how long? Outcome

Add anything else you would like to include and think might be important.

If, in order to help you, it is appropriate to send reports to other agencies or professional persons, or to contact other agencies or professional persons for additional information, please indicate your permission by signing below.

I authorize and request (fill in name of clinician or clinic) to obtain and/or exchange pertinent medical/educational information. I understand that all information will be kept confidential.

Signed: _____

Date: _____

If signed by person other than client, please state name and capacity of that person:

_____

_____

Please return this completed form at least 2 weeks before your evaluation.

Figure 7.2.—*continued*

lems. It also allows the clinician to learn ahead of time whether the client referred for stuttering has a different or an additional disorder. The form gives the clinician information about the extent to which stuttering, if that is the problem, affects the client's life.

ATTITUDE QUESTIONNAIRES

We assess clients' communication attitudes through observations, interview questions, and questionnaires. Because we want to be able to review the questionnaires before our diagnostic interview, we prefer to send them to clients and ask them to complete and return them before the interview. Otherwise, clients can complete them when they arrive for an evaluation before we interview them. Before an interview, we prepare follow-up questions based on information from the questionnaires to further explore the client's attitudes. The questionnaires are described in the section on Feelings and Attitudes.

Assessment

INTERVIEW

We begin by welcoming the client and reviewing the procedures we will use to evaluate his problem—interviewing him about his stuttering and his feelings and attitudes, videotaping and audiotaping his speaking and reading, and examining what he does when he stutters and determining whether he can change it. This, we explain, will be followed by an analysis of the information and a concluding interview in which we will share our diagnosis with him and discuss the things that can be done about his problem. We also must remember to have the client complete any questionnaires we haven't already obtained. We then begin our interview with an open-ended question such as, "What is the problem that brings you here today?" or "Why don't you tell us about your stuttering?" The first question might be used if we don't know what is motivating the client to come for an evaluation at this time; the second question when we already know, from prior information, why the client has come right now.

Once the client has had a chance to describe his speech problem, we ask further questions to try to get a deeper understanding. Following are typical questions and a brief commentary about each. Sometimes we group several questions together—a question to start the client talking about a particular topic and follow-up questions to be asked if the first question doesn't elicit some desired information.

1. **When did you begin to stutter? How has the way you stutter changed over the years?**
   We realize that, in answering the first part of this question, the client may be just reporting what his parents told him about his stuttering. The accuracy of his response may be questionable, but at least we will learn his perception of the onset. The second part of the question—about changes over the years—may reveal what kinds of things affect the way a client stutters. Does he stutter more severely because of a recent job change or because of a threat to self-esteem, such as a divorce or loss of employment? Less frequently, we may find out that the client began to stutter in late adolescence or adulthood. If so, we would want to consider the possibility of neurogenic or psychogenic stuttering, which is discussed briefly in the section on diagnosis.

2. **What do you believe caused you to stutter?**
   This may give some insights about motivation. For example, one client reported that her mother and several brothers stuttered and that her stuttering was therefore a genetic problem that could not be helped. This led us to confront the issue of whether or not she could change early in treatment.

   We also find sometimes that clients have misinformation about possible causes of stuttering that we can correct, thereby changing some of our clients' attitudes about their problem. We have met clients who come to therapy believing that their problem is entirely psychological. As they learn our view of stuttering, they are relieved to know that we believe they can modify their speech without long-term psychotherapy.

3. **Does anyone else in your family stutter?**
   We might find that a parent stutters. This is of interest because a parent's attitudes about his or her own stuttering may have had a profound effect on the client. Moreover, knowing about other family members who stutter and how they have responded to it may help us develop a better understanding of factors related to this client's stuttering. This may be useful in treatment. For example, someone we are interviewing may have had a parent who stuttered but never talked about it. We might then want to explore whether the individual we are working with feels especially ashamed of his stuttering or whether he feels it gives him an important bond with the parent.

4. **Have you ever had therapy for your stuttering? What did the therapy consist of? How effective do you think it was?**
   This information is important in planning therapy. For example, if a client had a type of therapy that he felt did not help, it would be unwise to put the client back into the same type of therapy. But if the client has had success with therapy and has regressed slightly or moved away before the treatment was finished, use of this type of therapy again may be most appropriate. It is important that the clinician be familiar with var-

ious types of therapy that clients may have undergone. Most current therapies emphasize either a stuttering modification or a fluency shaping approach.

5. **Has your stuttering changed or caused you more problems recently? Why did you come in for help at the present time?**
   The responses to these questions allow us to see the current problems faced by the client. Usually, we also get some inkling of the client's motivation. For example, the client may have been offered a promotion if he can improve his speech, or he may have recently learned of the treatment program and is hoping for some relief of a longstanding problem.

The following four questions about the client's pattern of stuttering are closely related to one another:

6. **Are there times or situations when you stutter more? Less? What are they?**
7. **Do you avoid certain speaking situations in which you expect to stutter? If so, which ones?**
8. **Do you avoid certain words that you expect to stutter on? Do you substitute one word for another if you expect to stutter? Do you talk around words or topics so you won't stutter?**
9. **Do you use any "tricks" to get words out? Escape behaviors?**
   These four questions will provide information that is useful in therapy planning. They tell us something about the client's most difficult situations, how he feels about them, and how he deals with them. This information may also corroborate what we learn from the questionnaires the client completed. It will also give us an idea of how aware he is of his stuttering behaviors.

10. **Have your academic or vocational choices or performance been affected because you stutter? How?**
    The client's answers will be used to help plan later stages of treatment in which new behaviors and new challenges are attempted. The answers may also prompt us to refer clients in later stages of treatment to an academic or vocational counselor to help them choose a more appropriate option for themselves.

11. **Have your relationships with people been affected because you stutter? How?**
    As in question 10, we can use this information to plan a hierarchy of generalization for a client, moving from easy to difficult social situations gradually if the client finds social interactions difficult. We also need to know how much a client blames his stuttering for any difficulties he has in social interactions. A client may be socially inhibited because he is sensitive and vulnerable to expected listener reactions. Such sensitivity can be assessed by observing his affect while stuttering. If he appears to be relatively unaffected emotionally by his stuttering, but professes to have difficulty relating to people, he may benefit from counseling or psychotherapy focused on resolving this interpersonal difficulty.
    The decision to refer an individual for psychotherapy as an adjunct to stuttering therapy usually is not made in the evaluation session. We need some time and a few therapy sessions to learn more about a person and to develop the needed trust for a successful referral. If we recommend psychotherapy too hastily, a client may feel we think his stuttering is too great a problem for one person to handle, perhaps an insurmountable problem. But if we work with him and he starts to make some progress before we refer, he will feel our support and he may be more likely to benefit from psychotherapy.

12. **What are your feelings or attitudes toward your stuttering? What do you think other people think about your stuttering?**

A client's responses will be used to help determine some of the foci of treatment, such as procedures in desensitization to decrease shame and guilt about stuttering. Perceptions about others' views of his stuttering may need to be confronted with various "reality-testing" tasks to find out what people really think.

13. **What are your family's (parents, spouse, children) feelings, attitudes, and reactions toward your stuttering and toward the prospect of your being in therapy?**

    This information could positively or negatively affect a client's motivation and may be an important consideration in planning therapy.

14. **Are there any additional things that you think we ought to know about your stuttering?**

    This gives the client a chance to get anything off his chest that he may be holding back, or it may be an opportunity for him to discuss things that occurred to him only after other questions were asked.

15. **Do you have any questions you'd like to ask us?**

    Sometimes an adult or adolescent has questions about stuttering that he has been reluctant to ask, and we can use this opportunity to answer them. On the other hand, a client may also want to ask about the length and type of treatment or other issues that we would rather deal with after our assessment is completed. In this case, we explain why we need to delay responding and keep the questions in mind to answer in the closing interview.

SPEECH SAMPLE

In this part of the evaluation, we assess our client's overt stuttering behaviors. Although we videotape and audiotape the entire evaluation, we pay particular attention to the taping of this section because we will need to analyze it carefully afterward. Clinicians use a variety of procedures for assessing overt stuttering. We next describe in detail the tool we currently use and then note other available options.

Stuttering Severity Instrument

The initial version of the Stuttering Severity Instrument (SSI), published in the *Journal of Speech and Hearing Disorders* (Riley, 1972), is illustrated in Figure 7.3. It has been used by many clinicians and researchers since its first publication. The most current version, the SSI-3 (1994), is commercially available with forms and a manual. Like its predecessors, the SSI-3 has some drawbacks. The sample of children and adults on which it was normed is not well described, the reliability of the present instrument is not strong, and its validity has not been convincingly demonstrated (McCauley, 1996).

In spite of these limitations, we find the SSI easy to use and effective in capturing the severity of overt stuttering behaviors as a composite of three important dimensions: frequency, duration, and physical concomitants. The SSI is one of the few measures of stuttering that has standardized procedures for gathering and scoring speech samples and the only one that includes the three dimensions just cited. In addition, we also assess speech rate from the speech and reading samples taken for the SSI, using procedures we describe in the section on speech rate.

For the SSI, Riley recommends using two 200-syllable samples: one of oral reading and one of conversation. We prefer to sample by time, but we make sure that each sample includes at least 200 syllables. We ask a client to read aloud for 3 minutes, using material believed to be at an appropriate level. Then, we ask him to converse about his job or school for 3 minutes of talking time. It is important to measure these samples accurately with a

STUTTERING SEVERITY INSTRUMENT (SSI)

Name _____   Date _____

I. Frequency

1. Job Task		2. Reading Task		3. Picture Task		
Percent	Task Score	Percent	Task Score	Percent	Task Score	
1	2	1	2	1	2	
2–3	3	2–3	3	2–3	6	
4	4	4–5	4	4	8	Frequency
5–6	5	6–9	5	5–6	10	Task Force
7–9	6	10–16	7	7–9	12	
10–14	7	17–26	8	10–14	14	(1 + 2, OR 3)
15–28	8	27+	9	15–28	16	
29+	9			29+	28	I. _____

II. Duration

Mean Length of Three Longest Stutters	Score	
Fleeting...	1	
½ second..	2	
1 full second....................................	3	Duration
2 to 9 seconds..................................	4	Score
10 to 13 seconds...............................	5	
30 to 60 seconds...............................	6	
More than 60 seconds..........................	7	II. _____

III. Physical Concomitants

Evaluating scale: 0 = None; 1 = Not noticeable unless looking for it; 2 = Barely noticeable to casual observer; 3 = Distracting; 4 = Very distracting; 5 = Severe and painful-looking.

Distracting sounds: Noisy breathing, whistling, sniffing, blowing, clicking sounds 0   1   2   3   4   5

Facial Grimaces: Jaw jerking, tongue protruding, lip pressing, jaw muscles tense......... 0   1   2   3   4   5

Head movements: Back, forward, turning away, poor eye contact, constant looking around.... 0   1   2   3   4   5

Movements of extremities: Arm and hand movements, hands about face, torso movements, leg movements, foot tapping or swinging 0   1   2   3   4   5

Physical Concomitants

(Total of four categories)

III. _____

Total Overall Score (TOS): I + II + III = _____

Children's Severity			Adult's Severity		
TOS	Percent	Severity	TOS	Percent	Severity
0–5	0–4	Very mild	0–16	0–4	Very mild
6–8	5–11	Mild	17–19	5–11	Mild
9–13	12–23	Mild	20–21	12–23	Mild
14–15	24–40	Mild	22–24	24–40	Moderate
16–19	41–60	Moderate	25–27	41–60	Moderate
20–23	61–77	Moderate	28–30	61–77	Moderate
24–27	78–89	Severe	31–33	78–89	Severe
28–30	90–96	Severe	34–36	90–96	Severe
31–45	97–100	Very severe	37–45	97–100	Very severe

Figure 7.3. The Stuttering Severity Instrument. (Reprinted with permission from Riley, G. (1972). A stuttering severity instrument for children and adults. *Journal of Speech and Hearing Disorders, 37,* 314-322. Copyright 1972, American Speech-Language-Hearing Association.)

stopwatch. In measuring the amount of speaking time in a conversational sample, we stop the watch whenever the client is not talking, but allow it to run during moments of stuttering. Short pauses (less than 2 seconds) are incorporated into the 3 minutes, but long formulation pauses (longer than 2 seconds) are excluded. With a little practice, starting and stopping a stopwatch during pauses and turn-switching become easy and natural.

Beginning clinicians should practice from taped samples to ensure that they are reliable before scoring a clinical sample. We usually videotape these samples and score them later. If they are audiotaped, the clinician must score the physical concomitants on line during taping because these are not accurately scored from an audio recording.

As noted earlier, we often gather more than one sample of spontaneous speech from adults and adolescents. A sample of speech during a telephone conversation in the clinic can be videotaped and scored using the SSI. A sample from the person's natural environment is usually audiotaped and scored, as described later, for both frequency of stuttering and speech rate.

The total overall score for the SSI is the sum of the three subcomponents measured: (*a*) Frequency is assessed as percentage of stuttering in reading and conversation. Riley originally used percentage of words stuttered, but currently uses the percentage of syllables stuttered, which is converted to the Task Score on the form. (*b*) Duration is assessed by estimating the length of the three longest blocks, calculating their mean duration, and finding the appropriate Task Score on the form. (*c*) Physical concomitants are assessed by adding the scale values of each subcomponent and deriving a total score. Percentiles and Severity ratings (e.g., mild, moderate, severe) based on total overall scores are given on the form. Clinicians should read Riley's directions on administering this measure in the *Journal of Speech and Hearing Disorders* (1972) or in the manual of the SSI-3 (1994) before using it.

When counting frequency of stuttering, we count as stutters: part-word repetitions, monosyllabic whole-word repetitions, prolongations, blockages of sound or airflow, and successful avoidance behaviors. Because we assess frequency as percentage of syllables stuttered, we assume that a syllable is stuttered only once. Thus, "Where is my ba-ba-ba-ba-ba-basketball?" is one stutter. "Where is my uh well my ba-ba-ba-ba-basketball?" is also one stutter, because we assume that the repetition of "my" and the use of "uh" as a postponement are part of the same stutter as the repeated first syllable, "ba." Occasionally, a word might have more than one stutter (e.g., "ba-ba-basketba-ba-ball). This presents no problem when counting frequency as percentage of stuttered syllables, because there is one stutter on the first syllable and one stutter on the third syllable.

We also compare a client's stuttering during reading with his stuttering during conversation. It is often true that, if stuttering is markedly worse during reading, the stutterer may be avoiding words he thinks he may stutter during conversational speech. It is important that clinicians select appropriate reading material for each client. Some may have reading problems, and if the material is above their reading level, stuttering may increase because their resources are stressed on the reading task.

The SSI is a measure we use when we first assess someone who stutters and when we evaluate progress at major intervals. There are other measures of stuttering that we use for different purposes, to capture different dimensions of the problem, which are described next.

Other Measures of Stuttering

We have found that if we are assessing stuttering frequently or are assessing samples that we cannot analyze visually, such as those audiorecorded by the client in his natural environment, we like to use a combination of frequency of stuttering (percent of syllables stuttered) and speech rate (syllables spoken per minute). These measures, first described in Andrews and Ingham (1971), taken together require much less time than the SSI.

When a detailed analysis of stuttering behavior is needed, Conture (1990) and other clinical researchers feel it is important to assess the types of disfluencies in the client's speech. Such analyses may be most appropriate when the clinician is trying to predict whether or not a child is at risk for persistent stuttering. In his text, Conture (1990) describes an evaluation procedure that calculates the percentage of each of seven categories of "within-word" disfluencies in a child's speech.

Starkweather (1991) has presented a case for capturing the amount of time that stuttering takes. This is done by totaling the duration of all disfluencies and pauses and dividing this total by the overall time spent in speaking, thus giving the clinician an impression of how much an individual's stuttering interferes with the rate of information flow.

As part of a determined effort to improve the reliability of stuttering measurement, Ingham (Ingham, Cordes, & Gow, 1993; Ingham, Cordes, & Finn, 1993) has developed a time-interval system of assessment. He and his coworkers have shown that when judges determine whether 4-second samples of speech contain stuttering, interjudge reliability is greater than when stuttering events are counted. The clinical usefulness of this procedure has not been determined.

Speech Rate

In addition to measuring stuttering using the SSI, we assess a client's speech rate. We and many other clinicians believe that speaking rate often reflects the severity of stuttering and concomitantly the effect it is having on communication. If a client's speech rate is markedly below normal, communication may be difficult for him.

Rate can be measured as either words or syllables per minute, depending on the clinician's preference. Some clinicians find it easier to calculate rate using words per minute because words are easily observable units. Others note that syllables per minute can be calculated more rapidly than words because clinicians can use the "beat" of syllables to count them "on-line" (i.e., while the speaker is talking). The syllables-per-minute approach also accounts for the fact that some speakers use more multisyllable words than others and might be penalized because their words may take longer to produce than those who use mostly one-syllable words.

No matter which method is used, the following rules can be used for counting words or syllables: Count only the words or syllables that would have been said if the person had not stuttered. Thus, if the person says, "My-my-my, uh, well my name is Peter," this should be counted as four words or five syllables because it can be assumed that the extra "my's" and the "uh" are part of the stuttering. If the person says, "When I went to Boston, I mean when I went to New York . . . ," and it does not appear that the person was postponing or using a "trick" to avoid stuttering, this would be counted as 13 words or 14 syllables because stuttering did not interfere with the utterance. Only words (or syllables in words) are counted: "uh" or "um" are not counted. "Oh" or "well" are counted, unless they are used as a postponement, starter, or other component of stuttering.

When words per minute are calculated, a transcript is made of a client's 5-minute sample of conversational speech, and his 5-minute reading sample is marked to indicate where he finished. The total number of words are counted, and this figure is divided by five to give a per-minute conversation or reading rate.

Normal speaking rates range from about 115 to 165 words per minute (Andrews &

Ingham, 1971).[2] Normal reading rates range from about 150 to 190 words per minute (Darley & Spriestersbach, 1978).

When syllables per minute are calculated, it is often easiest to use an inexpensive calculator to count syllables cumulatively as they are spoken (although this takes some practice). Before the speaker begins, push the "1" key, then the "+". When the speaker starts speaking, depress the "=" key for each syllable spoken or read. The cumulative total appears in the readout window.[3] We think it is easier to count syllables by reading a transcript of the conversational sample aloud slowly and pushing the "=" key for each syllable spoken; inexperienced raters should learn to count syllables first from a transcript. An experienced rater can assess conversational speech rate directly from a tape recording by pressing the "=" key for each syllable spoken. If this procedure is used, it is wise to recheck your counts to ensure accuracy.

Normal speech rates in syllables range from 162 to 230 syllables per minute, with a mean of 196 (Andrews & Ingham, 1971). Normal reading rates are about 210 to 265 syllables per minute.

Pattern of Disfluencies

Throughout our evaluation of adult or adolescent stutterers, we observe the pattern with which the client stutters. For example, we try to determine roughly what proportion of core behaviors are repetitions, prolongations, and blocks, respectively. During blocks, where and how does the person who stutters shut off airflow or voicing? What are his escape and avoidance behaviors? Is he able to tolerate being in a block, or does he speak in an unusual or vague way to avoid stuttering? More detail on various escape and avoidance patterns can be found in Chapter 5.

As we explore the behaviors that constitute a client's stuttering, we comment on his behaviors, question him about how typical this sample of stuttering is, and ask about the escape and avoidance behaviors we see. If the client doesn't seem too uncomfortable confronting his stuttering, we ask him to teach us how to stutter as he does and we work together, with both the client and ourself emulating his various types of stuttering. This need not be an exhaustive exploration because we will do much more in treatment. Here, we are trying to begin three tasks: (a) model an "approach" attitude toward stuttering, showing our calmness and objectivity in the face of behaviors that the client may have felt to be shameful, perhaps terrifying; (b) study the client's emotional reaction when he is face to face with his stuttering (and perhaps reduce some of his fear); (c) teach both of us about what he does when he stutters so that he may learn how to change it.

Trial Therapy

We try therapy techniques with clients during the assessment session for several reasons. First, we get an idea of how he responds to different approaches, giving us information to use if we recommend treatment. Second, trial therapy helps us make a differential diagnosis between typical stuttering and stuttering that has an immediate neurological or

---

[2] All rate figures given in this section are for adults.
[3] Although many calculators require pressing the "1," then the "+" then the "=" button repeatedly to count cumulatively, others will count cumulatively when the "1" is pressed, followed by repeated pressing of the "+" button. Some experimentation may be necessary to find the appropriate sequence on your calculator. Some of the more expensive calculators cannot be used to count cumulatively because of the types of microchips used in them.

psychological basis. Third, it gives the client a taste of things to come, providing hope and motivation to follow through on treatment.

We begin with *stuttering modification,* which can be done easily in the context of studying disfluency patterns as previously described. In fact, this exploration with a client of his stuttering is a condensed version of the first stage of stuttering modification. Once a client is able to emulate his stuttering to a small degree, we carry out stuttering modification trial therapy by coaching him through this sequence: (*a*) "freezing" during the moment of a stutter, maintaining the level of physical tension and the posture with which he was stuttering; (*b*) becoming aware of what he is doing in terms of physically tensing muscles, holding his breath, pushing against jammed postures; (*c*) changing the elements that are maintaining the stutter by releasing the excess physical tension, moving structures that are held rigid, or allowing himself to breathe. We may stop here with clients who are unable to do this (*c*) or do it only with difficulty.

With clients who seem able to make these changes easily, we go one step further. We ask them to hold onto the stutter, which by now has become voluntary, and prolong the airflow or voicing for several seconds and then produce the remainder of the word slowly. If a client is able to do this with our coaching, we ask him to do it while reading without our coaching. This is enough. No matter how much or how little our client is able to do, we want to stop when he is feeling successful.

We now turn to fluency shaping trial therapy. We begin by reducing our own speech rate as we describe to a client the aim of this exercise—to produce words very, very slowly. We use a written sentence that begins with a vowel or a glide, going over it word by word, teaching him to use a gradual and gentle onset of voicing and to stretch each sound, whether vowel or consonant. The clinician needs to provide a good model for each word and give constant feedback. When words are produced slowly enough, with each part of the speech production system—respiration, phonation, and articulation—moving in slow motion and without excess tension, fluency results. When the client produces each word of the sentence this way, he is coached to produce the entire sentence, linking each word to the next. Breath supply is monitored so that pauses for breath are taken whenever the client would take a breath naturally. Again, modeling and frequent feedback are vital.

As an example, the sentence, "Apples are a red fruit," should take from 15 to 20 seconds to produce, with a pause for a new breath after the word "a". The /p/ in "Apples," the /d/ in "red," and the /t/ in "fruit" all should be produced without stopping the airflow, making these plosives sound like fricatives.

If clients are particularly adept at this, they can be taken all the way to saying short sentences in conversational speech that are produced in this slow, fluent way. Clients who have difficulty doing this should be coached only through the production of the short, written sentence, and care should be taken to see that they stop before experiencing notable failure.

FEELINGS AND ATTITUDES

A variety of questionnaires can be used to assess various aspects of a stutterer's feelings and attitudes about communication and stuttering. We obtain information about the client's communication attitudes with the Modified Erickson Scale of Communication Attitudes (S-24) (Andrews & Cutler, 1974). This questionnaire has been normed on both stutterers and nonstutterers (Fig. 7.4). Guitar and Bass (1978) studied a sample of 20 individuals treated by a fluency shaping program; they found that if communication attitude, as measured by the S-24, doesn't change during treatment, likelihood of relapse

MODIFIED ERICKSON SCALE OF COMMUNICATION ATTITUDES (S-24)

Name: _____   Date: _____   Score: _____

Directions: Mark the "true column with a check (✔) for each statement that is true or mostly true for you and mark the "false" column with a check (✔) for each statement which is false or not usually true for you.

	TRUE	FALSE
1. I usually feel that I am making a favorable impression when I talk.	_____	_____
2. I find it easy to talk with almost anyone.	_____	_____
3. I find it very easy to look at my audience while speaking to a group.	_____	_____
4. A person who is my teacher or my boss is hard to talk to.	_____	_____
5. Even the idea of giving a talk in public makes me afraid.	_____	_____
6. Some words are harder than others for me to say.	_____	_____
7. I forget all about myself shortly after I begin a speech.	_____	_____
8. I am a good mixer.	_____	_____
9. People sometimes seem uncomfortable when I am talking to them.	_____	_____
10. I dislike introducing one person to another.	_____	_____
11. I often ask questions in group discussions.	_____	_____
12. I find it easy to keep control of my voice when speaking.	_____	_____
13. I do not mind speaking before a group.	_____	_____
14. I do not talk well enough to do the kind of work I'd really like to do.	_____	_____
15. My speaking voice is rather pleasant and easy to listen to.	_____	_____
16. I am sometimes embarrassed by the way I talk.	_____	_____
17. I face most speaking situations with complete confidence.	_____	_____
18. There are few people I can talk with easily.	_____	_____
19. I talk better than I write.	_____	_____
20. I often feel nervous while talking.	_____	_____
21. I find it hard to make talk when I meet new people.	_____	_____
22. I feel pretty confident about my speaking ability.	_____	_____
23. I wish that I could say things as clearly as others do.	_____	_____
24. Even though I knew the right answer, I have often failed to give it because I was afraid to speak out.	_____	_____

Data on the "Modified Erickson Scale of Communication Attitudes"

I. Answers (Andrews and Cutler, 1974)

Score 1 point for each answer that matches this:

1. False	7. False	13. False	19. False
2. False	8. False	14. True	20. True
3. False	9. True	15. False	21. True
4. True	10. True	16. True	22. False
5. True	11. False	17. False	23. True
6. True	12. False	18. True	24. True

II. Adult Norms (Andrews and Cutler, 1974)

	Mean	Range
Stutterers	19.22	9–24
Nonstutterers	9.14	1–21

Figure 7.4. Erickson S-24 Scale of Communication Attitudes. (Reprinted with permission from Andrews, G., & Cutler, J. (1974). Stuttering therapy: The relation between changes in symptom level and attitudes. *Journal of Speech and Hearing Disorders, 39,* 312–319. Copyright 1974, American Speech-Language-Hearing Association.)

within 12 to 18 months increases. Ingham (1979) disputed this finding, but Young (1981) confirmed it using a reanalysis of the original data. New data by Andrews and Craig (1988) also supported the relationship between normalizing attitudes on the S-24 and long-term outcome.

We also use questionnaires to assess a client's tendency to avoid stuttering, using the avoidance scale of the Stutterer's Self-Rating of Reactions to Speech Situations (Johnson, Darley, & Spriestersbach, 1952). This scale, which we refer to as the SSR, assesses the client's tendency to avoid specific speaking situations (Fig. 7.5).

Our research suggests that clients with avoidance scale scores higher than 2.56 before treatment may be more likely to have an appreciable level of stuttering 1 year after treatment with fluency shaping therapy than are clients with lower scores (Guitar, 1976). Thus, we suggest that clinicians use a client's avoidance scale score to guide them in choosing whether to use fluency shaping alone or to combine fluency shaping with stuttering modification.

We also may use Perceptions of Stuttering Inventory (PSI) (Woolf, 1967) to examine a stutterer's perception of the presence of struggle, avoidance, and expectancy of stuttering (Fig. 7.6). Woolf suggests that the PSI can be used to help a stutterer view his problem more objectively, to develop treatment goals, and to assess progress. We find that the avoidance section of the PSI complements the avoidance scale of the SSR because the SSR focuses more on situations and the PSI deals more with stuttering behaviors.

Another measure of attitude that has been shown to predict long-term outcome is the locus of control of behavior scale (Craig, Franklin, & Andrews, 1984). This scale assesses the extent to which a client believes he controls his own behavior: whether the control is "internal" or "external" (Fig. 7.7). Scoring adds the points for each item, and higher scores reflect greater "externality." Because the values of items 1, 5, 7, 8, 13, 15, and 16 are reversed to minimize the effect of social desirability in responding, the scores on these items are transposed (change a "5" to a "0", a "4" to a "1", and so on) before totaling the score. This scale is given just before treatment, then again immediately after treatment. Studies have shown that clients who did not decrease their locus-of-control scores more than 5% from pretreatment to post-treatment are in danger of relapse (Craig & Andrews, 1985; Craig, Franklin, & Andrews, 1984).

Andrews and Craig (1988) reported that two measures of attitude, combined with a measure of stuttering behavior, are useful in predicting relapse after fluency shaping treatment. They found little relapse among those stutterers who met these three goals by the end of treatment: no stuttering on telephone calls to strangers, a score of 9 or below on the Modified Erickson Scale of Communication Attitudes (see Fig. 7.4) , and locus-of-control score reductions greater than 5%. Their assessment of relapse was based on a single telephone call with a stranger 10 to 18 months after treatment, and relapse was considered to be more than 2% of syllables stuttered on the call.

OTHER SPEECH AND LANGUAGE BEHAVIORS

As we interact with a client during the interview, we informally assess his comprehension and production of language, his articulation, and voice. We also screen his hearing. If we suspect that there is an articulation, language, or voice problem, we follow up with further evaluations of the suspected areas. Adolescent language assessment procedures can be found in McLoughlin and Lewis (1990); those for articulation can be found in Hoffman, Schuckers, and Daniloff (1989). We let a client's concern about other disorders guide us in treatment. If, as we have found occasionally, a stuttering client also lisps, we discuss it with him. If he is not concerned, we don't feel it is necessary to treat that prob-

STUTTERER'S SELF-RATING OF REACTIONS TO SPEECH SITUATIONS

Name _____ Age _____ Sex _____
Examiner _____ Date _____

After each item put a number from 1 to 5 in each of the four columns.

Start with the right-hand column headed Frequency. Study the five possible answers to be made in responding to each item, and write the number of the answer that best fits the situation for you in each case. Thus, if you habitually take your meals at home and seldom eat in a restaurant, certainly not as often as once a week, write number 5 in the Frequency column opposite item No. 1, "Ordering in a restaurant." In like manner respond to each of the other 39 items by writing the most appropriate number in the Frequency column

Now, write the number of the response that best indicates how much you stutter in each situation. For example, if in ordering meals in a restaurant you stutter mildly (for you), write number 2 in the Stuttering column.

Following the same procedure, write your responses in the Reaction column and, finally, write your responses in the Avoidance column.

Numbers for each of the columns are to be interpreted as follows:

A. Avoidance
1. I never try to avoid this situation and have no desire to avoid it.
2. I don't try to avoid this situation, but sometimes I would like to.
3. More often than not I do not try to avoid this situation, but sometimes I do try to avoid it.
4. More often than not I do try to avoid this situation.
5. I avoid this situation every time I possibly can.

B. Reaction
1. I definitely enjoy speaking in this situation.
2. I would rather speak in this situation than not speak.
3. It's hard to say whether I'd rather speak in this situation or not.
4. I would rather not speak in this situation.
5. I very much dislike speaking in this situation.

C. Stuttering
1. I don't stutter at all (or only very rarely) in this situation.
2. I stutter mildly (for me) in this situation.
3. I stutter with average severity (for me) in this situation.
4. I stutter more than average (for me) in this situation.
5. I stutter severely (for me) in this situation.

D. Frequency
1. This is a situation I meet very often, two or three times a day or even more, on the average.
2. I meet this situation at least once a day with rare exceptions (except Sunday perhaps).
3. I meet this situation from three to five times a week on the average.
4. I meet this situation once a week, with few exceptions, and occasionally I meet it twice a week.
5. I rarely meet this situation—certainly not as often as once a week.

(continued)

Figure 7.5. Stutterer's Self-Rating of Reactions to Speech Situations. (Reprinted with permission from Johnson, W., Darley, F., & Spriestersbach, D.C. (1952). *Diagnostic manual in speech correction.* New York: Harper & Row. Copyright 1952 by Harper & Row. Copyright renewed 1980 by Edna B. Johnson, Frederick L. Darley, and Duane C. Spriestersbach.)

	Avoidance	Reaction	Stuttering	Frequency
1. Ordering in a restaurant.	____	____	____	____
2. Introducing myself (face to face).	____	____	____	____
3. Telephoning to ask price, train fare, etc.	____	____	____	____
4. Buying plane, train, or bus ticket.	____	____	____	____
5. Short class recitation (10 words or less).	____	____	____	____
6. Telephoning for taxi.	____	____	____	____
7. Introducing one person to another.	____	____	____	____
8. Buying something from a store clerk.	____	____	____	____
9. Conversation with a good friend.	____	____	____	____
10. Talking with an instructor after class or in his or her office.	____	____	____	____
11. Long-distance phone call to someone I know.	____	____	____	____
12. Conversation with my father.	____	____	____	____
13. Asking girl for date (or talking to a man who asks me for date.	____	____	____	____
14. Making short speech (1–2 minutes).	____	____	____	____
15. Giving my name over telephone.	____	____	____	____
16. Conversation with my mother.	____	____	____	____
17. Asking a secretary if I can see the employer.	____	____	____	____
18. Going to house and asking for someone.	____	____	____	____
19. Making a speech to unfamiliar audience.	____	____	____	____
20. Participating in committee meeting.	____	____	____	____
21. Asking the instructor a question in class.	____	____	____	____
22. Saying hello to friend passing by.	____	____	____	____
23. Asking for a job.	____	____	____	____
24. Telling a person a message from someone else.	____	____	____	____
25. Telling a funny story with one stranger in a crowd.	____	____	____	____
26. Parlor game requiring speech.	____	____	____	____
27. Reading aloud to friends.	____	____	____	____
28. Participating in a bull session.	____	____	____	____
29. Dinner conversation with strangers.	____	____	____	____
30. Talking with my barber/hairdresser.	____	____	____	____
31. Telephoning to make appointment or to arrange to meet someone.	____	____	____	____
32. Answering roll call in class.	____	____	____	____
33. Asking at a desk for book or card to be filled out, etc.	____	____	____	____
34. Talking with someone I don't know well while waiting for bus, class, etc.	____	____	____	____
35. Talking with other players during game.	____	____	____	____
36. Taking leave of a host or hostess.	____	____	____	____
37. Conversation with friend while walking.	____	____	____	____
38. Buying stamps at post office.	____	____	____	____
39. Giving directions to a stranger.	____	____	____	____
40. Taking leave of a girl/boy after date.	____	____	____	____
Totals	____	____	____	____
Averages (divide total by # of answers)	____	____	____	____

Figure 7.5.—*continued*

PERCEPTIONS OF STUTTERING INVENTORY (PSI)

The symbols S, A, and E after each item denote struggle (S), avoidance (A), and expectancy (E). In practice, these symbols are not included in the Inventory, but are listed on a separate scoring key.

Name _____ Age _____ S A E

Examiner _____ Date _____ # _____

% _____

Directions

Here are 60 statements about stuttering. Some of these may be characteristic of your stuttering. Read each item carefully and respond as in the examples below.

Characteristic
of me

_____ Repeating sounds

Put a check mark (✔) under "characteristic of me" if repeating sounds is part of your stuttering; if it is not characteristic, leave the space blank.

"Characteristic of me" refers only to what you do now, not to what was true of your stuttering in the past and which you no longer do, and not what you think you should or should not be doing. Even if the behavior described occurs only occasionally or only in some speaking situations, if you regard it as characteristic of your stuttering, check the space under "characteristic of me."

Characteristic
of me

_____ 1. Avoiding talking to people in authority (e.g., a teacher, employer, or clergyman). (A).

_____ 2. Feeling that interruptions in your speech (e.g., pauses, hesitations, or repetitions) will lead to stuttering. (E).

_____ 3. Making the pitch of your voice higher or lower when you expect to get "stuck" on words. (E).

_____ 4. Having extra and unnecessary facial movement (e.g., flaring your nostrils during speech attempts). (S).

_____ 5. Using gestures as a substitute for speaking (e.g., nodding your head instead of saying "yes" or smiling to acknowledge a greeting). (A).

_____ 6. Avoiding asking for information (e.g., asking for directions or inquiring about a train schedule). (A)

_____ 7. Whispering words to yourself before saying them or practicing what you are planning to say long before you speak. (E).

_____ 8. Choosing a job or hobby because little speaking would be required. (A).

_____ 9. Adding an extra or unnecessary sound, word, or phrase to your speech (e.g., "uh," "well," or "let me see") to help yourself get started. (E).

_____ 10. Replying briefly using the fewest words possible. (A).

_____ 11. Making sudden, jerky, or forceful movements with your head, arms or body during speech attempts (e.g., clenching your fist, jerking your head to one side). (S).

_____ 12. Repeating a sound or word with effort. (S).

_____ 13. Acting in a manner intended to keep you out of a conversation or discussion (e.g.,

(continued)

Figure 7.6. Perceptions of Stuttering Inventory. (Reprinted with permission from Woolf, G. (1967). The assessment of stuttering as struggle, avoidance, and expectancy. *British Journal of Disorders of Communication, 2,* 158–171.)

being a good listener, pretending not to hear what was said, acting bored, or pretending to be in deep thought). (A).

_____ 14. Avoiding making a purchase (e.g., avoiding going into a store or buying stamps in the post office). (A).

_____ 15. Breathing noisily or with great effort while trying to speak. (S).

_____ 16. Making your voice louder or softer when stuttering is expected. (E).

_____ 17. Prolonging a sound or word (e.g., m-m-m-m-my) while trying to push it out. (S).

_____ 18. Helping yourself to get started talking by laughing, coughing, clearing your throat, gesturing, or some other body activity movement. (E).

_____ 19. Having general body tension during speech attempts (e.g., shaking, trembling, or feeling "knotted up" inside). (S).

_____ 20. Paying particular attention to what you are going to say (e.g., the length of a word, or the position of a word in a sentence). (E).

_____ 21. Feeling your face getting warm and red (as if you are blushing) as you are struggling to speak. (S).

_____ 22. Saying words or phrases with force or effort. (S).

_____ 23. Repeating a word or phrase preceding the word on which stuttering is expected. (E).

_____ 24. Speaking so that no word or sound stands out (e.g., speaking in a singsong voice or in a monotone). (E).

_____ 25. Avoiding making new acquaintances (e.g., not visiting with friends, not dating, or not joining social, civic, or church groups). (A).

_____ 26. Making unusual noises with your teeth during speech attempts (e.g., grinding or clicking your teeth). (S).

_____ 27. Avoiding introducing yourself, giving your name, or making introductions. (A).

_____ 28. Expecting that certain sounds, letters, or words are going to be particularly "hard" to say (e.g., words beginning with the letter "s"). (E).

_____ 29. Giving excuses to avoid talking (e.g., pretending to be tired or pretending lack of interest in a topic). (A).

_____ 30. "Running out of breath" while speaking. (S).

_____ 31. Forcing out sounds. (S).

_____ 32. Feeling that your fluent periods are unusual, that they cannot last, and that sooner or later you will stutter. (E).

_____ 33. Concentrating on relaxing or not being tense before speaking. (E).

_____ 34. Substituting a different word or phrase for the one you had intended to say. (A).

_____ 35. Prolonging or emphasizing the sound preceding the one on which stuttering is expected. (E).

_____ 36. Avoiding speaking before an audience. (A).

_____ 37. Straining to talk without being able to make a sound. (S).

_____ 38. Coordinating or timing your speech with a rhythmic movement (e.g., tapping your foot or swinging your arm). (E).

_____ 39. Rearranging what you had planned to say to avoid a "hard" sound or word. (A).

_____ 40. "Putting on an act" when speaking (e.g., adopting an attitude of confidence or pretending to be angry). (E).

_____ 41. Avoiding the use of the telephone. (A).

_____ 42. Making forceful and strained movements with your lips, tongue, jaw, or throat (e.g., moving your jaw in an uncoordinated manner). (S).

Figure 7.6.—*continued*

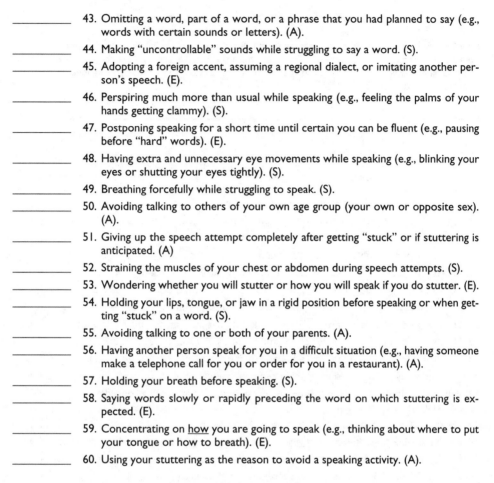

_____ 43. Omitting a word, part of a word, or a phrase that you had planned to say (e.g., words with certain sounds or letters). (A).

_____ 44. Making "uncontrollable" sounds while struggling to say a word. (S).

_____ 45. Adopting a foreign accent, assuming a regional dialect, or imitating another person's speech. (E).

_____ 46. Perspiring much more than usual while speaking (e.g., feeling the palms of your hands getting clammy). (S).

_____ 47. Postponing speaking for a short time until certain you can be fluent (e.g., pausing before "hard" words). (E).

_____ 48. Having extra and unnecessary eye movements while speaking (e.g., blinking your eyes or shutting your eyes tightly). (S).

_____ 49. Breathing forcefully while struggling to speak. (S).

_____ 50. Avoiding talking to others of your own age group (your own or opposite sex). (A).

_____ 51. Giving up the speech attempt completely after getting "stuck" or if stuttering is anticipated. (A)

_____ 52. Straining the muscles of your chest or abdomen during speech attempts. (S).

_____ 53. Wondering whether you will stutter or how you will speak if you do stutter. (E).

_____ 54. Holding your lips, tongue, or jaw in a rigid position before speaking or when getting "stuck" on a word. (S).

_____ 55. Avoiding talking to one or both of your parents. (A).

_____ 56. Having another person speak for you in a difficult situation (e.g., having someone make a telephone call for you or order for you in a restaurant). (A).

_____ 57. Holding your breath before speaking. (S).

_____ 58. Saying words slowly or rapidly preceding the word on which stuttering is expected. (E).

_____ 59. Concentrating on <u>how</u> you are going to speak (e.g., thinking about where to put your tongue or how to breath). (E).

_____ 60. Using your stuttering as the reason to avoid a speaking activity. (A).

Figure 7.6.—_continued_

lem. If, however, he feels that an articulation, language, or other problem handicaps him communicatively, we treat that problem also.

Sometimes we place a voice problem in a separate category. We find that some stutterers may be hoarse, but suspect this may be the result of laryngeal tension related to stuttering. If stuttering treatment is successful, the hoarseness may disappear. Again, we take our cue from the client. If the problem bothers him and isn't remediated by treatment, we address it in therapy. If hoarseness is of recent origin and not associated with the acute stage of a cold, we may refer him for an otolaryngological examination to rule out serious laryngeal pathology.

OTHER FACTORS

In this section, we discuss evaluation of the following factors: intelligence, academic adjustment, psychological adjustment, and vocational adjustment. Each of these factors can affect the treatment of an adult or adolescent stutterer and therefore must be considered in planning therapy.

If a stutterer has below-normal intelligence, he may have difficulty following the regimen of a typical therapy program. Usually, the clinician knows beforehand if a stutterer scheduled for an evaluation has below-normal intelligence. Adolescent stutterers in

LOCUS OF CONTROL OF BEHAVIOR SCALE

Directions: Below are a number of statements about how various topics affect your personal beliefs. There are no right or wrong answers. For every item there are a large number of people who agree and disagree. Could you please put in the appropriate bracket the choice you believe to be true? Answer all the questions.

0	1	2	3	4	5
Strongly disagree	Generally disagree	Somewhat disagree	Somewhat agree	Generally agree	Strongly agree

1. I can anticipate difficulties and take action to avoid them........................... ( )
2. A great deal of what happens to me is probably just a matter of chance............... ( )
3. Everyone knows that luck or chance determines one's future....................... ( )
4. I can control my problem(s) only if I have outside support. .... ( )
5. When I make plans, I am almost certain that I can make them work. .... ( )
6. My problem(s) will dominate me all my life..................................... ( )
7. My mistakes and problems are my responsibility to deal with...................... ( )
8. Becoming a success is a matter of hard work; luck has little or nothing to do with it. .... ( )
9. My life is controlled by outside actions and events............................... ( )
10. People are victims of circumstance beyond their control......................... ( )
11. To continually manage my problems I need professional help..................... ( )
12. When I am under stress, the tightness in my muscles is due to things outside
    my control. .... ( )
13. I believe a person can really be the master of his fate. .... ( )
14. It is impossible to control my irregular and fast breathing when I am having difficulties... ( )
15. I understand why my problem(s) varies so much from one occasion to the next........ ( )
16. I am confident of being able to deal successfully with future problems............... ( )
17. In my case, maintaining control over my problem(s) is due mostly to luck............. ( )

Figure 7.7. Locus of Control of Behavior Scale.

schools are usually identified as mentally handicapped if they are, and they are likely to be in a special class. Adults, too, are usually identified as mentally handicapped if this is the case, because either the referral source will indicate this or because a guardian will have filled out the case history form.

Problems of academic adjustment in an adolescent stutterer usually become apparent from either the original referral or interviews with the child's teachers as part of the evaluation process. These interviews are described in more detail in the section on the Elementary School Child. An example of poor academic adjustment relevant to stuttering is a student's conflict with a teacher who insists on oral presentations that the student is unwilling to do.

As stated in Chapter 2, there are no group differences between stutterers and nonstutterers in their psychological health. However, we sometimes see stutterers who do not function well in their environments. They may be unable to achieve a satisfying marriage. They may be unable to hold a job, or they may be socially withdrawn. The clinician needs to be alert to the effect that adjustment problems may have on treatment. If psychological problems are suspected of interfering with treatment progress, the clinician may wish to refer these clients for a psychological evaluation. In such cases, the clinician should take care to ask professional colleagues for recommendations of the most effective psychotherapists in the area.

Psychological problems that are relevant to stuttering also may become apparent during the interview when the onset of stuttering is explored. Sudden onset after a psychological trauma, particularly if onset is in late adolescence or adulthood, may indicate psychogenic stuttering. We have found that, if the psychological effects of the trauma have subsided, an adolescent or adult client may respond well to our integrated approach to treatment described in Chapter 9. If it is clear that psychological factors are still affecting the client's speech and behavior, or if there is doubt, we refer the client for a psychological evaluation. Unless the disorder is psychosis, in which case stuttering therapy is not recommended, a client with a psychological problem may respond well to a combination of psychotherapy and stuttering therapy.

INTERVIEW WITH PARENTS OF ADOLESCENT

When we evaluate an adolescent stutterer, we want to talk with his parents to obtain more background information about the child, to give them an opportunity to express their concerns and feelings privately, and to let them know what we will be doing.

We begin the initial interview by asking the parents to describe the problem as they see it. We encourage them to express their fears, concerns, and frustrations, and we listen carefully. We try to get an understanding of how their child functions within his family. We usually ask questions such as these: "What is his stuttering like at home?" "How does he seem to feel about it—is he embarrassed or does he show fear of talking or anger?" "How do you feel about it?" "What are your and other family members' reactions to it—what do you do when he stutters?" "Has he been seen anywhere else for therapy?" "If so, what were the results?" Although parents may ask what can be done to help their child and what they should do, we prefer to wait until after we've seen the youngster before answering these questions.

Adolescents strive to become more and more independent from their parents. Therefore, we find that therapy works best if an adolescent is treated as an adult. We begin fostering independence by first talking to the teenage client separately from his parents so that he can give us his own view of the situation and how he views the prospect of treatment. After this and after our meeting with the parents, we meet with the parents and the teenage client together to seek mutual agreement about their respective roles in treatment. This is often an important time. It serves to let the youngster know that we respect his ability to work independently from his parents, and it serves to let the parents know that they can be most helpful by being supportive but not directive.

Diagnosis

After we gather the information just described, we need to integrate the material to determine whether the client stutters and, if so, what treatment level is appropriate. Typically, teenage clients are advanced stutterers; however, some are still in the intermediate stage. Let us consider first the possibility that a teenager turns out *not* to be a stutterer.

In rare cases, teens who are normally but highly disfluent, may be referred by teachers, employers, or friends. Most have phrase repetitions, circumlocutions, revisions, and hesitations—the types of disfluencies we described in Chapter 5 as normal. These types of disfluencies are observed relatively infrequently after children's elementary school years. However, some adolescents and adults may simply be at the disfluent end of the continuum of normal fluency. In addition to differences in the type and number of disfluencies, secondary behaviors and negative feelings and attitudes will be absent. Our role in such cases is to explain to the individual and to the referring person (when there is one) that this kind of speech is normally disfluent and need not be of concern. It might be emphasized to the referring source of an adolescent that excessive attention to these disfluencies may be more harmful than helpful.

Another need for differential diagnosis, besides in instances of normal disfluency, is in cases in which cluttering, neurogenic disfluency, and psychogenic disfluency need to be distinguished from stuttering. Moreover, it is also necessary to rule out the disfluency caused by word-finding difficulties that we might find in persons with a learning disability.

Some of the salient features of cluttering in adults and adolescents are rapid, sometimes unintelligible speech, frequent repetitions of syllables, words, or phrases, lack of awareness or concern about speech, disorganized thought processes, and language problems. Cluttering sometimes coexists with stuttering, and both disorders may respond to a highly structured, fluency shaping approach for treatment. The book *Cluttering* by Deso Weiss (1964) is a prime source for diagnostic and treatment information. An excellent chapter by David Daly (1993), "Cluttering: Another fluency syndrome" in the book *Stuttering and Related Disorders of Fluency* describes assessment and therapy procedures. Kenneth St. Louis and Florence Myers (1997) have recently published a chapter describing evaluation and treatment of cluttering in its pure form as well as when it occurs simultaneously along with learning disabilities and with stuttering.

Neurogenic disfluency in the adolescent or adult is usually the result of stroke, head trauma, or neurological disease. Symptoms are likely to be repetitive disfluencies, but may include blockages as well. Because stuttering commonly begins in childhood, if a client reports onset of stuttering after age 12, a neurogenic-based disorder is a possibility. A chapter by Nancy Helm-Estabrooks (1986), "Neurogenic Stuttering in Adults," in *The Atypical Stutterer,* discusses diagnostic signs and treatment possibilities. In almost all such cases, the onset of neurogenic-based fluency problems are clearly linked to a well-defined episode of acquired neurological damage.

Disfluency that begins in adolescence or adulthood can also result from psychological trauma. Carole Roth, Arnold Aronson, and Leo Davis (1989) indicate that psychogenic disfluency often arises during periods of "environmental stress or interpersonal conflict." They found that these fluency difficulties were often accompanied by what appear to be neurological signs such as weakness, numbness, tingling, and seizure-like activity. In fact, many of their subjects had neurologic damage. Disfluencies included repetitions, prolongations, blocks, secondary behaviors, and feelings and attitudes similar to those of stutterers. Psychogenic disfluency was generally found to be amenable to traditional psychotherapy and stuttering treatment approaches, both during a diagnostic interview and later during treatment. In our own experience, however, not all psychogenic disfluency responds to treatment. In one case of a man who had been mute for several years before beginning to show symptoms of severe stuttering, we were unable to make any change in his disfluencies using slow speech, singing, and delayed auditory feedback. Further information about psychogenic disfluency can be obtained from another article about this disorder, by Mahr and Leith (1992). In summary, when late-onset disfluencies are seen and are associated with psychological stress and conflict and the onset of a psychiatric condition, psychogenic disfluency should be suspected. Traditional treatments, such as those described in Chapters 8 and 9 may or may not be helpful. The patient should be referred for both psychological and neurological assessment, so that treatment needed in these areas will be provided.

When the clinician determines that stuttering treatment would be appropriate for a client, whether the stuttering had a typical onset during early childhood or whether it has another etiology, the focus turns to a consideration of what level of treatment to select for the client. As we said earlier, adult and adolescent stutterers are most likely to be at the advanced developmental and treatment level. Signs of this level include the core behaviors of repetitions, prolongations, and blocks, all with tension, secondary behaviors of escape and avoidance, and negative feelings and attitudes about communication in general and stuttering in particular.

DETERMINING DEVELOPMENTAL/TREATMENT LEVEL

The determination of a developmental/treatment level for an adolescent or adult stutterer is based largely on the client's age. Intermediate and advanced treatment approaches are well suited for stutterers whose core behaviors are blocks, who have escape and avoidance as secondary symptoms, and whose attitudes about speech are relatively negative. A stutterer suited to advanced level treatment will usually have more entrenched negative attitudes about speech and himself as a speaker simply because he has been stuttering longer. The major difference between intermediate and advanced treatment levels is that more independence and responsibility are required of clients at the advanced level. Consequently, clinicians ordinarily place adult clients at the advanced level, but determine an adolescent's placement based on how much responsibility he can take for self-therapy.

Intermediate Stuttering

The stutterer who is at the intermediate level will probably be younger than 14. His stuttering pattern will be characterized by escape and avoidance behaviors and considerable tension on blocks, prolongations, and repetitions. He will also be avoiding some speaking situations. Moreover, his feelings and attitudes, as revealed in the interview with him and with his parents and teachers and reflected in questionnaires, will suggest many negative speech attitudes.

Advanced Stuttering

The individual who fits into the advanced developmental/treatment level is 14 years or older and sufficiently mature to handle the assignments used in advanced treatment. His stuttering pattern is similar to the intermediate stutter's, but his patterns of avoidance and escape may be more habituated (i.e., patterns appear to be highly automatized and rapidly performed). He will probably avoid difficult speaking situations whenever possible as well. We also often find strong negative self-concepts and anticipated negative listener reactions. An advanced stutterer may feel, for example, "I must be awfully incompetent to talk like this" or "People think I'm dumb because I stutter."

Closing Interview

We assume here that our client is a stutterer. By this point in the evaluation, we have a pretty good picture of his stuttering and where we will start therapy. We begin by summarizing our impression of his stuttering pattern (core and secondary behaviors) and his attitudes and feelings. One of our aims is to let him know we understand him and understand why he does what he does. We feel it is important to let him know that, given his level of stuttering, it is no surprise that he would use the various secondary behaviors and avoidance tactics that he does. We accept these behaviors rather than criticize them. We then let him know that we feel we can work with him to help him discover other ways to respond. We ensure that he feels he will not be alone, that we will be working alongside him, and that we will gradually give him more and more responsibility to work on his own.

We then outline the particular type of therapy we have chosen. Afterward, we may give an adult client an assignment to begin the process of his taking responsibility for part of his treatment. This will also take advantage of the fact that many adult clients are highly motivated to change at the time they come for an evaluation. We generally don't do this with adolescents, but there are exceptions. Some adolescent clients are reluctant, rather than highly motivated, because of the desire to close ranks with their peers and distance themselves from adults. With adolescents, we often end our evaluation session by striking a bargain to try at least four sessions of therapy before they make a decision about treatment. We may also give them the booklet, *Do You Stutter: A Guide for Teens* (Fraser & Perkins, 1987) and the video, *Do You Stutter: Straight Talk for Teens* (Guitar & Conture, 1996) so they can read about therapy on their own and develop realistic (and motivating) expectations about its potential outcome.

At the end of the closing interview, we ask a client if he has any questions about the evaluation. We also try to answer questions asked in the initial interview that we postponed for response until after the evaluation. Adult and adolescent clients sometimes ask how long treatment will take. This is a reasonable question, given that they need to budget time and money to undertake treatment. We have no easy answer for this difficult question. With appropriate cautions about individual differences and unexpected issues, we reply that with hard work and a willingness to tackle their fears, we believe that considerable progress can be made with a year of treatment.

ELEMENTARY SCHOOL CHILD

Preassessment

CASE HISTORY FORM

This form is shown in Figure 7.8 and is the same one we use for preschool children. Of course, many of the questions about speech and language development will be difficult for parents to recall. We should not be too concerned about this for the elementary school-age child, but we should probe for other speech and language delays that may be maintaining factors in an this child's stuttering. An important section on the form for this age child deals with how the problem has changed since it was first noticed, what has been done about it, and how others have reacted to it. In addition, the section on educational history lets us know ahead of time if the child is having problems in school. We discuss this at greater length in the section that follows on academic adjustment.

Assessment

PARENT INTERVIEW

We begin by describing the course of the evaluation, getting some history of the child's problem, and enlisting parents' help in identifying what they believe will enable the child to deal with his problem. We use essentially the same questions as those used for the preschool child's parents (see the section on interviewing parents of the preschool child). However, we sometimes ask parents of a school-age child about his school experiences.

Note: Please complete and return this form before your appointment. Thank you.

Speech Clinic
Stuttering Case History Form—Child and Preteen

Date: _____
Child's name: _____
Address: _____
_____   Tel: _____
Date of birth: _____   Place of birth: _____
Medicaid # _____   Referring physician: _____
Child lives with: Own parents: _____   Other relative: _____
           Foster parents: _____   Institution: _____
(If other than own parents, give name/s):
_____
Referred by: _____
Teacher's name: _____
School (if applicable): _____   Age: _____
School placement or grade level _____
Name of person completing this form: _____
Relationship to child: _____

FAMILY

<u>Father:</u>
  Name: _____   Age: _____
  Living with the family? _____   Occupation: _____
  Employed by: _____
  Educational level _____
  Telephone (home): _____   (Work): _____
  Social Security #: _____

<u>Mother:</u>
  Name: _____   Age: _____
  Living with the family? _____   Occupation: _____
  Employed by: _____
  Educational level _____
  Telephone (home): _____   (Work): _____
  Social Security #: _____

<u>Brothers and sisters:</u>
  (Name)   (Age)   (Name)   (Age)

  _____ _____ _____ _____

  _____ _____ _____ _____

<u>History of Stuttering</u>
Give approximate age at which stuttering was first noticed. _____
Who first noticed or mentioned the stuttering? _____
In what situation was the stuttering first noticed? _____
Describe any situations or conditions that might be associated with the onset of stuttering.
_____
Under what circumstances did the stuttering occur after initial onset?
_____
Were the first signs of stuttering (check all that apply):
    A. Repetitions of the whole word? (boy-boy-boy) _____
    B. Repetitions of the first letter? (b-b-b-boy) _____
    C. Repetitions of the first syllable? (ca-ca-cat) _____
    D. Complete blocks on the first letter? (b. . .oy) _____

(continued)

Figure 7.8. Case history form for school-age and preschool children.

    E. Prolongations of the vowel? (caaaaaaaat) _____

    F. Visible attempt to speak (e.g., mouth movement) but no sound forthcoming? _____

Was the stuttering always the same, or did it occur in several different ways? _____ If it occurred in different ways, how were they different from one another? Describe. _____

_____

Approximately how long did each block (on one word) seem to last? _____

Was the stuttering easy or was there force at the time when the stuttering was first noticed? _

_____

Were the words that were stuttered at the beginning of sentences, or were they scattered throughout the sentence being said? _____

_____

When stuttering first began, was there any avoidance of speaking because of it? Give examples, If any. _____

_____

At the time when stuttering was first noticed, what was the child's reaction?

    Awareness that speech was different? _____   Surprise? _____

    Indifference? _____   Anger or frustration? _____

    Fear of stuttering again? _____   Shame? _____

    Other? Describe. _____

What attempts have been made to treat the stuttering problem (either formally or informally)?

_____

Does the child have articulation or pronunciation problems in addition to stuttering? If so, please describe. _____

_____

Development of Stuttering

Since the onset of stuttering, has there been any change in stuttering symptoms? Check those that are appropriate.

    Increase in number of repetitions per word _____

    Change in amount of force used _____   (Increased? _____   Decreased? _____

    Increase in amount of stuttering _____

    Increase in length of block _____

    Periods of no stuttering _____;   longer periods of stuttering? _____

    More precise in speech attempts _____

    Lowered voice _____

    Slower speech rate _____

    Change in location of force when stuttering (if voice has been present) _____

    Looking away from the listener _____

    Describe any of the above that apply _____

_____

Were there any periods (weeks/months) when the stuttering disappeared? _____

_____

Were there any periods (weeks/months) when stuttering increased? _____

_____

Can you give any explanation for these "worse" periods? _____

_____

Are there any situations that are particularly difficult? If so, describe. _____

_____

List any situations that never cause difficulty. _____

_____

Answer "yes" or "no" to the following as they apply to your (your child's) stuttering.

    Do you stutter when you—

    Talk to young children? _____   Say your name? _____

    Answer direct questions _____   Talk to adults, teachers? _____

    Use new words that are unfamiliar? _____   Use the telephone? _____

    Read out loud? _____   Recite memorized material? _____

Figure 7.8.—*continued*

Ask questions? _____ Talk to strangers? _____
Speak when tired? _____ Speak when excited? _____
Talk to family members? _____ Talk to friends? _____
Do you know any stutterers? _____ Describe your relationship. _____

Do you feel that stuttering interferes with your (your child's) daily life? _____ Social relationships? _____ Success in school? _____

Medical, Developmental, and Family History
Describe mother's health during pregnancy and birth history (i.e., complications). _____

Describe any development problems during infancy or early childhood (i.e., late in walking, feeding problems, food allergies, late in talking) _____

Do you think the child's speech and language development was unusually rapid or delayed? If so, please describe. _____

List all illnesses, injuries, and operations:

Name	Date	Fever	Complications	Treatment	Name of Physician

List all present physical disabilities. _____
Any chronic illnesses, allergies, or physical conditions? _____

Vision normal? _____ Hearing normal? _____
Do other members of the family have speech, language, or reading problems or learning disabilities? If so, please describe. _____

Are any family members left-handed, or do they use both right and left hands equally well? ___

Does the child or other family members show artistic talent or interest? _____

Do any family members talk very rapidly? If so, who? _____

School and Social History
Favorite subjects or activities in school _____
Difficult subjects _____
Hobbies _____ Sports _____
Leisure time activities _____
What specific questions do you have about your child that you would like us to try to answer? (Use back of sheet if necessary.) _____

What goals would you like to see accomplished as a result of this evaluation?
_____
_____

(continued)

Figure 7.8.—*continued*

If, in order to help your child, it is appropriate to send reports to other agencies or professional persons, or to contact other agencies or professional persons, please indicate your permission by signing below.

I authorize and request [fill in name of clinician or clinic] to obtain or exchange pertinent medical/educational information. I understand that all information will be kept confidential.

Name: _____

Relationship to child: _____

Date: _____

Return this completed form at least 2 weeks before your evaluation. You may mail it to [fill in name of clinician or clinic]

Figure 7.8.—*continued*

Does he like school? Does his speech seem to bother him in school? Do you think he stutters more at school than he does at home? Has he gotten therapy in his school?

As we ask parents questions dealing with the child's home environment and school, we listen for answers that may help us understand why the child's stuttering has persisted into elementary school. Here are some of the questions we ask ourselves as we try to integrate the information we are getting: Does this child believe that talking is hard? Does he feel that he has to change to make his speech acceptable to listeners? Have the parents conveyed their high expectations by giving approval only for above-average behavior?

We also need to remember that these parents are probably doing their best with the expectations with which *they* grew up. One of the most important things clinicians can do in a parent interview is to convey an acceptance of the parents as they are and point out the helpful things they have done for their child.

TEACHER INTERVIEW

The more assistance we can get from a child's teachers, the more we can help the child. We need to approach teachers with respect for their heavy responsibilities and their concern for their students, including the one with whom we are working. But we also should anticipate that they may neither understand nor know what we do to help a child who stutters. As we talk with the teacher, we should try to sense what they might like to know about stuttering and our treatment approach. The following questions serve as a guideline for the types of things we want to find out:

1. **Does the child talk in class? Does he stutter? What is his stuttering like? How does he seem to feel about his stuttering and about himself as a communicator?**
   Here we are trying to determine how much the child stutters in class and whether his stuttering might keep him from talking as much as he might otherwise. We may also get a flavor of how the teacher feels about the child and his stuttering.
2. **Does stuttering interfere with the child's academic progress?**
   This question is obviously related to the previous one about how much he talks in

class despite his stuttering. But it also may give us some information about how much he may be avoiding oral performance. We need to ask about disparities between oral and written performance; a big disparity may suggest that he declines to talk or says "I don't know" even when he knows the answer.

3. **Do other children tease him about stuttering?**

   Most children who stutter in school get some teasing, and we need to find out how extensively he is teased and how it affects him.

4. **How does the teacher feel about stuttering and how does he or she react to it?**

   We often are able to get this information indirectly, from what he or she may have said before, but, if not, we should ask directly. The teacher is also likely to ask how he or she *should* respond to stuttering, an important issue because the teacher's response often influences how the class responds. This and other issues related to the child's speech in the classroom are discussed in Chapter 11.

CLASSROOM OBSERVATION

In addition to the information obtained through teacher and parent interviews, some direct observation can help clinicians understand the severity of the child's stuttering and the degree to which it interferes with his academic adjustment. In many cases, if a child is to receive services in the schools, the clinician must establish that the child's stuttering is interfering with his academic performance. What better way to verify this than by first-hand observation of a child in the classroom?

Arrange with the teacher to come to the classroom at a time when the child is likely to be participating in class. Observe unobtrusively, if possible, the performance of the class. By observing the class when many students are participating—not just when the child you are seeing is talking—you do not call as much attention to his speech.

CHILD INTERVIEW

After we obtain the parents' consent to evaluate a child, we ask the child to come to the treatment room where we talk with him for a while. School-age clients sometimes tell us that it helps just to have someone to talk to about stuttering and other things that are bothering them. This can occur only after a trusting relationship is established, and this first interview is the first step in building that relationship.

In our first encounter, it is important for the child to sense that we are genuinely interested in him as well as his stuttering. We usually begin by asking him what he likes to do, with whom he likes to play, and who is in his family. Then we tell him a little about ourselves and how we work with children who sometimes get stuck on words. As he talks, we note whether he stutters or not and how he stutters. When a child's body language and behavior tell us he's comfortable in the situation, we talk to him about his speech. The following questions are not asked in machine-gun style, one right after another, but over a session or two. Often, it is more effective to make the question a comment, such as phrasing the first question below as: "Sometimes kids have trouble getting words out. Words just seem to stick a little bit." Then, leave some silence to see if the youngster will talk about his own speech.

1. **Does the child think that he has any trouble talking?**

   We rarely see school-age stutterers who are unaware of their difficulty. However, if a child regards his problem as minor or seems genuinely unaware of a problem, we try to avoid giving it undue emphasis or create an unfavorable attitude about it. Thus, our first talk with a child is usually low key, and if he truly doesn't seem to be bothered by his stuttering (although his parents and teachers are), we respect his perception and try to treat it as a relatively minor problem, but remain aware that the child may be much more bothered by his stuttering than he wishes to let on at first.

2. **How does the child describe the problem? When does it happen? What is it like at different times?**

   We are looking for several things here. One is to learn the words that the child uses to describe his stuttering so that we can use them when talking with him about it. We also find out if the child is unaware of some of his stuttering behaviors and if they seem to be too painful for him to face, or if he just doesn't like to talk about them. Even more important, these questions let the child know the clinician really wants to understand his problem.

3. **Does he use any helpers or "tricks" to get words out? Does he avoid certain words?**

   With this question, we can convey that we understand what some people often do when they stutter. We can also let the child know that we are nonjudgmental about the "tricks" he uses, by conveying acceptance and interest in his descriptions. In addition, we are also exploring which level the child's stuttering has reached by determining if he is using escape and avoidance behaviors.

4. **Are certain speaking situations more difficult? Does he avoid them?**

   Again, this question helps us to understand what the child is experiencing, while conveying that understanding.

5. **Does anyone ever tease the child about his speech? Who? How does he feel about it? How does he react?**

   Many children who are teased are not willing to talk about it straightaway with someone they don't know well. So this question is a "feeler," and if the child denies being teased, the clinician should not dwell on it now.

6. **How does the child feel about his speech?**

   It is the unusual child who can describe how he feels. To help a child express feelings about stuttering, we may suggest some possibilities by asking, "Does it make you mad sometimes?" or "Do you wish you didn't get stuck?" Don't be surprised if the child says it doesn't bother him, because a child's feelings may have been rejected, perhaps unintentionally, by adults. They may say, for instance, "You don't need to feel that way," or "Why do you let it bother you?" An effective clinician will show the child that whatever he feels is okay, that she is really trying to understand. A real discussion of feelings probably won't begin until a child learns to trust the clinician deeply. But, in this first interview, we may be able to infer what some of the feelings are and, from that, understand how far the child's stuttering has advanced.

   Another avenue to feelings is through drawing pictures. For some children, drawing with crayons or magic markers makes it easier to talk about feelings. The child doesn't have to look directly at the clinician, and his self-consciousness may be decreased somewhat by his focus on the drawing. We simply suggest to a child that both of us draw whatever we would like and as we are drawing, we talk about feelings. If this is going well, we can bridge the gap between the drawing and the talking by suggesting that the child might want to draw a picture of what stuttering is like or of what he feels when he stutters. We have found that this technique can make extensive discussion of feelings much easier for some children. In some cases, children have used their drawings when they talked about stuttering with their class.

7. **How do the child's parents feel about his speech? What do they do when he stutters?**

   This helps us determine what sort of learning experiences the child may have been going through at home. One parent may be much less accepting of a child's stuttering than the other. Whatever we determine may help us to enlist the parents' participation in treatment.

8. **Ask the child, "Can you think of anything else important for me to know about you or about the trouble you sometimes have when you talk?"**

   This is a chance to let the child know that we are interested in him and that we value his ideas.

SPEECH SAMPLE

Pattern of Disfluencies

During interviews with teachers, parents, and the child himself, as well as from the speech samples described here, we extract information about when and how the child stutters. The elementary school child is likely to show beginning or intermediate stuttering, so we want to know as much as possible about the amount of tension in the child's stuttering, the escape behaviors he uses, and the extent to which he avoids words and situations. As with adults or adolescents who stutter, we use this information not only to decide at which developmental/treatment level to place the child, but we also use it, when appropriate, to plan the process of unlearning conditioned responses that once created and now maintain the pattern of stuttering.

Stuttering Severity Instrument

We need a sample of conversational speech and a sample of reading from which to calculate a SSI (Stuttering Severity Instrument). The administration and scoring of the SSI are described in a preceding section in this chapter on the adolescent and adult. It should be noted that there is a separate scoring system for children. With an elementary school child, we tape-record him talking for 5 minutes about school and other activities. We prefer not to turn on the tape recorder the moment the child first walks into the room. Instead, we talk for a few minutes, then ask the child if he would mind if we record our conversation as we talk. Then, we record a sample that includes, optimally, 5 minutes. If only 3 minutes of the child's speech are available, that is acceptable, but we do not advise using less than that. We also record a sample of the child reading for approximately 3 minutes.

Speech Rate

In addition to using these samples for calculating the SSI score, we also use them to assess the child's speaking rate. The purpose of assessing rate is to get some idea of how much the child's stuttering is interfering with the rate of speech he is normally using. As we help the child manage his stuttering, we should expect a steady increase in his speech rate toward normal levels. In the section on evaluation of adolescent and adult stutterers, we described how to calculate speech rate in either words or syllables per minute. The normal rates for school children in Vermont, measured in syllables per minute, are given in Table 7.1. These rates were obtained in children's conversations with a clinician about Christmas, hobbies, school, and home activities. They were calculated by including normal pauses in their conversation, but excluding long pauses (longer than 2 seconds) for thought. It is reasonable to expect children's speech rates in other states will be similar.

Table 7.1. Speech Rates for School Children

Age (yr)	Range in Syllables per Minute
6	140–175
8	150–180
10	165–215
12	165–220

FEELINGS AND ATTITUDES

A fair measure of a child's feelings and attitudes is the clinician's judgment, which usually improves as she gets to know the child better. Nevertheless, the clinician should be able to get a pretty good indication of the child's feelings and attitudes from the first interview. Some indications will result from the clinician's discussion with the child about his feelings, and some will result from observations of his behavior. Watch how the child responds when asked about his stuttering and note how much he avoids stuttering. When the child does stutter, observe how calm he is and how good his eye contact is.

After the clinician has gotten to know the child a bit, she may want to administer a paper and pencil assessment of attitude. In Figure 7.9, we present an attitude scale we have occasionally used to assess children's communication attitudes, the A-19 scale (Guitar & Grims, 1977). This scale consists of questions that we have found will distinguish between children who stutter and children who do not. Hence, if treatment is effective, a child's attitude about communication may change, although this has not been established by research.

In addition to the A-19, the Communication Attitude Test (CAT) (Fig. 7.10), which was developed by Brutten, has been tested on normal children (Brutten & Dunham, 1989) and shown to differentiate them from stuttering children (De Nil & Brutten, 1991). Both tests are probably ineffective if given before a trusting relationship with the client has developed.

OTHER SPEECH AND LANGUAGE DISORDERS

In our discussion of the preschool child, we described the importance of screening language, articulation, and voice. The same variables should be assessed in the elementary school child, although if this child has a language or articulation (and, to a lesser extent, voice) problem, it may have been diagnosed previously and the child may be in therapy. If so, the clinician should seek out details of any current or previous therapy. We have previously suggested articulation assessment procedures that would be appropriate for the elementary school child. Language assessment for this age child is well described in Lund and Duchan (1988) and Wiig and Semel (1984).

If a child has received articulation or language therapy in the past, the clinician should determine the type of treatment the child received and how he responded. Did he overcome his articulation or language difficulties? Did his stuttering first appear or worsen during treatment? If so, the clinician should pay particular attention to indications that the child may think of himself as a poor speaker and may believe that speaking is difficult. The interviews and questionnaires we suggested in this section will help the clinician explore this possibility, and the therapy approaches described in Chapters 11 and 13 are designed to help a child regain confidence in his ability to speak.

A-19 Scale for Children Who Stutter

Susan Andre and Barry Guitar
University of Vermont

Establish rapport with the child, and make sure that he or she is physically comfortable before beginning administration. Explain the task to the child and make sure he or she understands what is required. Some simple directions might be used:

"I am going to ask you some questions. Listen carefully and then tell me what you think:
Yes or No. There is no right or wrong answer. I just want to know what you think.

To begin the scale, ask the questions in a natural manner. Do not urge the child to respond before he or she is ready, and repeat the question if the child did not hear it or you feel that he or she did not understand it. Do not re-word the question unless you feel it is absolutely necessary, and then write the question you asked under that item.

Circle the answer that corresponds to the child's response. Be accepting of the child's response because there is no right or wrong answer. If all the child will say is "I don't know" even after prompting, record that response next to the question.

For the younger children (kindergarten and first grade), it might be necessary to give a few simple examples to ensure comprehension of the requited task:

a.	Are you a boy?	Yes	No
b.	Do you have black hair?	Yes	No

Similar, obvious questions may be inserted, if necessary, to reassure the examiner that the child is <u>actively</u> cooperating at all times. Adequately praise the child for listening and assure him or her that a good job is being done.

It is important to be familiar with the questions so that they can be read in a natural manner.

The child is given 1 point for each answer that matches those given below. The higher a child's score, the more probable it is that he or she has developed negative attitudes toward communication. In our study, the mean score of the K through 4th grade stutterers (N = 28) was 9.07 (S.D. = 2.44), and for the 28 matched controls, it was 8.17 (S.D. = 1.80).

Score 1 point for each answer that matches these:

1. Yes	10. No
2. Yes	11. No
3. No	12. No
4. No	13. Yes
5. No	14. Yes
6. Yes	15. Yes
7. No	16. No
8. Yes	17. No
9. Yes	18. Yes
	19. Yes

(continued)

Figure 7.9. A-19 Scale of Children's Communication Attitudes. (Reprinted with permission from Susan Andre.)

A-19 SCALE

Name _____   Date _____

1. Is it best to keep your mouth shut when you are in trouble?	Yes	No
2. When the teacher calls on you, do you get nervous?	Yes	No
3. Do you ask a lot of questions in class?	Yes	No
4. Do you like to talk on the phone?	Yes	No
5. If you did not know a person, would you tell your name?	Yes	No
6. Is it hard to talk to your teacher?	Yes	No
7. Would you go up to a new boy or girl in your class?	Yes	No
8. Is it hard to keep control of your voice when talking?	Yes	No
9. Even when you know the right answer, are you afraid to say it?	Yes	No
10. Do you like to tell other children what to do?	Yes	No
11. Is it fun to talk to your dad?	Yes	No
12. Do you like to tell stories to your classmates?	Yes	No
13. Do you wish you could say things as clearly as the other kids do?	Yes	No
14. Would you rather look at a comic book than talk to a friend?	Yes	No
15. Are you upset when someone interrupts you?	Yes	No
16. When you want to say something, do you just say it?	Yes	No
17. Is talking to your friends more fun than playing by yourself?	Yes	No
18. Are you sometimes unhappy?	Yes	No
19. Are you a little afraid to talk on the phone?	Yes	No

Figure 7.9.—*continued*

OTHER FACTORS

Other factors can influence the outcome of treatment. We recommend evaluating all factors that may have precipitated or are maintaining a child's stuttering, so that they may be included in the overall treatment plan.

Physical Development

Our main concern in this area is that motor development may lag behind language development. A child with a speech-motor delay may benefit from fluency shaping therapy that helps him coordinate respiration, phonation, and articulation, thereby reducing stuttering. He may also benefit from stuttering modification procedures that help him learn to stutter easily and openly, rather than becoming tense and frustrated, if his fluency breaks down under stress. This child's treatment should also focus on building self-esteem, which may be low in children who are not well coordinated.

Cognitive Development

We need to find out whether or not the cognitive stresses of school are increasing the general demands experienced by the child. This is discussed further in a following section on

Name _____   Age: _____
                                          Sex: _____
                                          Grade: _____

Communication Attitude Test
Gene J. Brutten, Ph.D.
Southern Illinois University

Read each sentence carefully so you can say if it is true or false <u>for you</u>. The sentences are about talking. If <u>you</u> feel that the sentence is right, circle true. If <u>you</u> think the sentence about your talking is not right, circle false. Remember, circle false if <u>you</u> think the sentence is wrong and true if <u>you</u> think it is right.

1. I don't talk right	True	False
2. I don't mind asking the teacher a question in class.	True	False
3. Sometimes words stick in my mouth when I talk.	True	False
4. People worry about the way I talk.	True	False
5. It is harder for me to give a report in class than it is for most of the other kids.	True	False
6. My classmates don't think I talk funny.	True	False
7. I like the way I talk.	True	False
8. People sometimes finish words for me.	True	False
9. My parents like the way I talk.	True	False
10. I find it easy to talk to most everyone.	True	False
11. I talk well most of the time.	True	False
12. It is hard for me to talk to people.	True	False
13. I don't talk like other children.	True	False
14. I don't worry about the way I talk.	True	False
15. I don't find it easy to talk.	True	False
16. My words come out easily.	True	False
17. It is hard for me to talk to strangers.	True	False
18. The other kids wish they could talk like me.	True	False
19 Some kids make fun of the way I talk.	True	False
20. Talking is easy for me.	True	False
21. Telling someone my name is hard for me.	True	False
22. Words are hard for me to say.	True	False
23. I talk well with most everyone.	True	False
24. Sometimes I have trouble talking.	True	False
25. I would rather talk than write.	True	False
26. I like to talk.	True	False
27. I am not a good talker.	True	False
28. I wish I could talk like other children.	True	False

(continued)

Figure 7.10. Communication Attitude Test. (Copyright 1985 Gene Brutten.)

29. I am afraid the words won't come out when I talk.	True	False
30. My friends don't talk as well as I do.	True	False
31. I don't worry about talking on the phone.	True	False
32. I talk better with a friend.	True	False
33. People don't seem to like the way I talk.	True	False
34. I let others talk for me.	True	False
35. Reading aloud in class is easy for me.	True	False

Score I point for each answer that matches these:

I. True	9. False	17. True	25. False	33. True
2. False	10. False	18. False	26. False	34. True
3. True	11. False	19. True	27. True	35. False
4. True	12. True	20. False	28. True	
5. True	13. True	21. True	29. True	
6. False	14. False	22. True	30. False	
7. False	15. True	23. False	31. False	
8. True	16. False	24. True	32. True	

In a study using this scale on Belgian children (De Nil and Brutten, 1990) mean score of a group of children who stutter (N = 70) was 16.7; mean score of a group of children who do not stutter (N = 271) was 8.71.

Figure 7.10.—*continued*

academic adjustment. If a child has academic difficulty or a learning disability, we may need to adjust our approach to treatment so that he understands our explanations and examples.

Social-Emotional Development

We are interested in how well the child fits in with his classmates, how comfortable he feels about talking and relating to others, and how often he feels a need to hide his stuttering. Some children are friendly and outgoing and are supported by their classmates, whether they stutter or not. These social skills are a positive factor in their prognosis for recovery from stuttering. Other children have not outgrown their self-centeredness, and stuttering compounds their self-concern and keeps them from relating easily to others. Such children need help in relating more easily to their classmates. Evaluation of this component can be done through teacher, parent, and child interviews; classroom observation may be helpful, too.

We are also concerned with the extent to which a child's home environment provides support and security. This information comes primarily from parent and child interviews. Parents often provide insight into conditions surrounding the onset of stuttering and conditions under which it gets better or worse. We sift through the evidence with the parents' help to determine whether there are things that can be done to improve the child's self-esteem. For some children, school psychologists have been helpful in building self-esteem and helping them improve their social adjustment.

Academic Adjustment

Parent, child, and teacher interviews let us find out how well the child is doing in school and how much he likes it. Stuttering may appear for the first time or worsen when a child is under the additional stress of learning many new things. For example, reading aloud in class when just learning to read may put substantial demands on a child's resources for language formulation and speech production. The child must make "second-order mappings of meanings and lexical units from speech" (Gibson, 1972) while simultaneously translating the written representation into units appropriate for speech production. Thus, some academic challenges may be more demanding for a child who stutters, and his stuttering in school should be understood in relation to this. In practical terms, the clinician can determine whether a child needs extra help in certain academic areas through discussions with his teachers about which speaking situations in school are most difficult. If the child has more difficulty in certain academic situations, these should be given extra attention when planning generalization of more fluent speech.

Diagnosis

At this point, we pull together the information we have collected from the case history, parent, teacher, and child interviews, speech samples, and classroom observations. We determine what developmental/treatment level the child's stuttering has reached, which will give us specific directions for the specific treatment. We also assess the various developmental and environmental influences that may still be operating on the child and make plans to alleviate those that can be changed and help the child cope with those that can't.

Most elementary school children are beginning or intermediate stutterers. As you will remember, beginning-level stuttering is characterized by physical tension, hurry, escape behaviors, awareness of difficulty, and feelings of frustration. The intermediate level also involves tension, hurry, escape behaviors, and frustration, but in addition avoidance behaviors are common as a result of fear and anticipation of stuttering. These levels were described in detail in Chapter 5. In addition to a child's stuttering behaviors and feelings, current developmental and environmental pressures must be considered in planning treatment. These pressures are uncovered from parent, teacher, and child interviews and the speech sample. Some of these pressures may be other speech and language disorders, motor problems, or pressures in the child's home. Some can be dealt with in our treatment, but others may require parent counseling or referral to other professionals.

Closing Interview

The closing interview provides an opportunity to summarize our immediate impressions for parents and make recommendations about treatment. It also gives us a chance to discuss the crucial role parents can play in reducing environmental pressures. We stay away from jargon. We let them know the many beneficial things they have done with their child's speech, and we assure them that the stuttering was not caused by anything they have done. Although some parents may have created conditions in which a child's predisposition to stutter has been transformed into a serious problem, it does not help to make an issue of this. Rather, we want to convince them that they are in a key position to help.

After describing clearly and in plain English what we observed about the child's stuttering, we summarize our thinking about appropriate treatment. We do this in only general terms because parents' main concerns at this time are not the details of treatment but about the prospects for their child's future. Therefore, we rely on our experience to describe likely outcomes. For example, we might say that a combination of many factors will determine the child's outcome. These include the natural increases in fluency that occur as a child matures, feelings of self-acceptance that a child develops when he finds that people accept him whether or not he has trouble with his speech, and his learning ways to speak more fluently. When we talk about the child's prognosis, we always want to include some aspect of the parents' role, such as their acceptance of the child's speech or their participation in treatment, as part of the formula for recovery.

After summarizing our impressions and describing some of the ingredients for recovery, we then discuss some of the things the parents can do to promote recovery. Specific suggestions depend on findings from our interviews, but the sections on parent counseling in Chapters 11 and 13 (on integrated approaches to beginning and intermediate stuttering) present general ideas for parents' involvement. Discussion of the family's involvement in therapy is the most important part of the closing interview and, in fact, may continue for several more meetings. If we treat the child directly and in a clinic rather than in a school setting, we meet with parents on a regular basis as part of treatment. In these meetings, we continue to help parents explore how various changes in the home environment can facilitate their child's fluency.

As we have said before, several aspects of an evaluation differ when we see a child in a school setting. School clinicians may not always be able to discuss the details of their findings with parents in person if parents are unable to come to the school. In such cases, which we hope will be infrequent, much of the continuing contact with the parents may have to be carried out by telephone. The closing interview follows a staffing team meeting concerning the child, in which teachers, other professionals, and parents discuss the child's speech and develop a treatment plan. The parents' permission to treat the child is then obtained. At this time or at a later parent counseling session, recommendations for environmental change are discussed. Many times a clinician can continue to meet with parents throughout treatment and to work with them to facilitate change in the child's speech. Our experience has been that many parents who are tentative at first become more involved in their child's treatment after the clinician has shown continued interest in the child and an accepting attitude toward the parents. However, there are other parents who, for one reason or another, do not become involved. In these cases, the clinician and others must try to provide some of the missing parent support. We try to give a child enough successful communication experiences to offset other environmental pressures that cannot be dealt with directly.

PRESCHOOL CHILD

Preassessment

CASE HISTORY FORM

This form, shown in Figure 7.8 (the same as that used for the elementary school child), is sent to the parents several weeks before the child's assessment. The case history informs the clinician about the parents' perception of the problem at present, as well as about onset and development. This information is used as a starting place for further questions during the parent interview.

TAPE RECORDING

We ask parents of a preschool child to send us an audiotape or videotape of their child speaking in a typical home situation, along with the case history form. This allows us to preview the child's speech soon after the parents have contacted us. In cases in which several weeks go by between the parents' contact and our evaluation, the child's stuttering may have diminished substantially and we may observe only a fluent cycle of the child's speech. In addition to previewing the child's stuttering, the tape often gives us a chance to learn a little about parent-child interactions.

Assessment

PARENT-CHILD INTERACTION

When possible, we observe one or both parents interacting with their child. We prefer to do this at the beginning of the evaluation for several reasons. First, parents may be less affected by our orientation toward stuttering, thereby giving us a more natural sample. Second, this interaction gives us a chance to see the child's stuttering first-hand. We can note, for example, how much the child seems aware of stuttering, how much accessory behavior there is, and whether or not the child appears embarrassed. These are not things that may be evident from an audiotape. Third, we can observe the ways in which the parents interact with their child. Do they interrupt? Do they correct? Do they talk at a fast rate, using complex vocabulary and syntax? These observations add to what we learned from an audiotape and provide a basis for planning our parent interview and recommendations for treatment.

The parent-child interaction can be done formally or informally. Some clinicians observe interaction in the waiting room and make only mental notes about it. Others who work in preschool programs may visit a child's home and arrange to observe parent-child interactions while they sit quietly in the same room. Still others, ourselves included, videotape the parents and child in a play-style interaction in a treatment room supplied with toys and games. When audiotaping or videotaping of these interactions is possible, this sample of the child's speech can be assessed as described in the later section on the speech sample.

PARENT INTERVIEW

We begin by letting parents know what we will be doing with them and their child during the evaluation. We assure them there will be a time at the end for us to share our opinions and recommendations. Sometimes during an initial interview, parents ask direct questions about things they may be doing wrong. We let them know that, in our view, stuttering is often the result of many factors acting together and that parents do not cause it. We rarely give advice—about what they should change or what they should do—until after we have interviewed the parents and assessed the child directly. In our experience, we are more accurate and parents are more receptive to recommendations if we delay discussion of what to do until after all available information has been pulled together in the closing interview.

We begin the initial interview by asking parents to describe the problem their child is having. We ask an open-ended question such as "Tell me about Billy's speech" or "Please describe Billy's speech and tell me what concerns you." When they have had a chance to share their concerns, we ask about the child's birth and development. We seldom ask all of the 19 questions that follow. Instead, we find out what we want to know during a discussion that is punctuated by both their questions and ours. We list these questions because we have found information in these areas to be helpful.

1. Were there any problems with your pregnancy or the birth of this child?
   Although there is little evidence that stutterers as a group have difficult birth histo-

ries, there is an increased incidence of stuttering among brain-damaged individuals. Thus, we are seeking to determine whether we should suspect the possibility of congenital brain damage. If a difficult pregnancy or birth is noted, we might examine the child's motor and cognitive development more closely. The case history form, which is completed before the evaluation, provides preliminary information about birth history that may or may not need to be followed up.

2. **What was the child's speech and language development like? How did it compare with siblings' development and with your expectations?**

   Because we believe that the first appearance of stuttering may be influenced by the "processing load" that language acquisition has on speech production, we think it is important to understand the course of a child's overall speech and language development. We explore the possibility that a child's language acquisition is proceeding so rapidly that the motor system cannot keep up with it. We also examine the possibility that a child's language development is delayed, and he is frustrated and finding it hard to talk. As mentioned in Chapter 2, there is some evidence that poorer language skills are predictive of persistent stuttering.

3. **Describe the child's motor development compared with that of his brothers, sisters, or other children.**

   We are interested in the parents' general impressions. Does this child seem to be developing motor skills like other children his age, or do his parents think he may be delayed? Some indicators of the normal range of gross and fine motor development, as well as personal-social and speech-language development, can be found in the Denver Developmental Screening Test (Frankenburg & Dodds, 1967).

   In our experience, many children who stutter appear to be slightly advanced in their language and, to a lesser extent, slightly delayed in their motor skills. Or, they may be well advanced in language but with completely normal motor skills. In either case, these children seem to benefit from models of speech produced at a slow rate. Other children who stutter may be delayed in several areas; they may need treatment for language and articulation that is integrated with therapy for stuttering.

4. **Have any other members of your family had speech or language disorders?**

   We ask this general question, then ask more specifically whether family members or other relatives have ever stuttered, had articulation or language disorders, or have been clutterers. To confirm that a disorder was a problem, we ask if the person ever received treatment. We use this information when we discuss stuttering as a disorder that may have predisposing factors. Handled tactfully, this discussion of predisposing factors helps parents realize that their child's stuttering was not something they caused. This, in turn, can help them be more effective in facilitating the child's fluency if they do not feel anxious about moments of stuttering because of guilt.

   If a parent stutters, or used to stutter, he or she may have strong negative feelings about the disorder, including guilt. Such feelings need to be discussed in the initial interview and throughout any treatment the child receives. The way in which a parent handles stuttering is also important because this behavior will serve as a model for the child. A parent who avoids words or otherwise tries to hide his stuttering is communicating an attitude to the child that may move the child to the intermediate level faster than if the parent accepts his stuttering, comments neutrally about it in front of the child, and uses facilitating techniques to handle it.

   If relatives of the child stutter, it is important to find out whether or not they recovered. Research cited earlier found that among children who were identified within 6 months of the onset of stuttering, those with relatives who did not recover from stuttering were more likely to have persistent stuttering than those with relatives who did recover.

After obtaining this background information, we turn to the onset and development of the child's stuttering.

5. **When was the child's disfluency first noticed?**
We have found that, if treatment is begun soon after the child starts to stutter—within a few weeks or months, rather than a year or more—we have a better chance of preventing negative feelings from building up, for both the parents and child. Therefore, we praise parents for bringing a child in promptly for an evaluation, if they have done so soon after they first sensed there was a problem. Another reason we want to know how much time has passed since onset is that most of the predictive information on chronicity of stuttering is based on children identified within 6 months of onset. For example, in a study by Yairi, Ambrose, Paden, and Throneburg (1996), children who recovered from their stuttering began to show a steady decline in stuttering within the 12 months after their stuttering was first identified. Children whose stuttering persisted for at least 3 years did not show such a decline. Therefore, knowing how long it has been since the onset of a child's stuttering helps us to make treatment decisions, based on findings that some children are likely to recover without therapy.

6. **Was anything special going on in the child's life when the stuttering started?**
This may provide some leads about the kinds of pressures to which a child may be vulnerable, which can help clinicians determine what changes the parents can make to reduce stuttering. Events that may contribute to the onset of stuttering include the birth of a sibling, moving to a new home, and growth spurts in language or cognition. Many times, there are no special circumstances at the onset of stuttering, which should be acknowledged to parents so they don't feel that they are to blame for the stuttering.

7. **What was the disfluency like when it was first noticed?**
Most stuttering begins with easy repetitions, although some children begin with prolongations and blocks as well. Some preliminary information suggests that when repetitions sound quite rapid (when the pause between repetition units is brief), a child is more likely to be stuttering rather than being normally disfluent (Allen, 1988; Throneburg & Yairi, 1994). These rapid-sounding repetitions may be predictive of persistent stuttering (Yairi, Ambrose, Paden, & Throneburg, 1996). This difference cannot be diagnosed accurately without instrumentation, but a practiced ear can help a clinician perceive the brevity of pauses between repetition units. This information should be used only in support of an overall pattern of findings that help the clinician decide whether or not to recommend treatment.

8. **What changes, if any, have been observed in the child's speech since stuttering was first noticed?**
The changes we are most interested in include frequency of disfluencies, types of disfluencies, and periods of remission. As indicated in the discussion of question 5, children whose frequency of stuttering disfluencies (part-word and single-syllable whole-word repetitions, prolongations, and blocks) does not decrease during the 12 months after onset are at risk for becoming persistent stutterers. In our clinical experience, if a child's physical tension and struggle during stuttering are increasing or if stuttering is becoming more consistent and less intermittent, the child is beyond the borderline level of stuttering and treatment should be considered.

We now turn to current observations of the disorder:

9. Does the child appear to be aware of his disfluency?

If the child appears to have no awareness, we are more likely to categorize him as normally disfluent or as a borderline stutterer than if he notices or seems concerned by his disfluencies. If he is aware that he has difficulty speaking or shows frustration, he may be a beginning stutterer. Note that such awareness may not be negative, but just a neutral level of awareness at early stages. Indications of the child's awareness include such things as his commenting on his stuttering, either when it occurs or at some other time, and the fact that other people have brought it to his attention. Awareness is also suggested if a child stops when he is disfluent and starts again or if he laughs, cries, or hits himself when he stutters. Even without any of these signs, a child may still be aware of his stuttering.

In some instances, preschool children may show more than just neutral awareness and frustration; they may show negative feelings about talking and may have fear of certain words. They may comment that they wished they could speak like someone else or may show some word avoidances.

10. Does the child sometimes appear to change a word because he expects to be disfluent on it?

Parents are usually able to guess this is happening because they can sense the child's apprehension about saying a word. We may also ask if the child changes words in midstream; that is, does he start a word, get stuck on it, and then change it? Both behaviors are not good signs and may indicate that the child is moving toward the intermediate stage of stuttering development.

11. Does the child seem to avoid talking in some situations, when he expects to be disfluent?

Again, this is something most parents know because they sense the child's fear of talking, and like the word avoidance discussed in question 9, this behavior may indicate an intermediate level of stuttering.

12. What do the parents believe caused the problem?

In some cases, parents may have ideas, which we believe are appropriate and accurate, about the possible cause of their child's stuttering. In other cases, parents' beliefs about causal factors may be incorrect, and we respond by providing more accurate information. We are particularly sensitive to whether or not parents blame themselves or each other for their child's stuttering. This is usually a good time to let the parents know that they are not to blame. We tell them that some children may have slight differences in their neurological organization for speech, which may emerge as stuttering during the normal stresses and strains of growing up and learning to talk. The parents should know that they didn't cause the child's stuttering, but they should also know that they can play a key role in the child's learning to deal with it.

13. How do the parents feel about the child's disfluency problem?

The kinds of feelings and attitudes we are looking for are: Do they feel concern? Guilt? Do they just assume the child will outgrow it? These parental feelings will obviously influence the child. Counseling may be needed to alleviate these feelings. If the parents feel guilty, counseling to relieve guilt is important. If the child is normally disfluent, but the parents are overly concerned, counseling can be directed at relieving this concern, so that the child himself does not become excessively concerned and develop stuttering.

14. What, if anything, have the parents done about the disfluency problem?

This question is aimed at finding out how the parents have responded to the child's disfluency. For example, have they asked the child to slow down or stop and say the word again? This will direct us in what we do in counseling. If parents are correcting the child, we may ask them first to observe, then participate in treatment soon after we begin, so that they may develop appropriate ways of responding.

15. **Has the child been seen anywhere else for the problem? If so, what were the outcomes?**

This information can be important in planning therapy and counseling parents. For example, if their family doctor has told them the child will outgrow stuttering, their experience needs to be dealt with, since they now are less convinced he will outgrow it. If the child has been in other treatment, it is important to know what advice the parents were given. Sometimes, parents have been given excellent advice but were not able to follow it. We need to find out why and to help them change their responses. We sometimes find that parents have had their child in successful therapy but have moved away and sought us out to continue the same kind of treatment. In these cases, we try to contact the previous therapist and explore with the parents what was done, so that we can continue to work in the same direction as before. In some cases, parents come to us seeking a second opinion, and we are able to reinforce what others have said, if we agree. In other cases, they may have been advised to ignore the child's stuttering, and we may tactfully discuss the possibility of going in an entirely different direction.

16. **When and in which situations does the child exhibit the most disfluency? The least disfluency?**

This information helps to identify fluency disrupters and fluency facilitators. We will want to use this information to help parents facilitate the child's fluency and have found it effective to point out, whenever possible, all the helpful things the parents are already doing. Just the awareness that their child's stuttering responds to environmental cues, and thereby has some logic to it, helps most parents to feel more competent to manage it.

After we believe that we understand a child's current stuttering behavior, we ask about social and emotional development.

17. **How does the child get along with his brothers and sisters and other children?**

We usually find that children who stutter relate fairly well to others, but we want to find out if a child's stuttering is interfering with his relationships. Sometimes, when asking this question, we learn about pressure and competition from siblings or teasing by a neighborhood bully.

18. **What is the child's personality and temperament like?**

Some children who stutter are more sensitive and fearful than other children. A child with this temperament may benefit from extra help in developing self-confidence.

We then finish with an open-ended question, like this:

19. **Is there anything else you can think of to tell us that will help us better understand your child's stuttering?**

Sometimes, it is not possible to direct questions to all areas of concern, and this question provides an opportunity for parents to provide information that we have not thought of asking.

CLINICIAN-CHILD INTERACTION

One of the most important parts of a preschool evaluation is the interaction between the clinician and the child. Here, the clinician can see firsthand what the child's disfluency is like, how he responds to various cues, and how well he can modify his disfluency. We always tape-record this interaction for later analysis because it is difficult to make notes as we interact. If videotape is available, it is preferable to audiotape because visual cues are often critical in determining a child's developmental/treatment level. If audiotape must be used, the clinician should make notes on visual aspects of the child's disfluencies.

We focus our interactions on toys or games that are suitable to the child's age. The Playskool farm or airport is a good example. We play alongside the child, letting him direct the action, commenting on what he's doing or playing with. We refrain from questions when we first start and talk in an easy, relaxed manner, much like we advise parents to do.

If a child is stuttering similarly to the way the parents described, we maintain the same speech style throughout the interaction. However, if a child is entirely fluent or normally disfluent and the parents have described behaviors typical of stuttering, we speed up our speech rate and ask many questions. Occasionally, we interrupt the child to elicit disfluent speech, which may be more characteristic. We do this to avoid misdiagnosing a child who is stuttering as a normally fluent speaker.

An adult client of ours described an experience that illustrates our concern. When she was 5, she stuttered quite severely, and her parents were understandably concerned. Seeking the best help, her mother took her to a famous midwestern university speech clinic for an evaluation. For reasons she never understood, she was relatively fluent throughout the entire evaluation. The clinicians observed her temporary fluency, and, despite her mother's protestations that her daughter stuttered at home, labeled her as a normal-speaking child and advised her mother to ignore any disfluency. Her disfluency gradually worsened, and she became a severe, chronic stutterer.

We realize that, even by putting pressure on the child, we may not elicit stuttering that the child has in other settings. Thus, the parents' report and recording made before the evaluation are of vital importance for a full understanding of a child's speech.

Talking About Stuttering

Before the clinician-child interaction, we try to determine whether the child is aware of his stuttering. If we think he isn't, we use observations of only nondirective play to assess his speech. If it seems clear from earlier information or our own observation that he is aware of his stuttering, we then try to determine how comfortable the child is in talking about his stuttering. Sometimes, we ask him if he knows why he has come to see us. Most children answer noncommittally, but some are very forthcoming and say something like, "Because I don't talk right." This gives us an opening to discuss his stuttering. It is also an important opportunity to let the child know that he isn't alone—that we know other children who get stuck on words and we are usually able to help them.

Some clinicians help a child to talk about his stuttering by first talking about another child who stutters (Bloodstein, personal communication, 1990). In discussing stuttering with a child, we usually try to use their vocabulary such as "getting stuck" or "having trouble on words." If the child indicates in his answer to why he came to the evaluation that he isn't interested in discussing stuttering, we drop the issue for the moment and return to playing. Then, later, we will insert a few normal-sounding disfluencies in our speech and comment that we sometimes have trouble getting words out. We might play some more, then insert a few more disfluencies and ask the child if he ever has trouble like this. As before, the child's answer will either indicate that he remains unwilling to discuss stuttering or will give the clinician an opening to discuss little by little the child's problem with disfluency. In summary, the goals of these attempts to discuss the child's disfluency with him are (a) to see if the child accepts himself and his disfluencies enough to discuss them and (*b*) to indicate to the child that he is not alone with the problem and that we may be able to help him.

A Child Who Won't Talk

At times, we may encounter a preschooler, especially a child who has trouble talking, who is reluctant to separate from his parents. This may occur after observing the parent-child interaction and we try to take the parents to another room for an interview while another clinician interacts with the child. A shy child may start to cry and cling to his parents. We would not force the child to separate. It is more important to have the child positively inclined toward the therapy situation than to have unpleasant memories of his first visit, even if we don't get all the information we want. In this situation, we talk with the parents in one part of the room while a clinician plays with the child in another part. We talk for a few minutes about general things, such as a typical day in their home or how they handle discipline, letting the child become familiar with the clinician with whom he's interacting. Then, we may suggest to the parents that we move to an adjacent room but keep the door open. With this arrangement, we usually can talk about sensitive matters without being overheard. An alternative would be to let the child follow, leaving the clinician and toys in the first room and both doors open. The child may then become bored with the room in which we are talking with his parents and wander back to the other room with the other clinician and the toys. In our experience, it is rare that a child has more than a momentary difficulty in separating from his parents.

Sometimes a child separates from his parents but won't interact with us during the evaluation. Under these circumstances, we avoid asking direct questions and take some time to play alongside the child, verbalizing as we do so. After several minutes, we usually find that the child relaxes and begins to speak spontaneously. After this continues for several more minutes, we begin more direct interactions by asking questions about the toys with which we are playing. Only after the child gets comfortable with us do we attempt to discuss his trouble talking, and then only if we're sure he is aware of his stuttering. With some children, we do not attempt to discuss stuttering. We always take our cues from the child and go slowly in this area. We can infer many things about a child's feelings from observations rather than direct questions.

A Child Who Is Entirely Fluent

Some preschool children who stutter may be entirely fluent during an evaluation. In these cases, there are several options. First, the tape recording we asked the parent to send us may have a good enough sample of stuttering to assess as the speech sample. Second, if the child is in a particularly fluent period, we may reschedule him for evaluation at a later time. If our recommendations to the parents enable them to change the environment enough in the meantime so that the child remains fluent, the parents may wish to postpone the evaluation until and if the stuttering returns.

SPEECH SAMPLE

This section describes how to analyze the sample of a preschool child's speech. Our procedures usually provide us with more than one speech sample to choose from: a tape recording the parents have sent in, the parent-child interaction, and the clinician-child interaction during the evaluation. We choose the sample that has the greatest amount of stuttering for the most detailed analysis, but we also note the extent of stuttering/fluency on the other samples.

Pattern of Disfluencies

In this analysis, we want information about whether or not the child is a stutterer and, if so, what developmental/treatment level he belongs in. We analyze the following six variables to begin this determination. Our choice of variables owes much to a number of authors who have written about the differential diagnosis of preschool stuttering (Adams, 1977; Curlee, 1984; Riley & Riley, 1979).

1. Frequency of disfluencies. This is calculated on the entire sample and is expressed as the number of disfluencies per 100 words (see Chapter 5 for details). Both normal disfluencies and those associated with stuttering are included in this count. Normally disfluent children usually have fewer than 10 disfluencies per 100 words.
2. Types of disfluencies. We identified eight types of disfluencies in Chapter 5: part-word repetitions, single-syllable word repetitions, multisyllable word repetitions, phrase repetitions, interjections, revisions-incomplete phrases, prolongations, and tense pauses. Children who are normally disfluent are likely to have more revisions and multisyllable whole-word repetitions. Below age 3½ years, they also have many interjections. Part-word repetitions, single-syllable word repetitions, prolongations, and tense pauses are more characteristic of stuttering children.
3. Nature of repetitions and prolongations. There are several dimensions to this variable. First, normally disfluent children are more likely to have only one extra unit in a repetition: li-like this. They may sometimes have two. But, as the number of repetition units increase, so does the likelihood that the child is stuttering. Second, we listen to the tempo of repetitions. If they are slow and regular, the child is more likely to be categorized appropriately as a normally disfluent speaker. If they are rapid or irregular, it is more likely that the child is stuttering. Third, we observe the amount of tension in both the repetitions and prolongations. Both visual and auditory cues help here; tension can be seen in facial expression and heard in increased pitch and more staccato voice quality. Children whom we would label as normally disfluent seldom show tension in their disfluencies.
4. Starting and sustaining airflow and phonation. The child whom we usually categorize as a stutterer often shows difficulty here. He may have abrupt onsets and offsets of words, especially repeated words, or momentary pauses with fixed articulator positions at the onset of words. Moreover, transitions between words may seem abrupt, jerky, or broken much of the time.
5. Physical concomitants. We look for physical gestures that accompany disfluencies, especially those that are timed to the release of a disfluent sound. Examples are head nods, eye blinks, and hand or finger movements. We also include such extra noises as the child gritting his teeth or clicking his tongue.
6. Word avoidances. Another sign we sometimes see in a disfluent preschool child that suggests that he stutters is word avoidance. This can be blatant, as when a child starts a word and then changes it, as in "pu-pu-pu. . . . dog," or it may be more subtle, as when saying "I don't know," when it's clear that he does know. We also ask about word avoidances when we interview the child's parents. When a clinician interacts with a child, she may sometimes miss avoidances in a live interaction, and it may take a viewing of the tape to pick them up. For example, after a recent evaluation, we noted on the tape a very subtle avoidance that we had completely missed in the face-to-face interaction. We had asked the child what he was going to dress as for Halloween. He pursed his lips for a "B," but when he couldn't say the word, he quickly sang "Na-na-na-na-na-na-na-nah! Batman!"

In our experience, if a child shows any of the characteristics of stuttering just described, he should be considered at least as a borderline stutterer. The presence of tension, stoppage of airflow or phonation, physical concomitants, or word avoidances would place him on a level above borderline. Details on this placement are given in the sections on diagnosis that follow.

Stuttering Severity Instrument (SSI)

By this time in an evaluation, we should have a fairly good indication as to whether or not the child is normally disfluent or is stuttering. If he is stuttering, we will want to obtain a standard sample of speech to analyze with Riley's SSI, shown in Figure 7.3 (see the adult and adolescent evaluation section for details on this reference). Riley suggests that any child below third grade should be asked to describe a set of pictures to provide a sample of 150 words for analysis. The child may also be engaged in conversation, and if this sample shows more stuttering than the picture description, it should be used for the analysis. We typically use a 5-minute sample, rather than a 150-word sample, because it is easier to interact naturally with the child for 5 minutes (which ensures a large enough sample) than to try to count words as we interact. Frequency of stuttering, mean duration of the three longest stutters, and physical concomitants are scored, and a total score is computed. The total score permits labeling severity from Very Mild to Very Severe.

Speech Rate

We assess the rate of preschool children's speech using the speech sample obtained for the SSI. Details on counting and timing procedures were given in an earlier section on assessment of speech rate of adults and adolescents. Speech rates for three age groups of nonstuttering preschoolers have been obtained by Rebekah Pindzola, Melissa Jenkins, and Kari Lokken (1989). Children in their study were asked a series of questions from the Developmental Learning Materials picture cards, and rates were obtained in syllables per minute (SPM) only. Their samples consisted of six males and four females in each of three age groups. They found the following: for 3-year-olds, 116 to 163 SPM; for 4-year-olds, 117 to 183 SPM; and for 5-year-olds, 109 to 183 SPM. Differences between age groups were not statistically significant, and no comparisons between males and females were made. Data on words per minute are not available, and more research is needed on speech rates of young children before conclusions can be drawn from assessments of the speaking rate of a potentially stuttering preschooler. In the meantime, if a child is stuttering and his speech rate is substantially below the range for his age, the extent to which stuttering is slowing his rate of speech may be a problem for listeners and for the child.

FEELINGS AND ATTITUDES

We assess a preschooler's feelings about stuttering by asking about them in the parent interview, by observing the parent-child interaction, and by bringing up the topic of stuttering, when appropriate, with the child in our interaction with him. Feelings and attitudes among preschoolers range from apparent unawareness of difficulty, to mild embarrassment, to extreme hypersensitivity. For example, a child may look slightly uncomfortable when we ask him why he's here, but he may venture that it's because he has trouble talking. At the other extreme, a child may cry at the prospect of talking about his speech and may be deeply embarrassed and uncommunicative even if we gingerly approach the topic of speech or "getting stuck." We are often able to learn a great deal by watching the tape of our interaction with the child. With the ability to devote our undivided attention to observing and replaying key segments, we find that taped interactions hold a rich payload of information about a child's feelings. The parent interview is also a valuable source for learning whether the child is simply frustrated or whether his feelings at times escalate into embarrassment and downright fear.

Assessment of the feelings and attitudes of a preschooler leads us to conclude tentatively whether the child (a) is unaware of his disfluencies; (b) is occasionally aware of them and, even then, is seldom and only transiently bothered by them; (c) is aware and frustrated by them; or (d) is highly aware, frustrated, and afraid of them. The amount of awareness and emotion that a child has about his stuttering is an important consideration in planning treatment, as we shall see.

OTHER SPEECH AND LANGUAGE BEHAVIORS

When we evaluate a preschool child's speech for stuttering, we also screen for possible articulation, language, and voice problems. In addition, we make sure that his hearing has been checked recently and, if not, arrange to have a hearing screening.

A child's language and articulation problems can usually be detected in the parent-child or clinician-child interactions that we record. When we suspect delays in these areas, we administer formal tests. The reader may wish to consult Bernthal (1994), Bernthal and Bankson (1998), Hoffman, Schuckers, and Daniloff (1989), or Weiss, Gordon, and Lillywhite (1987) for testing articulatory and phonological disorders, and Paul (1995) for assessment of language problems. We discuss the management of concomitant articulation and language disorders in the chapter on our treatment of beginning stuttering.

Our view of the relationship between language and stuttering, described in Chapter 3, is that one of the pressures on a child who stutters may result from language that is significantly advanced over motor development. Thus, in evaluating a child's language and articulation, we explore the possibility that his language is above age expectation. In addition, we observe and question parents about his general motor development and intelligibility of speech.

When language development outstrips motor development, there may be a risk that the child will try to produce long sentences at an adult pace with a speech system better suited to a child's slower rate. The child's motivation to speak quickly may come from his own eagerness to express his complex thoughts, or it may come from his parents' pleasure at his adult-like speech. When we assess a child who stutters and who also has advanced expressive language for his age, we train parents to use a slower speech rate when speaking to the child, with the expectation that this model of a slower rate will influence the child to produce speech more slowly, thereby putting fluency within his reach. In such cases of advanced language, we also explore ways in which the family may inadvertently be putting pressure on the child's language skills by stimulating language development.

Verbal activities that some parents most enjoy with their children, such as puns and other word play, as well as teaching them exotic multisyllabic words, may convey to the child that the parents place high value on verbal ability. For most children this would be an incentive to develop their verbal skills. For children struggling with fluency, parents' pride in their verbal proficiency may only elicit feelings of shame at their ineptitude.

As we review our observations of a child's speech and language, we consider not only the possibility that the child's language is advanced relative to average speech motor abilities, but also the possibility that he has markedly delayed motor abilities. A few children have motor problems that impair their coordination of respiration, phonation, and articulation with language production. Many are aware that speech is difficult for them and have already felt frustration and shame—not just about stuttering, but about the way they speak and the way they perform many other fine motor tasks. Therefore, we think it is important to improve their feelings about themselves as talkers as we work on their speech motor skills. These children seem to benefit especially from models of slow speech as well as specific activities that teach them to speak more slowly.

In addition to exploring the possibility of language and articulation difficulties, we also want to assess a child's voice. A hoarse voice may be especially significant in a preschool stutterer because it may be a sign that the child is increasing tension in his laryngeal muscles to cope with stuttering. We look closely at how the child is handling his blocks and listen for signs of excess laryngeal tension, such as pitch rises and hard glottal attacks. Because many of the techniques we use in treatment of stuttering focus on gentle onset of phonation and a relaxed style of speech, we usually don't treat voice separately from stuttering. However, if a child has voice problems other than hoarseness or if hoarseness does not diminish with stuttering therapy, clinicians may want to refer the child to an otolaryngologist and follow a treatment approach such as those suggested by Boone and Mc-Farlane (1988) and Colton and Casper (1996).

OTHER FACTORS

In Chapter 3, we described a number of possible developmental influences on stuttering. In this section, we review them briefly so that they may be recognized if they are important in a particular preschool child's stuttering. Because much of this information is usually obtained from the parent interview, the reader may wish to consult Chapter 3 for further details about developmental influences before planning or conducting a parent interview.

Physical Development

We like to ascertain what the child's general physical development was like, in terms of both gross motor skills and oral motor development. Most children learn to walk at about 1 year but usually do not learn to walk and talk at the same time. If the child we are evaluating was delayed in walking, but average or advanced in talking, we may explore the possibility that his stuttering was exacerbated by delayed motor development.

Cognitive Development

Here we want to rule out retardation, which is associated with increased disfluency problems. We also want to know if the child may be going through a period of intense cognitive growth that might hypothetically take a temporary toll on fluency.

Social-Emotional Development

As a child grows, various tensions develop between him, his parents, and his siblings. Between ages 2 to 3 and 4 to 5 years, many children may display negativism in ways that are felt throughout the family. When we ask a child's parents about conditions surrounding the onset or worsening of a child's stuttering, we explore social-emotional factors, as well as other environmental and developmental factors.

In Chapter 3, we described various life events that may affect a child's stuttering. We now examine the life events surrounding the onset of stuttering to see if upsetting events or ongoing situations may be linked to the child's stuttering. Some events, like the birth of a sibling, are happy ones, but they can create disturbances in the psychological balance of a family.

Speech and Language Environment

We have referred to this factor before, but here we are explicit: many children have their hands full trying to compete verbally with fast-talking, articulate adults. Children who stutter may find this particularly hard. We listen to the tape sent by the parents and watch parent-child interactions carefully for indications of a complicated verbal environment that may be like rough water to a new swimmer.

Diagnosis

We now turn to the task of pulling together all of the information we have gathered and making a diagnosis of a young client's problems. We have to decide whether or not the child needs treatment and, if so, for which level of stuttering should he be treated. These decisions are made on the basis of data from all the sources assessed in the evaluation: the case history, home tape recording (if available), observation of parent-child interaction (if possible), parent interview, and clinician-child interaction.

DETERMINING DEVELOPMENTAL/TREATMENT LEVEL

We may categorize a preschool child as normally disfluent, a borderline stutterer, a beginning stutterer, or, in rare cases, an intermediate stutterer. In the following paragraphs, we present brief reviews of each level but recommend reading the relevant sections of Chapter 5 for details.

Normal Disfluency

All of the following characteristics for this level must be met for the child to be considered normally disfluent: The child will have fewer than 10 disfluencies per 100 words. These disfluencies will consist of mostly multisyllable word and phrase repetitions, revisions, and interjections. When the disfluencies are repetitions, they will have two or fewer repeated units per repetition. The repetitions will be slow and regular in tempo. All disfluencies will be relatively relaxed, and the child will seem hardly aware of them and will certainly not be upset when he is.

A child may be considered borderline or above if he has any of the characteristics that are described in following paragraphs. Place him at the level—borderline, beginning, or intermediate—that has the child's more salient characteristics.

Borderline Stuttering

The child we place in this category shows more than 10 disfluencies per 100 words. They may be part-word repetitions and single-syllable word repetitions, as well as prolongations. Repetitions may be more than two per instance. Disfluencies will be loose and relaxed.

Beginning Stuttering

The key features at this level are the presence of tension and hurry in the child's stuttering. They may take the form of rapid, abrupt repetitions, pitch rises during repetitions and prolongations, difficulty starting airflow or phonation, and signs of facial tension. The beginning stutterer shows that he is aware of his stuttering and may be quite frustrated by it. He may use a variety of escape behaviors, such as head nods or eye blinks, to terminate blocks.

Intermediate Stuttering

The child we place at this level will have most of the characteristics of the preceding levels plus avoidance behaviors. He avoids words and situations and feels both fear and shame about stuttering.

Although we use information from all sources to determine a child's level, we have found that our own observations of parent-child and clinician-child interactions provide the most reliable data. Although parents are helpful in describing long-term changes in their child's stuttering, they frequently miss many avoidance behaviors, such as starters, circumlocutions, and postponements, which are critical indicators of the more advanced levels of stuttering. Parents' reports do provide at least as much information about a child's feelings and attitudes as we usually gather in observing interactions in the clinic. Thus, parent reports and our own observations provide valuable, complementary data. A vital adjunct to direct observations are videotapes of parent-child and clinician-child interactions. We sometimes revise our initial determination of a child's developmental/ treatment level after viewing videotapes of the interactions we have already directly observed.

ASSESSING OTHER FACTORS

In addition to determining how far a child's stuttering has advanced, we assess developmental and environmental factors that may be affecting his fluency. This information is critical for treating a preschool stutterer and for counseling his parents. The reader who is familiar with Chapter 3 can draw from the case history, parent interview, and parent-child interaction relevant information with which to formulate tentative hypotheses about developmental and environmental factors.

In a child whom we categorize as normally disfluent, we often find that spurts in physical, cognitive, or linguistic growth may be related to the appearance of disfluencies. We look for these and other changes in a normally disfluent child's life to help explain to a parent why disfluencies may be occurring or increasing during this period.

In children who have borderline, beginning, or intermediate stuttering, we look for evidence of language growth outstripping motor development or other developmental asymmetries or delays. These may be especially important to consider in working out a tentative treatment program. We are also sensitive to environmental factors, either normal or unusual, that may be putting enough pressure on a child to precipitate stuttering. The areas we examine most often are the parents' communication models and their standards for the child's speech and language. Do they talk fast and use complex language? Do they frequently correct their child's speech or encourage his use of more advanced language than he typically uses? We also note such events as the birth of a sibling or a pending divorce, which could be creating the kind of anxiety or insecurity that appears to increase stuttering in some children.

Once we draw together these fragments of data and make some tentative conclusions about the child's speech and how to treat it, we meet with the parents in a counseling and treatment-planning session, which ends the evaluation.

Closing Interview

We begin by describing characteristics of the child's stuttering that we observed in parent-child and clinician-child observations. We stay away from jargon as we briefly describe the child's behaviors, review the important information the parents provided in the case history and interview, and estimate how serious the child's problem is. If stuttering is a serious concern, we say so. If the parents have expressed feelings of guilt about their child's stuttering, we again reassure them that they aren't to blame for the problem but that they will be crucial in helping us to resolve it and in helping their child to respond to his stuttering in a healthy way. At this point, it is important to describe appropriate treatment approaches—environmental changes, indirect treatment, direct treatment—which differ, depending on the developmental/treatment level of the child's problem.

NORMAL DISFLUENCY

If we believe the child's speech is normally disfluent, we deal with the parents' concern rather than the child's disfluencies. In some cases, we give parents information about normal disfluency, such as the following: During the preschool years, many normal children pass through periods of disfluency. Interjections, revisions, pauses, repetitions, and prolongations are common during these periods. Their disfluencies are usually fewer than 10 per 100 words spoken. Interjections and revisions are more common than part-word repetitions, which usually have only 1 or 2 units repeated per disfluency. Normally disfluent children are largely unaware of their disfluencies, don't develop reactions to them, and gradually outgrow them.

In other cases, we might offer parents the following analogy to help them understand their child's disfluent speech: Learning to speak is like learning many other skills, such as riding a bike or learning to skate. A learner falls down a lot in the early stages. We try to use analogous situations in the parents' own lives to help them realize the value of an accepting environment. Parents who are concerned about their child's normal disfluencies are reassured when they find out that it is normal. In those rare cases in which parents are still not convinced that their child's speech disfluencies are normal, we teach them to slow their speaking rates, simplify their language, and relieve other pressures that we mutually agree to change. Then, we set up further appointments to help them make these changes.

We keep the door wide open for all parents of normally disfluent children. This reassures them that help is near at hand, that we realize it is possible their child might develop stuttering someday, and that we will help them if that happens.

BORDERLINE, BEGINNING, OR INTERMEDIATE-LEVEL STUTTERING

For children whom we evaluate within 12 months of the onset of stuttering, we have some preliminary information to help us decide which children should begin treatment and which can be followed for a period of time without treatment. Table 7.2 lists some of the characteristics of those children who have a high probability of recovery without treatment. Children whose stuttering-like disfluencies (part-word and single-syllable word repetitions, prolongations, or blocks) are decreasing during the first 12 months after onset are likely to recover. If other factors in Table 7.2 also characterize the child, the likelihood of recovery may be increased.

We believe that any child we diagnose as a borderline, beginning, or intermediate stutterer should either be treated or followed up carefully for several months. For those children close to onset whose stuttering is diminishing and whose families are not overly concerned, we stay in contact by telephone for several months. When families are highly concerned or when a child's stuttering is not decreasing, we begin treatment as soon as possible.

Our closing interview with these parents is usually the first of many sessions we will spend together. Consequently, we don't need to accomplish everything in this meet-

**Table 7.2. Factors That May Be Associated With Increased
Likelihood of Recovery From Stuttering Without Treatment**[a]

Factor	Comment
1. Decrease in stuttering-like disfluencies during the 12 months after onset	This is an important predictor of recovery. It applies to children with borderline, beginning, and intermediate-level stuttering.
2. Female	Evidence suggests females are more likely to recover.
3. No relatives who stutter; or relatives have recovered from stuttering	Preliminary evidence suggests that persistent stuttering may run in families.
4. Good language and articulation skills	Both receptive and expressive language skills should be considered. Evidence of early phonological problems may predict persistent stuttering.
5. Good nonverbal intelligence scores	Children with persistent stuttering had normal, but slightly lower nonverbal skills.
6. Outgoing, carefree temperament	Our clinical experience suggests these children who begin to stutter often outgrow it.

[a]*When a young preschool child is assessed within 1 year of stuttering onset.*
*Factors 1 to 5 are based on evidence cited in Andrews et al. (1993) and on studies of Yairi & Ambrose (1992) and Yairi, Ambrose,
Paden, & Throneburg (1996).*

ing. Because treatment of any preschool stutterer is largely focused on the home environment, we often begin our discussion with things the parents can do at home. Chapter 14 contains more suggestions for parents about ways in which changes in the environment may reduce pressure on their child. Refer to that chapter to see how you may help parents reduce environmental pressures. We may also discuss only general principles and let the parents decide on specific stresses. We encourage them to select only a small number of potentially critical situations to work on. We find that if parents see success at first, they will be highly motivated to continue the changes they have started.

We also give parents reading material to help them better understand stuttering and what they can do to help their child. We have found that two recent publications by the Stuttering Foundation of America provide a good basis for ongoing discussions. These are *Stuttering and Your Child: Questions and Answers* (Conture & Fraser, 1989) and *If You Think Your Child Is Stuttering* (Guitar & Conture, undated). We may also give parents an excellent publication from the National Easter Seal Society, *Understanding Stuttering: Information for Parents* (Cooper, 1979). In addition, two videotapes are available for interested parents: *Childhood Stuttering: A Videotape for Parents* (Conture, Guitar, & Williams, 1996) and *Preventing Stuttering in the Preschool Child: A Video Program for Parents* (Skinner & McKeehan, 1996).

After brainstorming with parents about changes they can begin to make, we also talk about appropriate treatment approaches. We give a brief overview of the goals of treatment and describe the important contribution the parents can make to the success of treatment. We then ask the parents if they have further questions and end by scheduling the next meeting.

Occasionally, we find that we are still undecided about our diagnosis when it is time for the closing interview. We may need time to review videotapes of interactions with the child. In such cases, we summarize the range of possibilities and give the parents something specific on which to begin work at home. Then, we schedule another meeting with them as soon as possible.

SUMMARY

In evaluating a client who may stutter, your task is to decide (*a*) if his disfluencies warrant treatment; (*b*) if so, what are the important characteristics of his history, current environment, speech behaviors, and reactions; and (*c*) what treatment do these characteristics indicate?

We have provided most of the tools needed to answer these three questions, but most critical is your judgment. Whether the person is to be treated as a normally disfluent speaker or as someone who stutters depends on your interpretation rather than a score. You must weigh what you see and hear to determine whether these things indicate stuttering, normal disfluency, or even another disorder. From the flood of information you have gathered, you must extract the essential characteristics that support your choice of treatment.

To hone your judgment, we urge you to make evaluations a continuing process. The procedures we have suggested for assessment and diagnosis in this chapter will give you a good start, but stuttering is highly variable, and no individual can be understood in an hour or two. Consequently, you will overlook an important element at times, and sometimes a vital clue will not be present in the sample of behavior you see during an evaluation. With good follow-up evaluation of a client—whether you treat him or not—you will be able to change decisions and redirect therapy as additional information and understanding become available.

STUDY QUESTIONS

1. In the section on evaluation of the adult and adolescent, what different pieces of information that you may gather from the interview questions help you to assess the client's motivation?
2. What various aspects of the client's behavior are assessed by the SSI?
3. Why is the client's speech rate assessed?
4. In what various ways do we assess the impact of the school environment on the school-age child who stutters?
5. How does the parents' role differ in the diagnosis of preschool versus school children?
6. What are the benefits of obtaining both a reading and a conversation sample with school children and adults?
7. Why is it useful to obtain tape recordings of a preschool child's stuttering before the evaluation, when this is not done for other age levels?
8. What questions in the interview of the parent of a preschool child assess (*a*) constitutional, (*b*) developmental and environmental, and (*c*) learning factors?
9. Name four of the seven variables we assess in the speech of a preschooler to determine his developmental/treatment level.
10. What are two reasons we suggest for continuing evaluation after the initial assessment of clients who stutter?

SUGGESTED READINGS

Culatta, R., & Goldberg, S. (1995). Culture and stuttering. In *Stuttering therapy*. Needham Heights, MA: Allyn & Bacon.

This chapter presents useful information not only on stuttering in different cultures, but, more important, about how differences in ethnic identity, religion, and gender may affect evaluation and therapy.

Emerick, L., & Haynes, W. (1986). *Diagnosis and evaluation in speech pathology,* **3rd ed. Englewood Cliffs, NJ: Prentice-Hall.**
The chapters on interviewing and on stuttering are particularly good. Emerick is an intuitive clinician and a down-to-earth writer. These chapters are filled with practical information, and they are highly digestible.

Guitar, B. (1981). Stuttering. In J. Darby (Ed.), *Speech evaluation in medicine.* **New York: Grune & Stratton.**
The sections on differential diagnosis of stuttering versus neurogenic disfluency, psychogenic disfluency, and cluttering will be especially useful to clinicians evaluating adult clients.

Guitar, B., & Belin-Frost, G. (1995). Stuttering. In S. Parker & B. Zuckerman (Eds.), *Behavioral and developmental pediatrics: A handbook for primary care.* **Boston: Little, Brown.**
This brief chapter for pediatricians summarizes key questions and important information for parents, criteria for referral, and initial treatment strategies.

Johnson, W., Darley, F., & Spriestersbach, D.C. (1952). *Diagnostic manual in speech correction.* **New York: Harper & Row.**
This manual is admittedly out of date, but its opening sections on the case history, particularly the description of interviewing techniques, are excellent.

Peterson, H., & Marquardt, T. (1990). *Appraisal and diagnosis of speech and language disorders,* **2nd ed. Englewood Cliffs, NJ: Prentice-Hall.**
The chapter on evaluation of fluency is authored by Harold Luper, who, like Emerick, was an experienced clinician and a fine writer. The section of this chapter on differentiating stuttering from normal disfluency is particularly good.

St. Louis, K. (Ed.). (1986). *The atypical stutterer.* **New York: Academic Press.**
This text contains interesting chapters on fluency disorders that are similar to stuttering, such as cluttering and disfluency associated with retardation. Therapy approaches for these other fluency disorders are also given.

8

Advanced Stutterer:
Stuttering Modification
and Fluency Shaping Therapies

In this chapter, we discuss the treatment of the advanced stutterer. Since most advanced stutterers are adults or high school students, we describe therapy procedures appropriate for these age groups. After reviewing the characteristics of the disorder at this level, we discuss stuttering modification and fluency shaping therapies. We conclude by comparing these two approaches on the clinical issues raised in an earlier chapter.

The advanced stutterer will exhibit any or all of the following core behaviors: part-word or monosyllabic word repetitions that contain excessive tension, prolongations that exhibit tension, and blocks. Secondary behaviors may include escape and avoidance behaviors such as starting behaviors, postponements, word substitutions and circumlocutions, and avoidance of speaking situations. The advanced stutterer will have a well-established self-concept as a stutterer, and he will evidence frustration, embarrassment, and fear relative to his stuttering.

STUTTERING MODIFICATION THERAPY

The two key elements in stuttering modification therapy for the advanced stutterer are (*a*) teaching the stutterer to modify his moments of stuttering and (*b*) reducing his fear of stuttering and eliminating the avoidance behaviors associated with this fear. These elements interact with each other. The better able a person is at modifying his stuttering, the more his fear and avoidance decrease. Likewise, the more he is able to reduce his fear and avoidance, the more easily he can modify his moments of stuttering.

To illustrate this approach, we describe Charles Van Riper's therapy for the advanced stutterer. Van Riper was a leading proponent of stuttering modification therapy, and his therapy is an excellent example of this approach. Other clinicians advocating stuttering modification therapy are also reviewed, and their therapy is briefly described.

Charles Van Riper: Fluent or Easy Stuttering

CLINICIAN'S BELIEFS

Nature of Stuttering

What position did Charles Van Riper take on the clinical issues we raised in an earlier chapter? With regard to the nature of stuttering, Van Riper (1982) saw stuttering as a disorder of timing. He believed that when a person stutters, a disruption occurs in the proper timing and sequencing of the muscle movements involved in producing a word. When this happens, the stutterer exhibits a core behavior, that is, a repetition, prolongation, or block. What accounts for this mistiming of motor movements involved in speech production? Van Riper suggested that this could be due to a constitutional predisposition that made an individual vulnerable to neuromotor breakdown under stress. According to Van Riper, secondary behaviors and negative feelings and attitudes are learned.

Speech Behaviors Targeted for Therapy

Stutterers exhibit mistimings in their speech, and Van Riper believed we should teach them how to cope with these disruptions. His solution was to teach the stutterer how to modify his hard, tense, struggled moments of stuttering into slow, easy, effortless ones. More specifically, the stutterer was to slowly work his way through each sound of the stuttered word. The transition from sound to sound was to be gradual. Van Riper wanted "the whole sequence to be slowed down, all sounds and transitions proportionally."[1] Articulatory contacts were to be light, not tense. Van Riper referred to this new way of stuttering as "fluent stuttering" or "easy stuttering."[2]

Fluency Goals

What were Van Riper's fluency goals for advanced stutterers? Van Riper said that, with therapy, a few advanced stutterers become normal speakers; that is, they exhibit spontaneous fluency all the time. However, in most cases, this does not occur. Thus, ideally, his

---

[1] Van Riper notes that some stuttering modification clinicians have clients prolong only the first sound of the word. Van Riper, however, believes it is better for a stutterer not to distort the motoric sequence of the word by using such prolongations.

[2] Sources for Van Riper's position on this and the remaining clinical issues were Van Riper, C. (1973). *The treatment of stuttering.* Englewood Cliffs, NJ: Prentice-Hall; and Van Riper, C. (1974). Modification of behavior. In *Therapy for stutterers* (pp. 45–73). Memphis: Speech Foundation of America.

goal was spontaneous fluency, but realistically, his goal for most advanced stutterers was controlled fluency or acceptable stuttering. These stutterers should use their new, easy, fluent stuttering to sound relatively fluent or, at least, to exhibit only a minimal level of stuttering.

Feelings and Attitudes

Van Riper believed it is very important to consider the feelings and attitudes of advanced stutterers about their stuttering in planning therapy. Because they have been stuttering for many years, he believed that most have developed strong feelings of frustration, fear, and shame focused around their disorder. Van Riper believed it is important to desensitize these stutterers to their stuttering and to other persons' reactions to it. By desensitization, Van Riper implied two things. On the one hand, he meant that the intensity of stutterers' negative feelings need to be reduced. On the other hand, he thought that stutterers need to be toughened to the experience of stuttering and to others' reactions to it. This may be just two ways of saying the same thing; namely, that these stutterers need to become less emotional about their stuttering. If this does not occur, Van Riper felt that advanced stutterers will not be able to modify their stuttering successfully. The reason is that like most people, stutterers cannot adequately control fine motor acts, such as modifying a moment of stuttering when they are wrought up emotionally.

Maintenance Procedures

Van Riper was very aware of the need to help advanced stutterers maintain the improvements they made during therapy. He put a great deal of emphasis on procedures or strategies to help them do this. In fact, one of his four phases of therapy, stabilization, is devoted to this goal. Van Riper developed a number of clinical procedures that he used during this phase. For example, he helped stutterers become their own speech clinicians. Since most of them will need to control their stuttering for a long time, possibly forever, they need to know what to do. He taught them how to keep their speech fears at a minimum and how to keep their stuttering modification skills intact. He also helped stutterers change their self-concepts from persons who stutter to persons who speak fluently most of the time but who occasionally stutter.

Clinical Methods

In terms of clinical methods, Van Riper's therapy could be characterized as a counseling/teaching mode of interaction. It can be implemented in either an individual or group situation. Even though the clinician has definite goals for a therapy session, it is loosely structured. Many times the clinician and client leave the clinical setting for real-life, speaking situations to achieve the goals of the day. The client also has daily therapy assignments that he performs on his own away from the clinic. These are then discussed with the clinician during a later therapy session. As a general rule, Van Riper has not stressed the collection of data in his discussion of therapy procedures.

CLINICAL PROCEDURES

Of all Van Riper's contributions to the field of stuttering, he is probably best known for the therapy procedures he developed for the advanced stutterer. In *The Treatment of Stuttering* (1973), he provided a comprehensive discussion of his therapy for the advanced stutterer. In the Stuttering Foundation of America booklet, *Therapy for Stutterers,* Van Riper (1974) provided a brief, but good, description of this therapy. A series of videotapes, also produced by the Stuttering Foundation of America, portrays Van Riper (1975b) doing therapy with an advanced stutterer; these will provide interested readers with insight into his clinical procedures. In this chapter, we draw on these sources for our presentation of his clinical procedures. We plan to describe his therapy in sufficient detail for you to understand his basic procedures. However, you may also wish to go to the above-mentioned sources for additional information.

Van Riper divided the therapy process into four overlapping phases: (*a*) identification phase, (*b*) desensitization phase, (*c*) modification phase, and (*d*) stabilization phase.

Identification Phase

In the identification phase, the stutterer identifies the core behaviors, secondary behaviors, and feelings and attitudes that characterize his stuttering. If the stutterer is to change, he must become aware of what to change. Clinical activities include oral reading, discussion, modeling of stuttering behaviors by the clinician, self-observation of stuttering in a mirror, and audio and video recordings (Fig. 8.1). During therapy sessions, the clinician is warm, understanding, and accepting of the client's stuttering behaviors and feelings. However, the clinician is also confronting and challenging when she suspects the stutterer is avoiding facing certain aspects of his problem. Yet, even at these times, her basic acceptance of the client allows him to become more comfortable with his stuttering. In other words, desensitization is already beginning to occur.

Van Riper recommended that components of a client's stuttering be identified in a hierarchical order from least to most difficult or stressful for the stutterer. Based on his experience, he recommends the following hierarchy. First, the clinician helps the stutterer identify easy stutterings in his speech. Most stutterers have some easy or effortless stutterings, which will become the target or goal behaviors of therapy. Next comes identification of escape behaviors, such as eye blinks and head nods during stuttering moments.

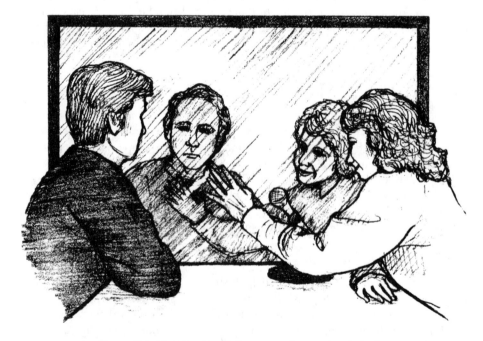

Figure 8.1. Identification of the core and secondary behaviors.

Then, Van Riper helped the stutterer identify avoidance behaviors such as postponements and starters, word and sound fears and avoidances, and situation fears and avoidances. After this, the stutterer studies his core behaviors and learns what he does when he stops the flow of speech with a block, a repetition, or a prolongation. Finally, he focuses on his feelings of frustration, shame, and hostility and initiates efforts to accept them.

These components of the stuttering problem are first identified in the clinic, then identified outside in the stutterer's own speaking environment. For example, if the goal were to help the stutterer become aware of his use of postponements, the clinician would first help the stutterer become aware of them while talking to her in the clinic. The stutterer would then be assigned to gather examples of postponements in his everyday speaking situations. From time to time, it would also be important for the clinician to accompany the client on some outside speaking assignments so that she may verify the validity of the stutterer's self-observations and reporting.

When the stutterer becomes able to identify and accurately discuss the various aspects of his stuttering, he is ready to move to the desensitization phase. At times, he may need to revisit the identification stage if and when his progress slows down.

Desensitization Phase

The goal of the desensitization phase is to reduce fears and other negative emotions, such as frustration and embarrassment, which are associated with a stutterer's speech. Van Riper also viewed it as "toughening" the stutterer to his stuttering. Specifically, Van Riper believed there are three features of the stuttering problem to which the stutterer needs to be desensitized. These are (*a*) the confrontation with the disorder, (*b*) the core behaviors, and (*c*) the reactions of his listeners. In other words, the stutterer needs to become more comfortable with or tolerant of each of these three aspects of his stuttering problem. The following are examples of typical procedures that could be used to desensitize the stutterer to each of the above three features.

Confrontation With the Disorder. Most advanced stutterers find it difficult to face up to the fact that they stutter. They tend to deny and run away from their problem. However, by enrolling in a therapy program and going through the identification phase that was just described, the stutterer has gone a long way toward confronting his problem. In other words, some desensitization to the disorder has already occurred. However, another strategy the clinician should suggest to help the stutterer confront his stuttering is self-disclosure. The clinician encourages him to be honest and open about stuttering, to let people know that he is involved in a stuttering therapy program. When he does this, she should reinforce this behavior with her enthusiastic approval.

Desensitization to Core Behaviors. The second target for desensitization is the core behaviors—the repetitions, prolongations, and blocks that characterize the stutterer's speech. Van Riper believed that for many stutterers these core behaviors are associated with feelings of frustration and fear. Stutterers need to build up their tolerance for them. One technique that Van Riper recommended is called *freezing*. Upon a signal from the clinician, Van Riper had the stutterer freeze his speech mechanism in the act of stuttering and continue the core behavior he was experiencing when the clinician signaled. If he were prolonging a sound, he should continue to do that. If he were repeating a syllable, he should continue repeating it.

These activities, like all desensitization activities, should be done in a hierarchical order, from the least to the most stressful. For example, a first step might involve the clinician's simulating the client's stuttering and freezing upon the client's signal. At these times, the clinician should remain relaxed as she voluntarily extends her simulation of the client's stuttering. When the client begins to freeze in his stutters, he should hold on to his stutters only briefly, and the clinician should remain calm, unhurried, and in no way punishing.

Over time, the clinician should have the stutterer extend his blocks for longer and longer periods of time and begin to introduce some impatience or other mildly aversive behavior into her responses. By experiencing these core behaviors over and over again, the stutterer becomes less emotional about or more tolerant of his core behaviors. In the videotape of Van Riper doing therapy, the fourth session provides excellent examples of how to desensitize the stutterer to his core behaviors.

Desensitization to Listener Reactions. One procedure that Van Riper used to desensitize the stutterer to listeners' reactions is pseudostuttering or voluntary stuttering. The purpose is to teach the client that he can stutter without becoming excessively emotional. By stuttering on purpose and observing his listeners, the stutterer will learn the following things. First, he will learn that most listeners are far more tolerant of stuttering than he thought. Second, he will learn that, even though he may encounter a negative reaction from a listener occasionally, he can remain relatively calm. Van Riper also recommends the use of hierarchies for pseudostuttering. At first, the stutterer's pseudostuttering consists solely of easy repetitions or prolongations. Gradually, his pseudostuttering is changed to approximate his own stuttering. At first, pseudostuttering is performed on nonfeared words, and later on feared words. Initially, pseudostuttering is practiced in the clinical setting with the support of a sensitive and understanding clinician.

The clinician should also engage in and share pseudostuttering with the client, both inside the clinic and later in outside speaking situations. While doing this, the clinician must remain calm and relaxed, so she must desensitize herself to her own fears of pseudostuttering by practicing. Only after much pseudostuttering in the company of the clinician will the stutterer be assigned to engage in pseudostuttering on his own in outside feared speaking situations. By going through this sequence of activities with the encouragement, sharing, and support of his clinician, the stutterer gradually becomes desensitized to listeners' reactions.

As the stutterer becomes less emotional about his stuttering and people's reactions to it, he is ready to move on to the modification phase of therapy.

Modification Phase

During the modification phase, the stutterer learns a new more fluent or easy way of stuttering. It is during this phase that stutterers learn to use Van Riper's well-known techniques of cancellations, pull-outs, and preparatory sets to modify stuttering (Fig. 8.2). However, before the clinician teaches these techniques, she must help the stutterer reduce or eliminate his postponement and avoidance of feared words and situations. She must convince the stutterer that if he is going to learn to stutter more easily, he must learn to tackle his feared words, and that he cannot run away from them. Fortunately, this task has been made easier because the stutterer has already gone through a great deal of desensitization. Nevertheless, the clinician will probably have to spend some time in helping the stutterer approach feared words rather than avoid them, before she tries to teach him cancellations, pull-outs, and preparatory sets.

Cancellations. Cancellations are the first step in the sequence of teaching the stutterer more fluent or easy ways of stuttering. To begin with, the stutterer needs to have a model of what easy stuttering sounds and feels like. During the identification phase, the clinician may have been able to help the stutterer identify some of his easy stutterings. If

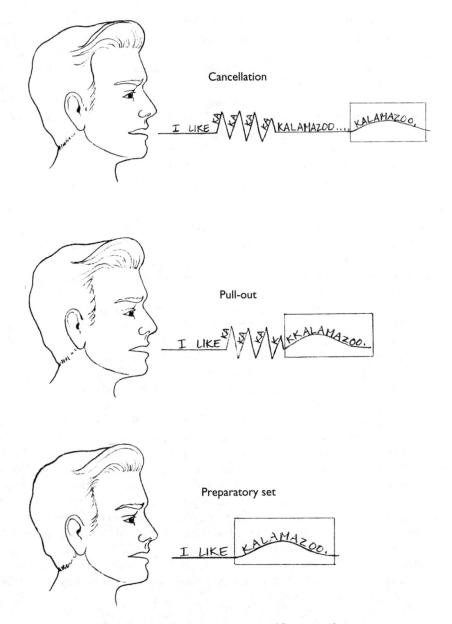

Figure 8.2. Van Riper's stuttering modification techniques.

so, these can be used as models. If the stutterer does not have any easy stutterings in his speech, the clinician will have to model them. What Van Riper has in mind is as follows. A word that is cancelled has to be said deliberately and in slow motion. Each sound of the word is to be produced slowly, and the transitions from sound to sound gradual. Articulatory contacts are to be relaxed or light. Once the stutterer can produce or model these easy stutterings on single words, he is ready to begin incorporating them into his speech. Cancellations are used for this purpose.

A cancellation goes as follows. After stuttering on a word, the stutterer pauses for a couple of seconds and then says the word a second time, but not fluently; this second time, he repeats the word using an easy stutter. The clinician should make sure that the stutterer completes the stuttered word fully the first time; he should not stop immediately following the moment of stuttering if the word is only partly finished. For example, if the stutterer says "B-B-Baltimore," he should finish the whole word "Baltimore" before pausing, rather than pausing after "B-B-Balt." The clinician should also insist that he not hurry his pause. It should be a deliberate pause during which the stutterer calms himself, analyzes the way in which he just stuttered, and prepares to use easy stuttering on the second attempt. Hierarchies are used in cancellations also. The stutterer first uses cancellations in the clinic with the clinician. Only after he uses them successfully in this context will he be given daily assignments to use them in outside speaking situations. Most people who stutter are very uncomfortable using cancellations in outside speaking situations.

In the 20-year follow-up session on the Van Riper videotape, the client indicates that he rarely used cancellations outside the clinic. They are therefore an excellent motivation for clients to move on to the next step in modification. Once the stutterer has shown that he can use cancellations reliably, he is ready to learn to use pull-outs.

Pull-outs. The second step in teaching the stutterer to use easy stuttering is pull-outs. Now, rather than stuttering the old way on the first attempt at a word, the stutterer is to catch himself while still in the act of stuttering and pull or ease himself out of the rest of the word. He uses the same behaviors that he has already learned; he freezes or extends the stutter until he feels he has voluntary control. That is, he says the rest of the word in slow motion. Movements from sound to sound should be gradual and articulatory contacts light. Once again, pull-outs are first used and practiced in the clinical setting before outside speaking situations are assigned. After the stutterer has mastered the use of pull-outs, he is ready to move on to preparatory sets.

Preparatory Sets. Preparatory sets are the third and final step in teaching the stutterer to use easy, fluent stuttering. As the stutterer scans ahead for feared words as he is speaking, he now prepares to use the same behaviors he used in cancellations and pull-outs. He starts the first sound of the word slowly and continues to work through all parts of the word at a reduced rate, using relaxed articulatory contacts. As before, preparatory sets are first practiced in the clinical setting and then in outside assignments.

In going through this sequence of teaching and practicing cancellations, pull-outs, and preparatory sets, Van Riper gradually modified the stutterer's old stuttering pattern into a fluent or easy form of stuttering. In operant conditioning terminology, this is a shaping procedure. Once the stutterer is using "prep sets" and pull-outs in most speaking situations and has a greatly increased amount of spontaneous fluency, he is ready for the last or stabilization phase of therapy.

Stabilization Phase

The goal of the stabilization phase is to help the stutterer solidify or stabilize his treatment gains. Van Riper has several subgoals he wants to achieve during this phase. The most important subgoal is to help the stutterer become his own therapist. The clinician needs to help the stutterer take responsibility for developing his own assignments based on his perceived needs. So, she now becomes more and more of a consultant, and the frequency of her contact with the client is slowly reduced. In time, the stutterer develops the ability and confidence to prescribe his own therapy activities.

Another subgoal of the stabilization phase is to make preparatory sets and pull-outs second nature to the client. When the stutterer first began using these techniques, they required a great deal of concentration. They need to become more automatic, which will require a great deal of practice using both techniques on feared words and in feared situations, in the clinic and in everyday speaking situations.

The stutterer also needs to work on extinguishing any residual speech fears. He should seek out remaining feared situations and use pseudostuttering in them. Another helpful technique for him would be to purposefully insert brief, easy, or fluent stutterings on non-feared words into his speech throughout the day.

Finally, Van Riper believed it is important to help the stutterer change his self-concept from that of a person who stutters to someone who speaks fluently most of the time but who occasionally stutters mildly. Self-concept change requires a series of steps that will involve considerable reality testing, but the day will come when the client feels he can manage on his own, and therapy will be terminated.

Other Clinicians

We now briefly comment on the clinical procedures of some other speech-language pathologists who advocate stuttering modification therapy for the advanced stutterer. This list of clinicians is not exhaustive, but their clinical procedures are representative of those in stuttering modification therapy. By being aware of the contributions of these writers, you will become more familiar with the stuttering modification literature.

OLIVER BLOODSTEIN

As discussed in a previous chapter, Oliver Bloodstein (1975) views stuttering as an anticipatory struggle reaction that is manifested as tension and fragmentation of the stutterer's speech. The original tension and fragmentation are the result of continued and severe communicative failures and pressures experienced by the young child.

Bloodstein's (1975) treatment goals for the advanced stutterer, or what he calls a "phase 4" stutterer,[3] are (*a*) the reduction of anxiety about stuttering and (*b*) the modification of stuttering behavior. His therapy sessions are loosely structured, and he does not emphasize data collection.

Bloodstein focuses on reduction of the advanced stutterer's anxiety for two reasons. First, it is often the most handicapping aspect of the problem. Second, if anxiety is not reduced, the stutterer will be unable to modify his stuttering behavior as effectively. Bloodstein does not believe it is possible to rid a client of all anxiety about stuttering; rather, he attempts to reduce anxiety as much as is reasonably possible. Typical procedures for reducing the stutterer's anxiety about stuttering include encouraging him to discuss his stuttering openly with others, helping him to evaluate his listeners' reactions realistically, and assisting him to overcome his use of avoidance behaviors.

In helping the stutterer learn to modify his stuttering, Bloodstein begins by teaching him to identify and relax the tension in his speech mechanism. Next, he teaches the stutterer to move through feared words in a forward-moving, integrated manner, thereby reducing the fragmentation in his speech. According to Bloodstein, the stutterer needs to learn to keep his speech mechanism moving forward in a deliberate, unhurried manner as he produces a stuttered word. Bloodstein notes that a few advanced stutterers become fluent speakers as a result of therapy. However, most are left with a residue of occasional mild disfluencies—in other words, acceptable stuttering.

---

[3] The terms "advanced stutterer," "beginning stutterer," and "intermediate stutterer" are not used by all clinicians. Thus, we had to determine comparable developmental/treatment levels of the other clinicians. Although comparisons are not always exact, we believe that they are close enough to make our discussions in this and the following chapters valid.

RICHARD BOEHMLER

Richard Boehmler's therapy (Boehmler, 1994; Starkweather, 1972) conceives of stuttering as a "speech-flow" disorder, a disruption in the normal processes of speech production and language formulation. Therefore, his therapy focuses on how and why a client's speech deviates from normal. This approach differs from most stuttering modification and fluency shaping therapies in teaching clients to make their speech more and more like normal speech, rather than using unusual or exaggerated styles of speaking. To make the procedures of therapy clearer, Boehmler helps the client to analyze his stuttering by placing the disfluencies into the following categories:

1. Simple syllable repetitions, which result from speaking too fast for language formulation speed
2. Glottal blocks, which reflect inappropriate breathing patterns
3. Articulatory blocks, which are caused by too much tension in articulators
4. Hypertension, which arises from anxiety about blocks and a lack of skills to cope with blocks

Boehmler believes that a person with advanced stuttering must become his own clinician early in therapy and discover for himself what he does to interfere with the normal flow of speech and how he can change his speech toward a normal flow. In helping clients achieve this, Boehmler has found that the following changes can be effective:

1. Decrease simple syllable repetitions, and speak more slowly.
2. Reduce glottal blocks by developing more effective breath control patterns for all utterances.
3. Make articulatory blocks more like normal speech, helping clients use only a normal amount of articulatory tension.
4. Decrease hypertension by reducing avoidance behaviors and teaching such block-coping skills as uttering a difficult word more slowly than usual.

EDWARD CONTURE

Edward Conture, in his book, *Stuttering* (1982, 1990), discusses stuttering therapy at different age levels. His therapy sessions appear to be loosely structured without heavy emphasis on data collection. In his chapter on the adult stutterer, he describes a stuttering modification approach for the advanced stutterer that has two goals: (*a*) identification and (*b*) modification. It is apparent from his writings that Conture believes it is important to be sensitive to an adult stutterer's feelings and attitudes about his stuttering and to discuss them; however, Conture does not have a separate goal for this purpose.

The intent of identification is to enable the stutterer to accurately and quickly identify when he is stuttering. Conture begins with "off-line" identification, which involves helping the stutterer identify moments of stuttering in recordings of other stutterers and then in recordings of his own speech. Next, Conture begins "on-line" identification by helping the stutterer identify his moments of stuttering as he is speaking. Once he is able to do this accurately and quickly, he is ready for modification.

Modification begins with the more easily recognizable stutters. Conture starts by helping the stutterer become aware of what he is doing when he stutters or what he is doing to "interfere with speaking." He then helps the stutterer modify this behavior by learning to reduce the duration of stutters by moving easily from one sound of a word into the next. After these skills are acquired in the clinic, they are practiced in speaking situations in the stutterer's own environment. Conture indicates that it will take much time and practice on the part of the advanced stutterer for these modification skills to become automatic. Thus, some advanced stutterers may become spontaneously fluent, but many will have to work for a long time to master controlled fluency or acceptable stuttering.

DAVID PRINS

In a recent chapter on the management of stuttering in adults, David Prins (1997) discusses stuttering as a learned defensive reaction to perceived interruptions in the flow of speech. To help stutterers manage their stuttering, Prins describes three phases of therapy: (*a*) exploring, understanding, and accepting responsibility for their speech behavior; (*b*) reducing emotional responses to stuttering; and (*c*) modifying stuttering so that it is loose and forward-moving, more like fluent speech. Prins' goal for clients is to "speak as fluently as they are able and have the will and motivation to do." Thus, a client could have spontaneous fluency, controlled fluency, or acceptable stuttering as a goal. Unlike other stuttering modification clinicians discussed in this section, Prins uses programmed instruction principles in much of his therapy and is a strong advocate of Bandura's (1977) cognitive therapy, especially modeling.

The goal of the first phase of therapy is to help stutterers become aware of "what they do and feel as they talk that inhibits and facilitates fluency" (Prins, 1997, p. 346). Prins wants clients to accept responsibility for their speech and to begin setting their own goals in therapy. To help clients achieve this goal, the clinician uses video equipment or a mirror to provide feedback and models of their stuttering to observe and examine. These activities are accompanied by a discussion of a client's stuttering behaviors, as well as the feelings and attitudes that accompany them.

In the second phase of therapy, *desensitization,* the goal is to reduce the intensity of the emotions that clients feel when they stutter. Using videotapes of themselves and other stutterers, clients learn to calm themselves when they stutter and convey this calmness to listeners. They learn new emotional responses to old cues of anticipated stuttering and discover that they can control not only how they feel, but also how they stutter. Hierarchies of more and more difficult situations are used to transfer these changes to clients' daily lives.

The goal of the final phase, *modification,* is a continuation of what clients were learning and practicing in the desensitization phase. The emphasis here is on acquiring a new motor response to the cues that triggered old stuttering patterns. With calmer emotional responses, clients find that they can say previously feared words in a smoother, looser, more fluent way. The clinician continues to use videotapes of other stutterers and of the clients to help them learn new motor responses and generalize them to more and more challenging speaking situations.

Prins' approach incorporates many of the elements of Van Riper's therapy within a structure for learning that is borrowed from Bandura's cognitive behavior modification.

JOSEPH SHEEHAN

Throughout most of his professional career, Joseph Sheehan (1953, 1975, 1984) viewed stuttering as an approach-avoidance conflict. According to Sheehan, the stutterer stutters whenever the drive to go ahead and talk is equal to the drive to hold back and avoid talking. Based on this theory, therapy for the advanced stutterer had twin goals: increasing a stutterer's approach tendencies and decreasing his avoidance tendencies. The primary emphasis, however, was on the reduction of avoidance.

Sheehan presents five phases of therapy: (*a*) the self-acceptance phase, (*b*) the monitoring phase, (*c*) the initiative phase, (*d*) the modification of pattern phase, and (*e*) the safety margin phase.[4] His therapy sessions are loosely structured or counseling in nature, and he places little emphasis on data collection.

The goal of the self-acceptance phase is for the client to accept himself as a stutterer. This does not mean that he must accept forever his stuttering as it now exists. This will change as therapy proceeds. During this phase, typical clinical procedures involve the stutterer using good eye contact with listeners and discussing his stuttering openly with friends and acquaintances.

During the monitoring phase, the client increases his awareness of his stuttering as he is doing it; he is not to modify or try to control it, just be aware of it.

In the initiative phase, the client seeks out feared situations and enters them, to say his feared words and stutter openly on them.

During the modification of pattern phase, the client learns to stutter openly and easily. Stuttering openly and easily, according to Sheehan, requires the stutterer to let his listener see and hear that he is having trouble saying a word. Sheehan recommends the use of a "slide" or a prolongation of the first sound of a word, followed by a smooth release into the next sound of the word. The stutterer is to use the slide on feared words as an alternative way of stuttering. A major element in this technique is holding on to the stuttered sound beyond the point at which it could be released and then sliding out only after tension is gone. This is often difficult, but it provides a great boost in fluency when done correctly.

The goal of the safety margin phase is the client's development of a tolerance for disfluency. He needs to become comfortable exhibiting more disfluency than he would naturally have. When a stutterer is comfortable putting more stuttering in his speech than he ordinarily would, he has developed a sense of security or "margin of safety." Sheehan recommends that the stutterer voluntarily stutter by using the slide on nonfeared words throughout his speaking day. The more this is done, the more solid his fluency will become. Although Sheehan believed that some advanced stutterers will become spontaneously fluent by doing this, most will have acceptable stuttering.

Summary of Stuttering Modification Therapy

At the beginning of this section on stuttering modification therapy for the advanced stutterer, we stated that this form of therapy was characterized by two key elements: (*a*) teaching the stutterer to modify his moments of stuttering and (*b*) reducing his fear of stuttering and eliminating the avoidance behaviors associated with this fear. Based on our description of Van Riper's clinical procedures and our overviews of Bloodstein's, Boehmler's, Conture's, Prins', and Sheehan's clinical procedures, it should be clear that each of these clinicians' treatments shares these two key components. The specific clinical procedures of these clinicians may vary, but they all share these two clinical elements.

Most of the stuttering modification clinicians use procedures that are compatible with our theoretical perspective on the nature of stuttering. In Chapter 4, we suggest that persistent stuttering may be associated with two factors: neuromotor instability or inefficiency for speech production and a temperamental predisposition to increased muscle

---

[4] For two excellent chapters on stuttering modification therapy, the reader is referred to Sheehan, J.G. (1975). Conflict theory and avoidance-reduction therapy. In J. Eisenson (Ed.), *Stuttering: A second symposium* (pp. 97–198). New York: Harper & Row; and Sheehan, J.G., & Sheehan, V.M. (1984). Avoidance-reduction therapy: A response-suppression hypothesis. In W.H. Perkins (Ed.), *Stuttering disorders* (pp. 147–151). New York: Thieme-Stratton.

tension, escape, and avoidance responses and vulnerability to emotional (classical) conditioning. We recommended that therapy deal with neuromotor breakdown by reducing the speed of speech production and treat the temperament factors by increasing approach (left hemisphere) emotions and decreasing avoidance (right hemisphere) emotions.

All the stuttering modification clinicians depicted here advocate slow, steady movements as clients work their way through feared words. Most (especially Sheehan) also recommend increasing clients' approach tendencies by means of techniques such as seeking out rather than avoiding feared words and situations and by increasing eye contact with listeners.

FLUENCY SHAPING THERAPY

The essence of fluency shaping therapy is that some form of fluency is first established in the clinical setting, reinforced, and gradually modified to approximate normal sounding conversational speech. The client's new fluency is then generalized to his everyday speaking environment. As a general rule, fluency shaping clinicians place little emphasis on reducing the stutterer's fear and avoidance of words and speaking situations.

We have chosen the fluency shaping approach of Megan Neilson and Gavin Andrews to illustrate this therapy. Andrews developed a fluency shaping program in the 1960s, training clients to talk to the rhythm of a metronome. Later, he and a former student, Roger Ingham, developed an approach borrowed from Israel Goldiamond, Ronald Webster, and others, which produced instant fluency in the clinic using slow, prolonged speech. The most recent version of the program has been "fine-tuned" by Megan Neilson, working with Andrews. We also describe several other fluency shaping clinicians' approaches to provide a broader understanding of fluency shaping therapy.

Megan Neilson and Gavin Andrews: Intensive Fluency Training

CLINICIAN'S BELIEFS

Nature of Stuttering

Neilson and Andrews have written extensively about their views of the nature of stuttering. In an article reflecting their joint research (Andrews et al., 1983), they described stuttering as a constitutionally based disorder of sensory-motor processing (the theory of stuttering as a reduced neural capacity for internal modeling in Chapter 2). They acknowledge that the severity of stuttering of an advanced stutterer is not determined by his basic constitutional disorder, but by an overlay of learned reactions. They believe that their treatment program trains clients to cope with their basic processing defect by learning to speak with highly conscious "smooth speech" skills, thereby developing more accurate internal sensory-motor models.

Speech Behaviors Targeted for Therapy

Neilson and Andrews teach "smooth speech" skills to help clients overcome their sensory-motor processing deficit. These skills include slower speech rate, relaxed breathing, easy phrase initiation, phrase continuity, proper phrasing and pausing, appropriate prosody, and effective presentation skills. These are taught first in the clinic and then used in more and more challenging speech situations. The details of each skill and the generalization procedures are discussed in the section on Clinical Procedures.

Fluency Goals

Neilson and Andrews believe that with diligent practice clients can achieve spontaneous fluency, but they are realistic enough to know that some clients will relapse or at least experience their former anticipation of stuttering. Consequently, they train clients to recover from a recurrence of stuttering after treatment by a brief return to the controlled fluency they learned in therapy. They also train clients to use controlled fluency if they anticipate stuttering.

Feelings and Attitudes

Neilson and Andrews and their coworkers have gathered evidence that clients' attitudes toward communication and their feelings about their ability to change predict the outcome of treatment. Consequently, their treatment program includes frequent opportunities for clients to experience successful communication in what were previously difficult situations, as well as to experience feedback regarding their ability to influence their own success. At the beginning and at the end of treatment, clients' feelings and attitudes are assessed by using the Modified Erickson Scale of Communication Attitudes and the Locus of Control of Behavior Scale (see Chapter 7). All clients participate in a cognitive component of therapy aimed at enhancing their perceptions of themselves as speakers and helping them realize that they are responsible for their fluency. Remedial work is offered to clients whose responses to these feelings and attitudes scales put them at risk for unsuccessful therapy.

Maintenance Procedures

The client returns to the clinic at 1-, 2-, 3-, 6-, and 12-month intervals after completing treatment to have his speech assessed in conversation and on recent audio recordings of phone calls he has made. Problems in maintaining fluency are addressed in group maintenance therapy, conducted once each month.

Clinical Methods

Neilson and Andrews use operant conditioning and programmed instruction techniques to establish fluent speech at a normal rate and to transfer it to a variety of situations in each client's home and work. Progress through stages of the program is determined by ongoing daily assessments of speech rate and fluency, accompanied by continuous feedback to the client. Data on attitudes and beliefs, as well as speech rate and fluency, are gathered at the beginning and end of treatment.

CLINICAL PROCEDURES

The program begins by giving the client a brief overview of stuttering, normal speech anatomy and physiology, and the 3-week treatment program.

Fluency in Statement

The client learns smooth speech at 50 syllables per minute (SPM), using:

1. Rate Control. Speech rate is reduced by extending the duration of all sounds (Fig. 8.3)
2. Breathing. Maladaptive breathing patterns are replaced by a relaxed, natural pattern.
3. Easy Phrase Initiation. Gentle onset of voicing and airflow and soft articulatory contacts are used for the first sounds of each phrase.

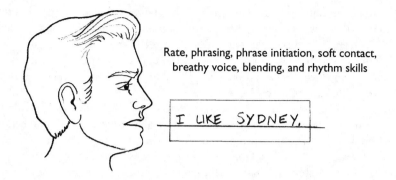

Rate, phrasing, phrase initiation, soft contact, breathy voice, blending, and rhythm skills

I LIKE SYDNEY,

Figure 8.3. Neilson and Andrews' fluency skills.

4. Phrase Continuity. The words in each breath phrase are produced as a single, joined unit with continuous movement and soft contacts of articulators, smooth elisions between words, and continuity of voicing and airflow.

When the client has progressed to 100 SPM, he learns three additional skills:

5. Phrasing and Pausing. The client learns to break speech into meaningful linguistic phrases, to pause for breathing, and to engage in speech planning in this break.
6. Prosody. Proper intonation, rhythm, and loudness are taught as soon as the client learns the first five skills.
7. Presentation. The client learns effective speaking styles incorporating appropriate eye contact and body language.

The sequence of activities for learning smooth speech begins with the client imitating the clinician's models of vowels, diphthongs, consonant-vowel combinations, words, and then short phrases. Using a training tape, the client drills on these utterances for several hours, then practices with the clinician in simple conversational interchanges that are limited to three-syllable long breath groups. At this speech rate using smooth speech techniques, the client is stutter-free.

Fluency Shaping

Starting at 50 SPM, the client learns to use smooth speech at gradually faster rates in steps of 10 SPM, until he is speaking fluently at the normal rate of 200 SPM. This is achieved through the use of "rating sessions"—group conversations in which each client has to speak a total of 7 minutes entirely free of stutters and at their prescribed rate. The clinician gives continuous feedback to each client about his rate and smooth speech techniques. If a client stutters, his speaking time is reset to zero and he must produce 7 minutes of fluent speech at the target rate to advance to the next level of the program.

In addition to clinician feedback, videotaping is used to hone clients' skills in self-assessment of their smooth speech techniques. Errors in breathing, smooth phrase initiation, and continuity are corrected early in the week devoted to fluency shaping, and conversational skills such as "presentation" are emphasized as the week goes on. By the end of the first week, all clients are speaking fluently in the clinic at a normal rate.

Transfer

During the week of fluency shaping, some transfer occurs by default when the client is in the home environment. Consequently, whenever a client speaks to family or friends, he is instructed to use smooth speech techniques at the speech rate last achieved in the clinic. At the end of the fluency shaping week, the client is taught coping skills to deal with anticipated stutters or to recover fluency after a stutter. These techniques, like Van Riper's "cancellations" and "preparatory sets," teach the client to respond to stutters by repeating a stuttered word with slow, smooth speech and to prepare for an expected stutter by "gearing down" to slower, smoother speech.

On each day of the second week of treatment, standard transfer activities are carried out between group rating sessions at both slow and normal speaking rates. Transfer activities, which must be completed with fluent, normal-sounding speech, include conversations with family, friends, and strangers, as well as phone calls, introductions, and shopping. The client tape-records transfer assignments and assesses them for fluency, rate, and normalcy before submitting them to the clinician for further evaluation. Once the assignments are completed satisfactorily, a group meeting is held with the client's friends and family to discuss his progress and to involve significant others in the client's transfer and maintenance.

In the third week, more difficult transfer activities are undertaken, involving speaking with peers and superiors at work, more introductions, giving a speech, and a conversation on a call-in radio show. This week also focuses on honing the client's self-evaluation, problem-solving, and self-reinforcement skills, all of which will be crucial for the client's success as his own therapist.

Maintenance Procedures

Maintenance activities, described earlier, consist of continued rating sessions at regular intervals at treatment end and include group sharing of advice. Clients are also urged to join a self-help group in which they practice skills and receive support.

Other Clinicians

As done in the stuttering modification section, we now provide brief overviews of the therapies that some other representative fluency shaping clinicians use for advanced stuttering.

EINER BOBERG AND DEBORAH KULLY

For a number of years, Einer Boberg and Deborah Kully (Boberg, 1984; Boberg & Kully, 1994) conducted intensive 3-week therapy programs during the summer at the University of Alberta in Canada. After Boberg's untimely death in 1995, Kully and Marilyn Langevin have continued this work. The program is divided into seven phases: (a) baseline, (b) identification, (c) early modification, (d) prolongation, (e) rate increase and cancellation, (f) self-monitoring and transfer training, and (g) transfer. Throughout this therapy program, Boberg and Kully put a great deal of emphasis on objective measurement of speech behaviors and the use of criterion levels for advancing the client from one phase to the next. Electronic counters and timers are used to aid in this process.

The baseline phase establishes a level from which to measure subsequent changes as the client moves through the program. During the identification phase, the client learns to accurately identify his moments of stuttering, both on-line while speaking and off-line, using audiotapes and videotapes. In the early modification phase, the client is introduced to the following fluency skills: prolongation, easy onset of phrases, soft contact on consonants, short phrases, and continuous airflow throughout the phrases. These skills are practiced first in vowels, then in consonant-vowel combinations, then in one- and two-syllable words, and finally in short phrases.

During the prolongation phase, the client speaks in a prolonged manner at approximately 60 SPM, incorporating the fluency skills learned in the previous phase. This slow, prolonged speech must be free of any struggle or tension. In the rate increase and cancellation phase, the client systematically increases his speaking rate in four steps from approximately 90 SPM to approximately 190 SPM. The criterion for moving from one rate to the next is less than 1% disfluency. Cancellation, a procedure in which the client smoothly repeats any syllable on which he struggles, is also introduced.

In the self-monitoring and transfer training phase, the stutterer learns to talk at normal speaking rates with less than 1% disfluency without any feedback from the clinician or electronic counters. Normal-sounding speech, or controlled fluency, is transferred from the clinic to a variety of nonclinical situations using a series of standard and personal assignments. Boberg and Kully (1994) sampled the speech of 17 adult and 25 adolescent clients 12 to 24 months after treatment ended and found that 69% had maintained a satisfactory level of fluency.

BRUCE RYAN

Bruce Ryan (1974) has been a pioneer in the development of stuttering therapy based on operant conditioning and programmed instruction. He organizes his treatment programs into three phases: (*a*) establishment, (*b*) transfer, and (*c*) maintenance. During therapy, Ryan continuously collects data on the client's speech performance, that is, his stuttered words per minute (SW/M) and his words spoken per minute (WS/M). These data are used to determine whether a client meets the criterion, usually 0 SW/M for a specified period of time, to move on to the next step of the program.

The goal of the establishment phase is to establish fluency with the clinician in the clinical setting. Ryan uses a number of establishment programs; however, he usually uses his delayed auditory feedback (DAF) program with adults. In this program, the DAF machine is used to help clients speak in a slow, prolonged, fluent manner. The delay times on the DAF machine are systematically reduced to allow the client to gradually increase his speaking rate by reducing the prolongation of speech sounds until he approaches a normal rate. In this program, Ryan sequentially moves the client through a series of steps, or delay times on the DAF machine, in each of the following three modes: reading, monologue, and conversation. The client begins with slow, prolonged, fluent oral reading that is gradually shaped into fluent conversational speech, or controlled fluency, in the clinical setting.

The goal of the transfer phase is to transfer the client's fluency from the clinical setting to a variety of other settings and people. To do this, Ryan uses a number of hierarchies, or sequences of speaking situations, ordered from easy to difficult, in which a client talks and meets the fluency criterion of 0 SW/M. The client obviously needs to be exhibiting spontaneous or controlled fluency, not acceptable stuttering, to meet this criterion.

The goal of Ryan's last phase, the maintenance phase, is for the client to maintain his fluency in all speaking situations for approximately 2 years and involves the client returning to the clinician for a series of maintenance checks.

GEORGE SHAMES AND CHERI FLORANCE

George Shames and Cheri Florance (1980) are authors of a fluency shaping program for adults that has as its goal "stutter-free speech." Their program is quite structured, but a little less so than that of the other fluency shaping clinicians. They obtain a substantial amount of data on their clients before, during, and after treatment. Shames and Florance divide their therapy into five phases: (*a*) volitional control, (*b*) self reinforcement, (*c*) transfer, (*d*) training in unmonitored speech, and (*e*) follow-up.

The goal of the first phase is for the stutterer to gain volitional control of his speech. The two skills that Shames and Florance believe are most important for the stutterer to acquire, if he is going to control his speech, are control of rate and continuous phonation. Shames and Florance use DAF to help clients learn these skills. They begin with the DAF machine set at its maximum delay and instruct the stutterer in the use of rate control and continuous phonation to produce slow, prolonged, stutter-free speech. Shames and Florance then gradually increase the client's speaking rate by systematically reducing delay times on the DAF machine. By the end of this phase, the client is producing stutter-free speech at a near-normal rate. In other words, he is using controlled fluency.

In the self-reinforcement phase, a client learns to monitor, evaluate, and reinforce himself for using stutter-free speech in the clinical setting. Administration of reinforcement is gradually shifted from the clinician to the client, and the reinforcement used by Shames and Florance is the opportunity for the stutterer to use brief periods of unmonitored speech. Thus, after a client engages in the work of monitoring his speech, he finds it rewarding to speak spontaneously and fluently for several minutes.

The third phase involves systematic transfer of monitored, stutter-free speech or controlled fluency into the client's environment. At first, this involves only a few situations each day, but by the end of this phase of therapy, it will involve the client using monitored, stutter-free speech for the entire day. Shames and Florance do not use hierarchies, as many clinicians do, to transfer monitored, stutter-free speech. Rather, they use a contract plan. The client prepares a daily contract that specifies the situations in which he will use monitored, stutter-free speech and then reinforces himself with unmonitored speech.

In the fourth phase, the client gradually replaces his monitored, stutter-free speech with unmonitored speech. Shames and Florance indicate that, by this time in treatment, the client's monitored, stutter-free speech and his unmonitored speech are both largely fluent. In other words, he is now exhibiting both controlled fluency and spontaneous fluency. The important difference is that the client finds the unmonitored speech to be much more reinforcing.

After completion of training in the unmonitored speech phase, the client is placed in a 5-year, follow-up program.

RONALD WEBSTER

Ronald Webster's (1974, 1979, 1980) Precision Fluency Shaping Program at Hollins College has received a great deal of national attention. Many people who stutter have come from across the country, including Annie Glenn, wife of the senator and former astronaut John Glenn, to participate in this 3-week intensive treatment program.

Webster believes that the core behaviors of stuttering reflect a discoordination of muscles for voicing and articulation and that these discoordinations have a physiological basis. He further believes that the stutterer's secondary behaviors and feelings and attitudes are most likely learned.

The goal of Webster's Precision Fluency Shaping Program is to teach clients to use fluency-generating target behaviors that, when used correctly, will result in fluency. The two most important target behaviors appear to be slightly increased syllable durations and gentle voice onset. The program begins by teaching the client to prolong or stretch syllables, using a stopwatch to measure their duration. The client is then taught to coordinate diaphragmatic breathing with these prolonged syllables. Gentle voice onsets are taught next, and a specially designed voice-onset computer, the Voice Monitor, is used to evaluate this target behavior.

After all the above target behaviors are established in syllables, they are practiced in one-syllable words; two-syllable words; three-syllable words; short, self-generated sentences; and finally, spontaneous conversation. As the length of linguistic units is systematically increased, the duration of the syllables is gradually reduced. Therefore, by the time the client is practicing his target behaviors in conversation, his speech rate has reached a slow-normal rate during his controlled fluency.

Now, the client is ready to transfer this controlled fluency to outside situations. This involves interactions with merchants: single-message telephone calls, single-message personal contacts, double-message telephone calls, double-message personal contacts, and multiple messages by both telephone and personal contact.

Webster uses a highly structured or programmed instruction approach to therapy. Every client goes through the same set of explicitly defined procedures. During the 3-week program, a typical client practices his fluency-generating target behaviors approximately 100 hours. Progress from one step of the program to the next depends on the client meeting specified criterion levels, and a record of correct and incorrect responses is kept for each step.

Summary of Fluency Shaping Therapy

When we began this section on fluency shaping therapy, we stated that the essence of this approach for the advanced stutterer is the establishment of some form of fluency initially in the clinical setting, which is reinforced and gradually modified to approximate normal-sounding speech. After the establishment of controlled fluency in the clinical setting, the client's fluency is generalized to the client's everyday speaking environment. We also said that, as a general rule, fluency shaping clinicians do not emphasize reductions of clients' fear and avoidance of words and situations; changes in fear and avoidance are assumed to occur as a by-product of clients' confidence in their controlled fluency. Based on our coverage of Neilson and Andrews' clinical procedures and on our brief descriptions of Boberg and Kully's, Ryan's, Shames and Florance's, and Webster's programs, it should be clear to the reader that all these clinicians share the previously discussed clinical beliefs.

COMPARISON OF THE TWO APPROACHES

Now that we have completed our descriptions of stuttering modification and fluency shaping therapies for advanced stuttering, we can compare these two approaches on the five clinical issues on which they often differ: (*a*) speech behaviors targeted for therapy, (*b*) fluency goals, (*c*) attention given to feelings and attitudes, (*d*) maintenance procedures, and (*e*) clinical methods. Table 8.1 summarizes the similarities and differences between these two therapy approaches.

With regard to targets for therapy, stuttering modification clinicians teach clients to modify moments of stuttering in ways that reduce their severity, whereas fluency shaping clinicians teach clients to use fluency enhancing skills to increase fluency. The goal of stuttering modification clinicians is spontaneous fluency for a few advanced stutterers, but for most clients, a realistic goal is controlled fluency or acceptable stuttering. Like stuttering modification clinicians, fluency shaping clinicians have spontaneous fluency as their goal for a few clients, but for most, the goal is controlled fluency. Acceptable stuttering is not a goal for any fluency shaping client.

Stuttering modification and fluency shaping clinicians differ sharply in their attention to targeting feelings and attitudes in therapy. Stuttering modification clinicians give considerable time and energy to reducing an advanced stutterer's negative feelings and atti-

Table 8.1. Similarities and Differences Between Stuttering Modification and Fluency Shaping Therapies for the Advanced Stutterer

Clinical Issue	Therapy Approach	
	Stuttering Modification Therapy	Fluency Shaping Therapy
Speech behaviors targeted for therapy	Moments of stuttering	Fluency skills
Fluency goals	Spontaneous fluency, controlled fluency, or acceptable stuttering	Spontaneous fluency or controlled fluency
Feelings and attitudes	Considerable attention given to changing feelings and attitudes	Little attention given to changing feelings and attitudes
Maintenance procedures	Emphasis on maintaining stuttering modification skills and changes in feelings and attitudes	Emphasis on maintaining fluency shaping skills
Clinical Procedures	Therapy characterized by loosely structured interaction	Therapy characterized by tightly structured interaction or programmed instruction
	Little emphasis on collection of objective data	Considerable emphasis on collection of objective data

tudes about his speech. They also stress the elimination of avoidance behaviors. In contrast, fluency shaping clinicians give relatively little attention to changing these feelings, attitudes, or avoidance behaviors, assuming they will change as fluency changes.

To help the client with advanced stuttering maintain improvement after termination of therapy, stuttering modification clinicians emphasize maintaining the reduction of negative feelings and attitudes and the elimination of avoidance behaviors. They also emphasize maintaining proficiency in the use of stuttering modification skills. In contrast, fluency shaping clinicians emphasize only the client's continuing proficiency in using fluency shaping or fluency enhancing skills.

It is on the last issue, clinical methods, that the two therapy approaches usually differ the most. Stuttering modification therapy is typically characterized by loosely structured sessions between clinician and client in a counseling/teaching types of interaction. Fluency shaping therapy, on the other hand, is characterized by tightly structured interactions between clinician and client in a programmed instruction format. These two approaches often differ as well with regard to data collection. Stuttering modification clinicians usually put little emphasis on collecting objective data, whereas fluency shaping clinicians generally put considerable emphasis on data for advancing clients through therapy and assessing treatment outcomes.

Even though stuttering modification and fluency shaping therapies differ to some degree on each of the five issues in the treatment of advanced stuttering, we believe that the two most clinically significant differences involve the speech behaviors targeted for therapy and the attention given to feelings and attitudes. Thus, when we discuss an integration of these two approaches in the next chapter, we concentrate much of our effort on the integration of these two aspects of therapy.

Because the two treatment approaches—stuttering modification and fluency enhancing—differ most at the level of advanced stuttering, it may be informative to look at them through the lens of our theoretical perspective. Our model of stuttering etiology proposes that most persistent stuttering, particularly in the advanced stutterer, is the result of two factors: neuromotor speech breakdown and a vulnerable temperament. Because persons who stutter may have differing proportions of each of these two components, different approaches may be needed for different clients.

Fluency shaping, with its emphasis on slow speech production, may be well suited for individuals who have less of the temperament component and more of the neuromotor breakdown component. In fact, some research suggests that clients who have relatively low scores on a measure of avoidance (Guitar, 1976) will gain substantial long-term benefits from fluency shaping. Stuttering modification therapies that emphasize exploration of and approach toward the stuttering as well as reduction of avoidance may be the best treatment for clients whose temperament makes them especially vulnerable to fear conditioning. On the other hand, clients who have more nearly equal proportions of both neuromotor breakdown and temperament components may be best served by approaches that integrate fluency shaping and stuttering modification, such as those described in the next chapter.

STUDY QUESTIONS

1. What are the two key elements in stuttering modification therapy for the client who stutters?
2. What are the goals for the following phases of Van Riper's therapy for the advanced stutterer: (a) identification phase, (b) desensitization phase, (c) modification phase, and (d) stabilization phase?
3. Briefly describe Van Riper's clinical procedures for advanced stuttering during the identification phase.
4. Describe one clinical procedure Van Riper uses to desensitize the client with advanced stuttering to each of the following features of the disorder: (a) confrontation with the disorder, (b) core behaviors, and (c) listener reactions.
5. Describe the following procedures Van Riper uses to modify advanced stuttering: (a) cancellations, (b) pull-outs, and (c) preparatory sets.
6. Briefly describe Van Riper's clinical procedures for the advanced stutterer during the stabilization phase.
7. Describe the key elements of fluency shaping therapy for the advanced stutterer.
8. List and explain the four smooth speech skills taught to clients at 50 SPM in Neilson and Andrew's program.
9. How do Neilson and Andrews incorporate operant procedures into their treatment program?
10. What procedures do Neilson and Andrews use to help clients prepare for maintenance of fluency after treatment? Can you think of other things they could do for this purpose?
11. Compare stuttering modification and fluency shaping therapies for the advanced stutterer on the following five clinical issues: (a) speech behaviors targeted for therapy, (b) fluency goals, (c) attention given to feelings and attitudes, (d) maintenance procedures, and (e) clinical methods.

SUGGESTED READINGS

Neilson, M., & Andrews, G. (1992). Intensive fluency training of chronic stutterers. In R. Curlee (Ed.), *Stuttering & related disorders of fluency.* (pp. 139–165). New York: Thieme.

The authors give a very detailed description of their fluency shaping treatment and provide many references for information about long-term outcome.

Onslow, M., & Packman, A. (1997). Designing and implementing a strategy to control stuttered speech in adults. In R. Curlee & G. Siegel (Eds.), *Nature and treatment of stuttering: New directions*. Boston: Allyn & Bacon.

These two authors use their years of experience with fluency shaping to develop individualized behavioral treatments for advanced stutterers. They place strong emphasis on using natural-sounding speech and maintenance strategies.

Prins, D. (1997). Modifying stuttering—The stutterer's reactive behavior: Perspectives on past, present, and future. In R. Curlee & G. Siegel (Eds.), *Nature and treatment of stuttering: New directions*. Boston: Allyn & Bacon.

This is an update of stuttering modification procedures for advanced stuttering. Prins provides insights into why past therapies of this type were effective and integrates these principles within a social cognitive model for treatment.

Sheehan, J.G. (1975). Conflict theory and avoidance-reduction therapy. In J. Eisenson (Ed.), *Stuttering: A second symposium* (pp. 97–198). New York: Harper & Row.

This chapter is a thorough presentation of Sheehan's stuttering modification approach for the advanced stutterer. Emphasis is placed on avoidance-reduction techniques.

Van Riper, C. (1973). Our therapeutic approach. In C. Van Riper, *The treatment of stuttering* (pp. 201–370). Englewood Cliffs, NJ: Prentice-Hall.

In the last half of this book, Van Riper presents a comprehensive presentation of his therapy for the advanced stutterer. For any serious student of stuttering modification therapy, these chapters are "must" reading.

Van Riper, C. (1974). Modification of behavior. In *Therapy for stutterers* (pp. 45–73). Memphis: Speech Foundation of America.

This is a brief but very good description of Van Riper's therapy for the advanced stutterer.

9

Advanced Stutterer: Integration of Approaches

Like many other clinicians, we adopt ideas and clinical procedures from both stuttering modification and fluency shaping therapies. We integrate these procedures so that clients learn skills to speak fluently but are also able to modify their moments of stuttering. We believe that in addition to changing speech behaviors, clients should reduce negative feelings and attitudes and eliminate avoidances. We describe our own clinical procedures in sufficient detail to allow clinicians to use them with their clients. We also briefly discuss the clinical procedures of other clinicians who integrate stuttering modification and fluency shaping therapies with the advanced stutterer.

Before we discuss our approach, it may be helpful to review the characteristics of the advanced stutterer. This client will be an adult or a high school student. Core behaviors will be part-word repetitions with excessive tension, vowel prolongations with excessive tension, and blocks. Secondary behaviors will be escape devices, starting behaviors, postponements, word avoidances, and situation avoidances. The advanced stutterer will evidence frustration, embarrassment, and fear about his stuttering and will have handicapping self-concepts.

OUR APPROACH

Clinician's Beliefs

In this section, we review our beliefs about advanced stuttering, with a special focus on aspects that are important considerations in treatment.

NATURE OF STUTTERING

As discussed in Section I, we believe that physiological predispositions for inefficient neural activation patterns and a vulnerable temperament interact with environmental influences to produce or exacerbate the core behaviors of stuttering. The child responds to these early core behaviors, or disfluencies, with tension and hurry. As the child continues to experience and react to core behaviors, he copes using a variety of escape and starting behaviors, which are reinforced through operant conditioning. During this same period, negative feelings, such as frustration, shame, and fear, become associated with stuttering. These feelings generalize through classical conditioning to more words and situations. Finally, the child begins to avoid feared words and situations, behaviors that are reinforced through avoidance conditioning. If these underlying processes continue until the individual has reached adolescence or young adulthood, the client will become an advanced stutterer.

Because increased tension, hurry, secondary behaviors, and feelings and attitudes are largely learned, we believe they can be unlearned or modified. Operant and classical conditioning principles are used in doing this. However, if predisposing physiological factors are contributing to these behaviors and because learning changes neural organization, *complete* unlearning may not be possible. So, we believe it is important to help the advanced stutterer to learn how to cope with these disruptions in speech, if he is going to maintain improvements in fluency.

SPEECH BEHAVIORS TARGETED FOR THERAPY

We believe that most advanced stutterers have acquired substantial tension and hurry responses with a considerable overlay of learned secondary behaviors. To cope with these learned behaviors and to speak more fluently, we believe it is beneficial for the advanced stutterer to modify moments of stuttering as well as use fluency enhancing skills. We believe that these two skills complement one another. For example, the slow movements and light articulatory contacts used in Van Riper's pull-outs or preparatory sets are identical with the slow, prolonged sounds and soft articulatory contacts involved in the skills of smooth speech. The only difference is that Van Riper's techniques focus on modifying stuttered words, whereas the development of smooth speech skills involves modifying the overall speech pattern. Thus, the stuttering modification clinician teaches the stutterer to modify words on which stuttering is anticipated or is occurring, and the fluency shaping clinician teaches the stutterer to modify the whole sentence in an effort to prevent stuttering from arising. So, why not teach the stutterer to do both (Fig. 9.1)?[1]

---

[1] As we (Guitar & Peters, 1980) have previously observed, stuttering modification and fluency shaping therapies often produce speech patterns that sound similar. As clients receiving either therapy become more fluent, "they pass through a stage of controlled fluency in which words are spoken with a prolonged, gradual onset. The pull-outs and preparatory sets of stuttering modification therapy may be indistinguishable from the gentle onsets or slow, prolonged patterns of some fluency shaping therapies."

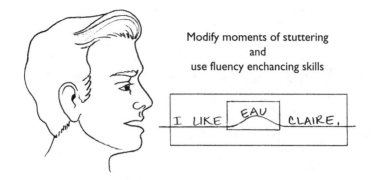

Figure 9.1. Integration of stuttering modification and fluency shaping therapies.

Whether the clinician is teaching the stutterer to modify given moments of stuttering or teaching him to use fluency enhancing skills, operant conditioning principles, especially reinforcement principles, are crucial in achieving either of these goals. In the Clinical Procedures section, we provide guidance in how to use positive reinforcement and response cost to shape slow, fluent speech into normal-sounding speech and to help the stutterer make his moments of stuttering easier and easier.

Finally, because the core behaviors may have a physiological basis, we believe that both stuttering modification skills and fluency enhancing skills are needed to help the advanced stutterer cope more effectively with physiological disruptions of speech. By using these skills, he will be able to maintain his fluency more effectively.

FLUENCY GOALS

The ultimate goal for an advanced stutterer is spontaneous fluency in all situations—in other words, normal speech. In our opinion, most advanced stutterers do not reach this level of fluency. After treatment, the client may have periods of spontaneous fluency lasting from a few hours to a month or more, but usually some stuttering returns, especially in stressful situations. At these times, we want the client to have three options available.

First, when the stutterer feels it is important to sound fluent, we want him to be able to successfully apply stuttering modification skills or fluency shaping skills or both to achieve controlled fluency.

Second, when he feels it is important to sound fluent but is unable to achieve controlled fluency, we want him to at least be able to apply and feel comfortable with combined stuttering modification and fluency shaping skills, which produce a modified level of stuttering that is close to fluent speech.

Third, when he feels it is not important to sound fluent and he does not want to put the effort into doing so, we would like him to be comfortable with acceptable stuttering so that he does not avoid speaking and is not embarrassed about his stuttering. These fluency goals seem realistic to us. Furthermore, in the final analysis, it will be the client who chooses which of the latter options he will use in a particular situation.

FEELINGS AND ATTITUDES

We believe that an advanced stutterer's avoidance behaviors and negative feelings and attitudes need to receive considerable attention in therapy (Fig. 9.2). He needs to eliminate the use of avoidances, because he will never reduce his fear of the words and speaking situations that he continues to avoid. In addition, it is very important that these fears,

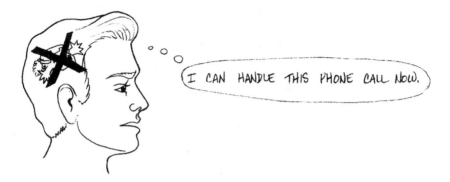

Figure 9.2. It is important to target feelings and attitudes.

not just avoidances, be reduced if the client is going to be successful in using either stuttering modification or fluency shaping techniques. Otherwise, fear will create excessive muscular tension, and he may be unable to alter his speech production toward fluency. We also believe that avoidances and speech fears need to be substantially reduced if the stutterer is going to maintain his improvement over the long run. If they are not significantly diminished, we believe they will become the seeds for relapse, which is so prevalent among advanced stutterers.

It is important for clinicians to understand classical conditioning principles when they attempt to eliminate the client's avoidance behaviors or reduce his negative feelings and attitudes. One strategy for changing classically conditioned responses is *counterconditioning,* which takes place when words and situations that elicit fear—the conditioned stimuli—are experienced over and over again in the presence of positive feelings. For example, when the stutterer confronts and explores his stuttering in the presence of an accepting and understanding clinician, counterconditioning occurs. The clinician's positive regard and reinforcement of this exploration decrease the stutterer's fears and negative feelings, a process that is also called *reciprocal inhibition.* Another approach, *deconditioning,* takes place when words and situations that elicit relatively low levels of fear are experienced over and over, in the absence of the feared consequences, until the fear becomes dissipated or extinguished. This is why we use hierarchies of least-to-most fearful stimuli in helping the client reduce negative emotions. By beginning with the client's least fearful words or situations and gradually working our way up the hierarchy, his fears are systematically reduced. Examples of these procedures are presented in the discussion of our clinical procedures.

MAINTENANCE PROCEDURES

We believe that effective maintenance depends on the client becoming his own clinician, beginning early in therapy. We help the client learn to evaluate his own performance in mastering stuttering modification and fluency shaping techniques and to monitor his speech fears and avoidances. We gradually shift more and more of the responsibility for therapy to the client as he improves. It is important for the client to have a realistic understanding of what he should expect in terms of long-term fluency. In other words, the client needs to understand the concepts of spontaneous fluency, controlled fluency, and acceptable stuttering in setting his own fluency goals. It is also important that the client comes to realize the relationship between the conscientiousness with which he practices what he has learned in therapy and the attainment of fluency goals.

CLINICAL METHODS

Our clinical procedures for the advanced stutterer are implemented primarily in a coun-seling/teaching type of interaction. The only exception is when we teach the fluency shap-ing or fluency enhancing behaviors (FEBs), in which we use a loose application of pro-gramming principles. We accompany our clients on many outside speaking assignments and also give them a great many outside speaking assignments to complete on their own. We have applied these clinical procedures in both individual and group therapy.

In terms of data collection, we measure clients' frequency of stuttering and speech rate before treatment begins and at the termination of treatment. At times, we measure their speech during each therapy session. This is especially true when teaching the client a new skill, such as fluency shaping or FEBs. We also attempt to assess our client's speech in his daily speaking environments and to evaluate his feelings and attitudes about his speech. The measures that we use were described in Chapter 7 in our discussion of as-sessment.

Clinical Procedures

We have been combining components of stuttering modification therapy and fluency shaping therapy in a number of ways in our clinical work for many years.[2] In the follow-ing pages, we describe what we are currently doing.

We believe it is important that treatment for advanced stutterers contain the follow-ing components or phases: (*a*) understanding and confronting stuttering, (*b*) reducing negative feelings and attitudes and eliminating avoidances, (*c*) using fluency enhancing skills and modifying the moments of stuttering, and (*d*) maintaining improvement. We usually sequence these components in the order listed but, at times, have found it bene-ficial for the third phase (using FEBs and modifying the moments of stuttering) to pre-cede the second phase (reducing negative feelings and attitudes and eliminating avoid-ances). This has been especially true with advanced stutterers who resist confronting their speech fears. This resistance is usually manifested by their being only nominally in-volved in therapy or missing many sessions.

We sometimes provide handouts developed by Theodore Peters to our clients for each of these phases. These are reproduced in the following sections and can be copied and changed to suit your clients' needs. We may also suggest other readings, which are noted in the appropriate places.

UNDERSTANDING AND CONFRONTING STUTTERING

The goal of this first phase is to help the client become more objective about his stutter-ing, to lift the cloud of anxiety and dread that surrounds stuttering when it remains mys-terious. Guiding the client through various experiences in getting to know his stuttering, accepting it, and feeling the clinician's acceptance of him, whether he is stuttering or not, fosters the development of objectivity. As this process goes on, the client becomes more optimistic about changing stuttering. He realizes that stuttering is made up of behaviors that he can potentially control, and he feels the clinician's belief in his ability to change. The similarities between what we do in this phase and what Van Riper does in his iden-tification phase are obvious.

---

[2] The reader is referred to Guitar, B., & Peters, T.J. (1980). The high school and adult stutterer. In *Stuttering: An integration of contemporary therapies* (pp. 31–47). Memphis: Speech Foundation of America for an ear-lier version of an integrated or combined approach to treatment for the advanced or adult stutterer.

When the clinician first meets the stutterer, she should be warm and friendly. Her behavior should convey that she is comfortable with stuttering, and she should be well prepared. By being thoroughly familiar with the goals and procedures of therapy, she will instill confidence in the client.

In the first therapy session, we give the client an overview of the stages of therapy and a glimpse of the activities in each stage. We emphasize that we will be working together as a team, at a pace that is appropriate for him. We stress that as treatment progresses, he will be asked to take a greater and greater role in planning his therapy. The balance between our support and the client's growing independence shifts gradually over the course of treatment, but we must plant the seeds for independence in the earliest sessions. In this therapy session, we remind the client that he must be sincerely committed to working on his stuttering if treatment is to be effective. He must understand that token efforts are a waste of time. Most clients are ready to work hard, especially at the outset of therapy, but a few hold back because they have failed before. These individuals may need some early successes if they are to complete the hard journey ahead.

Understanding the Speech Mechanism

It is a common mistake to assume that clients know the functions of the respiratory, laryngeal, and articulatory systems of speech. In fact, most clients are unaware of how they talk. Therefore, before we begin to focus on what the client may be doing when he stutters, we help him realize what he's doing when he's fluent. We usually begin by giving a brief overview of breathing for speech, phonation, voiced versus voiceless sounds, and how the articulators produce different sounds. Next, we have the client experiment with his respiratory, laryngeal, and articulatory systems in producing voiceless airflow, then voiced airflow. Then, we add various articulations to voiceless and voiced airflows to help him learn the feel of each part of his speech mechanism.

After this work on fluent speech, we have the client explore what he may do at each level—respiratory, phonatory, and laryngeal—when he stutters on various sounds. Often, what may start out as an imitation of a stutter turns into a real one. This can turn into some real gains if we are able to use this opportunity to help the client feel what he's doing with his speech mechanism as he stutters. This may go on for one or two sessions, depending on his tolerance for exploring stuttering and our ability to help him feel comfortable as he "touches" what has previously been repugnant to him.

After this exploration of the speech mechanism, we move into exploration of stuttering. We have the client read the "Understanding Your Stuttering" handout, which appears below. If he is like most stutterers, he will have questions or will comment on some of his own behaviors that are described in the handout. The clinician should answer his questions carefully and enthusiastically reinforce any insights shared about his own speech. Then, we can begin to help him catalogue and confront the components of his stuttering.

UNDERSTANDING YOUR STUTTERING

We want to better understand your stuttering, and we want you to do the same. You may not know what you do or how you feel when you stutter. Because it's unpleasant, you have probably attempted to hide it from yourself as well as from others. Let's begin to explore your stuttering by discussing the following components of the problem. Once you explore and better understand your stuttering, it will lose its mystery, and you will be less uncomfortable with it.

Core Behaviors

These are the repetitions, prolongations, and blocks (getting completely blocked on a word) that you have. These are the core or heart of the problem. Core behaviors were the first stuttering behaviors you had as a child.

Why do you have these core behaviors? An increasing amount of research suggests that persons who stutter may have "timing" problems related to the control of the speech mechanism. For fluent speech to occur, muscle movements involved in breathing, in voice production (voice box), and in articulation (tongue, lips, jaw) must all be well coordinated. Evidence suggests that persons who stutter experience a lack of coordination between these muscle groups during speech. Furthermore, the research implies that these physical timing problems are so slight that they show up as stuttering only when feelings and emotions are strong enough to cause a breakdown in the coordination of the speech mechanism. We know that our ability to perform any physical skill can be affected by our emotions at the time. When our feelings and emotions are strong, they usually interfere with our performance. This is especially true with regard to the fine coordinations of the speech mechanism in the person who stutters. In therapy, we will teach you techniques to cope more effectively with these core behaviors.

Secondary Behaviors

Secondary behaviors are tricks or crutches that you use to avoid your stuttering or to help you get a word out. They are behaviors you have learned over the years to help you cope with the core behaviors. They can be unlearned. There are different types of secondary behaviors. Which of the following do you use?

Avoidance Behaviors

The general category of avoidance behaviors covers all the things you might do to keep from stuttering. Word and situation avoidances include substituting words, rephrasing sentences, not entering feared speaking situations, pretending not to know the answer. You might also use "postponements," such as pausing before a difficult word or repeating another word or phrase over and over before trying to say a word on which stuttering is expected. Another avoidance trick some stutterers use is called a "starter." This is when you might say a sound or word quickly just before a difficult word, as in saying "umwould you like to go to a movie?" Hand or body movements might be used in the same way.

Escape Behaviors

These behaviors are things the stutterer does to get out of a word once he is stuttering, such as a head nod, jaw jerk, or eye blink. You may have developed escape behaviors that are so subtle that you don't notice them anymore. Some of them might be called "disguise behaviors" because they are attempts to hide your stutter as it is happening. These include covering your mouth with your hand or turning your head when you stutter.

Feelings and Attitudes

When you began to stutter as a child, you were probably unaware of your stuttering. However, because you have been stuttering for many years, you may have had many frustrating and embarrassing speaking situations. Consequently, if you're like most stutterers, you have probably developed or learned some negative feelings and attitudes about your speech. You may feel embarrassed, guilty, fearful, or even angry. Fear is the most common. Stutterers typically fear certain speaking situations and certain sounds or words. What feelings and attitudes do you have regarding your stuttering? As part of your therapy, we will help you reduce these unpleasant feelings and attitudes.

With our help, explore and describe the various components of your stuttering problem. Before you can change something, you need to understand what you are changing.

After the client has asked questions about the handout and shared insights that it may have provided, we go through each section of the handout together, cataloguing various aspects of the client's stuttering. This may take several sessions. It is important that the stutterer become familiar with the components of his stuttering, because if he is going to change, he needs to know what to change. Part of the work will involve questioning the client about his stuttering to help him understand the nature of each component. We may imitate the client's stuttering and ask whether we are stuttering as he does, putting him in the role of teacher for a moment and reassuring him that we are not afraid to share his stuttering. We may also have the client watch himself in the mirror as he talks, or we may replay videotapes or audiotapes of his stuttering to identify and confront some of the core and secondary behaviors he uses. This level of self-confrontation can be difficult for many clients. So we always wait until we are sure that the client is emotionally ready before using the mirror or tape playback, which we do only briefly at this stage of treatment.

As with other difficult tasks, we model the task, voluntarily stuttering ourselves before asking the client to do it. Because good therapy is often confrontational, even painful at times, we must be sure that the client feels our support and acceptance as we progress. As noted earlier, counterconditioning of negative emotions is a powerful component of therapy for persons with advanced stuttering. As we push the client to be in touch with his emotions surrounding his stuttering, we must provide a highly accepting and supportive environment to countercondition his negative emotions.

REDUCING NEGATIVE FEELINGS AND ATTITUDES AND ELIMINATING AVOIDANCES

The goal of this second phase of therapy is to help the stutterer reduce fear and other negative emotions associated with stuttering. In fact, some of this fear reduction is introduced earlier in therapy when we help clients gain a better understanding of stuttering. We have adopted some guiding principles from the literature on the treatment of phobias, particularly those treatments that reduce fear by exposing the human or animal subject to the feared object and prevent his avoidance (Mineka, 1985).

Applying this research to our therapy, we find that fear can be reduced more quickly if (*a*) the client stays in contact with a moment of stuttering for a relatively long period of time, holding onto a stutter rather than rushing through it; (*b*) therapy is conducted by a clinician who is not afraid of stuttering; and (c) the client approaches and explores a moment of stuttering with curiosity and interest. These are essentially the techniques pioneered by Van Riper and Johnson more than half a century ago.

As well as reducing the client's fears, we want to help him change his attitudes about his speech. We want him to become more open and accepting of his disfluency. In addition, we want him to eliminate his use of speech avoidance behaviors.

We have organized this phase of therapy into the following four techniques: (a) discussing stuttering openly, (b) deliberately using feared words and entering feared situations, (c) freezing or holding on to moments of stuttering, and (d) using voluntary stuttering.

Discussing Stuttering Openly

We usually begin this second phase by encouraging the stutterer to discuss his stuttering openly with others. We have found the following handout helpful in introducing this activity.

DISCUSSING STUTTERING OPENLY

One way to become more comfortable with your stuttering is to discuss it openly with your family, friends, and acquaintances. When you get to the point of being open about your stuttering, you will lose much of your fear of it and be more relaxed. In most cases, your listeners know you stutter, you know you stutter, but nobody ever says anything about it. It's like the ostrich sticking his head in the sand in the face of danger, pretending it's not there. You would feel much more comfortable about your stuttering if you could talk about it openly. Your listener would also be more comfortable if you were open and at ease with your stuttering. Your listener often takes his cue from you regarding how to respond. If you look uncomfortable, he will probably be uncomfortable, but if you are open and comfortable with your stuttering, your listener will probably be at ease.

How can you be more open about your stuttering? Tell family and friends that you are in therapy and explain what you are doing in therapy and why you are doing it. After you have talked about it, encourage them to ask you questions about it. Create an opportunity to let them know how you would like them to respond to your stuttering. For example, some of your family and friends may finish words for you when you stutter. Let them know if you would rather just have them wait until you're finished. Or, some of your listeners may look away when you stutter. If this makes you uncomfortable, as it does most people who stutter, let your listeners know it is helpful if they can keep eye contact even when you stutter.

Another good practice is to make comments about your stuttering. If you feel like it, you can make a funny comment about your stuttering to put yourself and your listeners at ease. For example, if you have to introduce yourself and you think you will stutter on your name, you can say, "Make yourself comfortable, it may take me a few minutes to say my name." Or, just comment casually on a hard block you've had by saying, "Whew, that was a hard one." The more you can do this, the less panicked you will feel when you stutter. Another opportunity for being open about your stuttering is when you are faced with a speech or a presentation to a group. Just before you begin your speech, let the audience know that you stutter. They'll find out anyway, but saying it up front will put everyone, including yourself, much more at ease.

A few advanced stutterers will find these assignments easy, but most will find them difficult. They will need considerable support from a clinician. We usually help the client make a list of situations in which he will begin to be open about his stuttering; then we model an example for him. If commenting on stuttering during a telephone call is on his list, we would call a store, pretend to stutter, and immediately make a comment, such as "Wow, looks like I'm really having some trouble today." Recently, when working with a young man who stutters, we had him videotape us as we interviewed three different people on a busy shopping street. After getting permission to videotape, we asked them a variety of questions about stuttering and found that each gave positive, supportive answers. Our client seemed impressed that the lay public was, after all, not so uptight about stuttering. Exercises such as the latter can help an individual test reality and find out that much of the anxiety and disapproval about stuttering is in his mind rather than in that of the listener.

Finally, as we help the client devise a variety of tasks to become more open about his stuttering, we ensure that the assignments are carried out in a hierarchical order from least to most stressful. This way the first task will be easy and give him confidence for later tasks. In psychological terms, reductions in negative emotions that are associated with less stressful tasks will generalize to more stressful tasks. Consequently, when the client gets to the more stressful tasks, these tasks will no longer be as difficult.

After the stutterer completes the assignments on his hierarchy, he should discuss their outcomes with the clinician, and she should give him a great deal of praise for confronting his fears and discussing his stuttering openly. At times, she may need to encourage or even push him to move on to the next step; however, she should be sensitive to the intensity of his feelings so that she does not expect too much too soon.

The stutterer will probably never completely finish this activity. That is, discussing his stuttering openly will be an important strategy for him to use, not only throughout therapy. It can also help him maintain his improved fluency long after therapy has ended. Thus, a clinician gets the client started on his hierarchy, then moves on to the next technique. The client continues to work on discussing his stuttering openly in outside assignments while also working on other techniques or procedures.

Using Feared Words and Entering Feared Situations

Again, we introduce this procedure by having the stutterer read the following handout.

USING FEARED WORDS AND ENTERING FEARED SITUATIONS

An important goal for you to achieve in overcoming your stuttering is to reduce your avoidance of feared words and feared situations. In the past, you have changed words that you were sure you would stutter on, and you have shied away from people and places that were very difficult for you. The problem is that avoidance perpetuates stuttering. To make real progress in therapy, you will need to change your "mind set" from one of avoidance to one of approach and seek out words you have stuttered on and situations you have found difficult in the past. This will become easier once you have mastered techniques to make your stuttering easier.

You can begin now to approach words and situations you previously avoided. Even though you may still stutter, the fact that you have an "approach" attitude will keep you from tensing and holding back as much as you usually do, and you will sometimes be surprised to find that you don't stutter as much as you expected to.

Starting today, stop substituting easier words for harder ones, stop rephrasing sentences to get around feared words, and stop pretending you don't know the answer to a question when you really do. Instead of using these tricks, say exactly what you want to say, even if you stutter. If you are afraid you will stutter on a word you are about to say, commit yourself to saying that word, even if you stutter. In time, you will find your old fears decreasing. With this decrease in word fears, you will find your word and sound avoidances decreasing and your fluency increasing as well.

From today on, you should try not to avoid talking while in the clinic. In fact, talk as much as you possibly can. If you want to talk about a topic or ask a question, do it. If you think you are going to stutter on a word, go ahead and stutter. In the long run, this is much better than avoiding or postponing. You will learn that you can tolerate your stuttering, you will be more comfortable with it, and gradually you will become more fluent.

Eliminate your avoidance of feared situations by talking in all those situations you have avoided in the past. Introduce yourself to strangers. Start using the telephone more than you usually would, and look for opportunities to speak in groups. If you are aware of any fear of a speaking situation, take that as a sign to approach and enter that speaking situation. Your willingness to speak in these situations will make things much easier for you in the long run. You will find your situation fears decreasing. Consequently, you will find your wanting to avoid these speaking situations also decreasing. A by-product will be increased fluency.

Besides not avoiding in the clinic, you should begin today to eliminate the use of word and situation avoidances in the real world. You will need to develop an approach set in your own speaking environment. We will help you set up a series of outside speaking assignments—from least fearful to most fearful—to help you overcome your use of avoidances. Now and then, old speech fears will be too strong; you will avoid, but come back the next day and try again. In time, you will find the old fears decreasing. Your tolerance for stuttering will increase. You will be more comfortable with yourself as a speaker, and you will be speaking more fluently. You will need to keep working on this approach attitude for a long time. It is important that you eliminate your avoidances—and keep them eliminated.

After the client has read the handout, the clinician should answer any questions he may have. She should then instruct him to try not to use any postponements or word avoidances when in therapy from then on. If he does, she should again remind him. When she sees him deliberately using a word that he appeared to want to avoid, she should strongly reinforce this approach behavior. The clinician can also set up activities in which the stutterer purposefully uses feared words that were previously identified. This may involve the stutterer's reading word lists or text loaded with his feared words or involve his making up sentences loaded with these words. The clinician should warmly praise him each time he does not postpone or avoid a feared word. She should remain calm when he stutters. She should also be sensitive to his feelings and let him know that she understands the frustration or anxiety he is probably experiencing. This will help him become more comfortable saying these words and will reduce his tendency to want to avoid them.

To help the stutterer eliminate his use of avoidances outside the clinic, the clinician needs to help him set up a hierarchy of the word and situation avoidances he commonly uses in daily life. Like all hierarchies, it should be sequenced from least to most difficult for the client. By using this strategy, the stutterer's fears will be kept to a minimum. A typical step in the hierarchy is the stutterer's deliberate use of certain feared words throughout the day. How often should he use these feared words? He has to use them over and over until he no longer wants to avoid them. Another step in the hierarchy involves the stutterer's entering situations that he usually avoids in daily life. Again, he should enter these situations often enough that he loses his motivation to avoid them. Many of the latter assignments can be done as the client goes through his daily routine. That is, they will not take any extra time. He just needs to answer the telephone, whenever it rings, with the feared "hello" or to introduce himself to a different person each day. Other assignments may have to be created, and the stutterer will need to go out of his way to perform them. For example, a stutterer may have to shop for an item whose name contains one of his feared sounds or fabricate reasons for making telephone calls to local businesses.

To help the stutterer get started on an outside hierarchy, it is helpful for the clinician to join him for some of the assignments. Thereafter, the stutterer completes the assignments by himself but discusses his progress and any problems with his clinician during regular therapy sessions. The clinician should make sure that he keeps on track in completing his hierarchy, and she should provide him with the necessary support, and possibly gentle nudging, to help him do so.

Like discussing stuttering openly, eliminating the use of avoidances is a strategy that the stutterer will use throughout therapy and beyond. So, once the stutterer has begun his outside assignments successfully, it is time to move on to the next procedure.

Freezing or Holding on to Moments of Stuttering

The next technique is referred to as freezing or holding on to a moment of stuttering. See the handout below.

FREEZING OR HOLDING ON TO THE MOMENT OF STUTTERING

The experience of being caught in a moment of stuttering—repetition, prolongation, or block—can be frustrating and scary. When your mouth doesn't do what you want it to, you feel out of control. If it goes on for several seconds and your listener is upset or impatient, you may feel devastated. As unpleasant as these core behaviors are, you need to increase your tolerance for them, to learn that you can experience them without panicking. Instead of avoiding them or hurrying to get out of them, you need to learn to experience them and remain calm, so you can change them.

How do you learn to remain calm while jammed (blocked) in a moment of stuttering? We use a technique called "freezing" or "holding on." By freezing we mean that when you are stuttering, and we signal, you are to hold on to that moment of stuttering until we again signal you to come out of it. If you are repeating a syllable, you are to continue repeating it; if you are prolonging a sound, you are to continue prolonging it; and if you are having a block, you are to maintain that phonatory arrest or articulatory posture. By experiencing these core behaviors over and over again while remaining relatively calm, you will find your tolerance for them increasing. You will no longer become fearful at the thought of getting stuck on a word. You will find the core behaviors becoming more relaxed, and that is the key to change.

> You will begin by holding on to a core behavior for only a brief period of time, possibly 1 or 2 seconds. When you get caught in a stutter, we will signal you to hold on to that stutter. You are to hold on to that core behavior and keep it going until we signal you to complete the word slowly. While holding on to the repetition, prolongation, or block, you are to try to be as calm as possible. Just experience the stutter and be as composed and relaxed as you possibly can be. As your tolerance increases, we will gradually increase the length of time you are to hold on to your stutters. Eventually, you will hold on to your stutters until the tension and struggle have dissipated and you can end them easily and slowly. This will involve your signaling yourself—and us—when you begin a stutter and when you will come out of a stutter. We will also have you watch yourself in a mirror and listen to yourself on a tape recorder as you are holding on to your stutters. Again, just experience your stuttering and try to be as calm as possible. Remember when you feel the tension ebb away, finish the word slowly and deliberately.
>
> By experiencing these moments of stuttering over and over again in this manner, you will gradually lose your fear of them. You will find yourself feeling more comfortable when you are talking, and you will be talking more fluently.

After the clinician has made sure that the stutterer understands the rationale and procedures involved in freezing, she explores with him the sequence of activities she and her client will follow. Freezing, like the other procedures in this phase of therapy, is implemented most effectively in a hierarchical order. Will the stutterer be able to stop in the middle of a block and hold on to it when the clinician signals, or will this be too stressful? Sometimes, the clinician first needs to put some stutterings into her speech and have the stutterer signal her to freeze. How long will the stutterer be able to hold on to a core behavior in the beginning? Will it be more unpleasant for him to watch himself in a mirror as he holds on to a block, or will it be more difficult to listen to himself on a tape recorder? After these questions are discussed and a hierarchy tentatively established, the clinician begins with the easiest task.

Suppose it was decided to begin by having the stutterer hold his stutters for 1 to 2 seconds. This activity would go something like this. Whenever the stutterer stutters during a conversation, the clinician signals him by raising her finger or touching his arm to freeze or to hold on to whatever he is doing at that moment. She has him hold his repetitions, prolongations, or blocks for only a second or two, then signals him to continue. If his tension and struggle have dissipated before the clinician's signal, the stutterer is to voluntarily keep his stuttering going until she signals. During these periods, the clinician remains calm and shows interest in what the stutterer is doing and encourages the stutterer to remain calm, too. If the stutterer appears to be frustrated, fearful, or angry, she verbalizes these feelings for him and accepts them. If the stutterer looks away when he is holding his stutters, she encourages him to maintain eye contact with her. She also strongly reinforces his successes in hanging on to his stutters. When the stutterer is successful with this activity, the clinician moves on to more stressful steps.

The more stressful steps include gradually increasing the duration with which the stutterer holds on to core behaviors. They also include having him assume responsibility for signaling when he begins and when he will end a stutter. He should wait until the tension and struggle have dissipated before he ends a stutter. These steps also include having the stutterer listen to himself on recordings and watching himself in a mirror as he holds on to moments of stuttering. Through each of these steps, the clinician continues to be understanding, accepting, and reinforcing of the stutterer's feelings and behaviors. By spending a number of sessions in the clinic engaged in such activities, the stutterer gradually loses much of the strong negative emotion associated with moments of stuttering; that is, he will become counterconditioned to his stutters. When this has occurred, it is time to move on.

Using Voluntary Stuttering

Voluntary stuttering can be a very potent procedure in the desensitization process. Every clinician should be familiar with it. Our handout explaining voluntary stuttering to the advanced stutterer follows.

USING VOLUNTARY STUTTERING

One of the most important goals for you to achieve in overcoming your stuttering is to reduce the negative feelings, such as embarrassment, fear, and shame, associated with it. The more embarrassed you are by your stuttering, the more fearful you are of getting jammed up in a stutter, and the more ashamed you are of your stuttering, the more you will try to hide the stuttering. The more you try to hide your stuttering, the more tense you become and the more you tend to stutter. This process needs to be reversed.

One way to reduce these feelings is to stutter voluntarily. If you are afraid of something and run away from it, you will always be afraid of it. The way to overcome fear is to confront it and discover that it's not as bad as you thought. By confronting your fear, you will learn that you are tougher than you think. By stuttering on purpose, first in easy situations and later in more difficult situations, you will learn that you can stutter without fear and shame.

You will begin using voluntary stuttering in the clinic. We will help you start by putting easy repetitions and prolongations in your speech on nonfeared words. Don't be alarmed if you stutter on some words on which you use voluntary stuttering. This is a common experience. Just keep on stuttering voluntarily until you can finish the word comfortably and without struggling. We will continue to practice this until you are able to remain calm while voluntarily stuttering here in the clinic.

The next step will involve you going with us out into the real world to do voluntary stuttering together. Again, you will use easy repetitions or prolongations with strangers on nonfeared words. You may be surprised that most people are accepting of stuttering and will wait for you to say what you want to say. A few may frown or try to finish your sentence for you, but these will be trophies to collect, listeners we can discuss together. While testing reality in this way, you will learn to tolerate your stuttering and any listener's reactions and stay cool.

You will also need to use voluntary stuttering in your own environment to reduce your old fears. Old feelings die slowly! However, if you conscientiously do voluntary stuttering sufficiently often over a long period of time, you will find your old fears decreasing. You will no longer be hiding your stuttering, you will be stuttering in a more relaxed way, and you will be talking more comfortably and fluently. When you are ready to do voluntary stuttering on your own in your everyday speaking situations, we will help you prepare assignments for yourself.

Upon being introduced to voluntary stuttering by their clinician, many stutterers believe their clinician must be crazy. After all, they came to therapy to rid themselves of stuttering, not to do more of it. At this point, the clinician needs to explain the rationale behind the use of voluntary stuttering. We often find the following analogy to be of help. Suppose a person wanted to overcome a fear of snakes. This could not be done by running away from them. Rather, the person would have to begin seeking out contact with snakes. The best way to do this would be to have the guidance of another person who was an expert on snakes and was not afraid. Then, the person's contact with snakes should come in a series of small steps.

For example, the first step might involve only looking at a harmless, little grass snake in a glass tank. The next step might be raising the lid on the tank. Next, the person might briefly touch the little snake. Then, the person might pick up the snake and hold it for a short period. Finally, this process would be repeated, over and over again with larger and more fearsome looking snakes until the person had overcome his fear of snakes.

This same process can be followed with stuttering. With the clinician's guidance, use of voluntary stuttering, and hierarchies, the stutterer will begin to stutter on purpose and learn that he has nothing to fear. The importance of a clinician who is comfortable with stuttering cannot be overemphasized, so clinicians need to desensitize themselves to stuttering by practicing voluntary stuttering until the experience of stuttering and listeners' reactions to it does not bother them.

After explaining the rationale behind voluntary stuttering, the clinician begins to teach the client how to stutter voluntarily. She models brief, easy repetitions or prolongations, while remaining calm and relaxed. Then, she encourages the client to attempt some voluntary stuttering and enthusiastically reinforces his efforts if he does. If he finds this too difficult, she can suggest that they do it together, with the stutterer imitating her voluntary stuttering. With this sort of modeling and support, most stutterers are able to do some voluntary stuttering within one session. The clinician continues to give the stutterer lots of praise for his courage in doing something he's afraid to do. She points out that what seemed so fearful before, no longer seems so.

After the client becomes comfortable using voluntary stuttering in the clinic, it is time to move out into the world. With input from the client, the clinician establishes a hierarchy of situations in which the stutterer can use voluntary stuttering. The beginning steps should always involve the clinician going into situations with the stutterer and using voluntary stuttering. She asks him to rate listeners on a scale that reflects a range of qualities. For example, a "1" might be someone who laughs or looks away, and a "10" might be someone who is attentive and listens patiently. The client may want to continue using this rating system when it is his turn to voluntarily stutter as well, because it can countercondition old emotions of feeling victimized and helpless.

The clinician voluntarily stutters in such situations as asking for directions from strangers or asking for information from store clerks, remaining calm as she does this. If all of her listeners are patient and understanding, she can ask the client to choose listeners who might be more difficult. After several of these are completed, it is the client's turn to stutter voluntarily with strangers. They continue to take alternate turns. This provides additional counterconditioning as the client and clinician compare their ratings of listeners and take turns choosing difficult listeners for each other. The stutterer's feelings of assertiveness and exploration usually increase, which diminishes feelings of fear and avoidance.

The clinician should be careful not to allow the client to get in "over his head" with listeners who may be too difficult. She should also lavish praise on each of the client's attempts, acknowledging how difficult it can be. She needs to be sensitive to how much he wants to discuss each event and provide the support needed. After a good workout with store clerks, for example, the clinician may suggest that they take a break for coffee or soda at a restaurant, where they can practice voluntary stuttering with the waitress and also enjoy the counterconditioning effects of drinking and eating while doing something that was previously unpleasant.

The client and the clinician should continue working together on voluntary stuttering until the client feels comfortable. Then the stutterer works his way up through the rest of the situations in his hierarchy on his own. He has to continue putting voluntary stuttering into his speech in each situation until his fear subsides before going on to the next situation. The clinician checks the client's progress during therapy sessions, commends him when he is successful, and supports, encourages, and counsels him when he runs into problems. Voluntary stuttering is a procedure that clients will continue to use throughout active treatment and maintenance. It is not an activity that will soon be discontinued.

By introducing and implementing the preceding four techniques, the clinician has the client on the way toward reducing negative feelings and attitudes toward his stuttering and eliminating his use of avoidance behaviors. It is an intensive counterconditioning/deconditioning process, which requires continued effort. The client will be rewarded as he finds his stuttering becoming more relaxed and briefer.

USING FLUENCY ENHANCING BEHAVIORS AND MODIFYING THE MOMENTS OF STUTTERING

The goal of this phase of therapy is to help the client integrate fluency shaping and stuttering modification skills. We now detail the two procedures that are the focus of this phase: (a) using FEBs and (b) modifying moments of stuttering.

We have sequenced these two skills in two ways. With clients who are already modifying their stuttering during initial stages of therapy, we typically teach stuttering modification skills first, then teach fluency shaping skills. However, with clients who are still not able to move through words easily and slowly, we begin with fluency shaping skills, then teach stuttering modification. Results seem to be equally effective. In the following sections, we describe the latter sequence.

Using Fluency Enhancing Behaviors

Fluency shaping clinicians, particularly Neilson and Andrews, have strongly influenced our thinking with regard to this procedure, which is apparent in the following handout.

USING FLUENCY ENHANCING BEHAVIORS (FEBS)

We know that stutterers can increase their fluency by modifying their speech patterns in certain ways. For example, one of the most common modifications that stutterers use is to slow down their rate of speech. Many stutterers have discovered on their own that if they speak more slowly, they will speak more fluently. Other techniques that stutterers have found helpful are to begin speaking with a gentle onset of voice after each breath, to use soft articulatory contacts, and to be highly aware of the feeling of movement of your articulators. We call these modifications or changes in the manner of speaking "fluency enhancing behaviors" (FEBs). Now let's talk about these FEBs in more detail.

The first FEB is "slower rate." There are at least two ways to use a slower rate. One way is to put more and longer pauses in your speech. The other way, which we prefer, is to prolong or stretch out the sounds in your words. We are not expecting you to speak abnormally slowly, but we are suggesting that you speak at a slow-normal rate when you want to increase your fluency.

The second FEB is the use of "gentle onsets." By gentle onsets we mean that after each breath you begin producing your voice slowly and with as little tension in your larynx (voice box) as possible.

The third FEB is "soft contacts." This can be achieved by moving your articulators (tongue, lips, jaw) in a slow, prolonged, and relaxed way. These articulatory movements should not be jerky, and you should not press hard with your tongue or lips. By using these FEBs, you will be able to feel the fluent movements of your articulators as you speak.

This brings us to the fourth FEB, "proprioception." You can get an appreciation of this by closing your eyes and pantomiming the words of a sentence. Feel the movement of your tongue, jaw, and lips and feel when your articulators touch. Proprioception is paying attention to the feel of your articulatory movements rather than the sound of speech. Try it in a sentence using normal speech with voicing rather than pantomime and just attend to the feeling of movement.

We're sure you're wondering how you are going to learn to use these FEBs. You'll begin by practicing at very slow speeds in the clinic, then gradually get up to a normal-sounding speed. Later, you can work on your FEBs outside the clinic, first with our help and then on your own. Eventually, these FEBs will be tools you will use for years to come to increase your fluency in certain speaking situations.

One word of advice in using these FEBs. You should not use them to hide the fact that you stutter. You should be open and honest about your problem. Let your listener hear and see you speaking slower and using gentle onsets and soft contacts. Be open about the fact that you are using these techniques to improve your fluency in a given speaking situation.

Teaching the client to use FEBs is most easily done by having him learn them while speaking very slowly and then gradually increasing his rate while retaining the FEBs. The instructions for fluency shaping trial therapy, given in Chapter 8, are useful for establishing the FEBs at a slow speed, so we have reproduced them here:

We begin by reducing *our own* speech rate as we describe to our client the aim of this exercise: to produce words very, very slowly. We use a written sentence beginning with a vowel or a glide. We teach our client, going over the sentence word by word, to use a gradual and gentle onset of voicing, and to stretch each sound, whether vowel or consonant. Once he can do this, we ensure that he can use light contacts, touching the articulators lightly without tension or pressure. Then, we work on proprioception—helping the client guide his speech by the feel of articulator movement rather than by auditory feedback.[3] We provide a model for each word and give constant feedback. When words are produced slowly enough with each part of the system—respiration, phonation, and

---

[3] Proprioception, as Van Riper (1973) conceived of it, may have elements of left hemisphere control in the sense that the deliberate and strongly voluntary movements that occur under proprioception may be associated with "approach" emotions, rather than "avoidance" emotions.

articulation—moving in slow motion and without excess tension, fluency results. When each word of the sentence has been produced in this way, the client is coached into producing the entire sentence, linking each word to the next, and maintaining gentle onsets, light contacts, and proprioception. Breath supply is monitored so that a pause for breath is taken whenever the client gets to the point in vital capacity when a breath would naturally be taken. Again, modeling and constant feedback are vital.

As an example, the sentence, "apples are a red fruit," should take from 15 to 20 seconds to produce, with a pause for a new breath after the word "a." The /p/ in "apples," the /d/ in "red," and the /t/ in "fruit" all should be produced without stopping airflow, making these plosives sound like fricatives. We make lists of sentences that use all the vowels and consonants in initial positions of phrases and have the client practice them until he is able to say each one completely fluently, using all of his FEBs. After the client masters speech at the sentence level, we move to structured conversation, in which we alternate taking conversational turns with him for trials of 1, 2, 3, 4, and 5 minutes. We record and play back samples of each trial and discuss with the client how well he is using his FEBs. We continue working at this very slow rate of conversation until we feel he has mastered it.

The client is now able to speak fluently for 5 minutes in a conversation, using good-quality FEBs with a speech rate of about 40 syllables per minute (SPM). We now undertake the process of helping the client learn to speak at gradually faster rates, using good-quality FEBs and remaining entirely fluent. To accomplish this, we take the client through 14 steps of conversational speech, each one slightly faster than the one preceding and entirely fluent. We set the target for the first step at 50 SPM ($\pm$20 SPM). We use a calculator and stopwatch, as described in Chapter 7, to assess the client's speech rate every minute. Whenever the client is speaking, we let the stopwatch run, stopping it for pauses of longer than 1 second or when we are talking. We count syllables on the calculator as he speaks, using its cumulative counting function.

When the client reaches the first minute, the calculator's count should be between 30 and 70 SPM. He should have had no stutters, and his FEBs should have been used consistently. If he stutters during that minute, we set the stopwatch at zero and start over. If the client is slightly over or under the target of 50 SPM ($\pm$20), we coach him during the next minute to be slower or faster, whichever is appropriate. If any of his FEBs is inconsistent or not of appropriate quality, we stop timing and instruct him for a moment in the element or elements he is not achieving adequately. Note that we provide a continuous model by using FEBs as we speak at the client's target rate whenever we are speaking to him.

Once the client has spoken for 5 consecutive minutes without stuttering and his overall rate is 50 SPM ($\pm$20), we move to the next step, which is 60 SPM ($\pm$20), and carry on as before. We continue this stepwise progression, increasing the rate by 10 SPM ($\pm$20) whenever the client has succeeded at the current step. This continues until the client has 5 minutes of fluent conversation at 180 SPM, which we consider to be normal rate, although slightly toward the slow end of the range. This progression from 40 to 180 SPM may take several hours and may be done intensively (Turnbaugh & Guitar, 1981) or at a once-a-week pace. This progression is essentially that described in detail in Neilson and Andrews (1993).

After the client completes the above establishment program and is speaking fluently at 180 SPM with the clinician, the clinician introduces the following two activities. She devotes about equal amounts of therapy time to each one, in parallel fashion. First, she begins to transfer the client's use of these FEBs to other locations and other people in the clinic. This is the first hierarchy that is used in transferring a stutterer's use of FEBs to his everyday speaking environment. Second, she introduces the stutterer to the next procedure, "stuttering easily." Before discussing stuttering easily, however, we have more to say about this first hierarchy.

We have found that hierarchies are very effective in helping the stutterer transfer his use of FEBs to everyday speaking situations. We typically use four hierarchies: (*a*) inside the clinic with the clinician, (*b*) outside the clinic with the clinician, (*c*) everyday speaking situations, and (*d*) the telephone. We discuss only the first hierarchy at this time, but we return to the remaining hierarchies after presenting the stuttering easily procedures.

The first hierarchy, inside the clinic with the clinician, involves varying the physical location and social complexity of therapy sessions in the clinic, which means conducting therapy in other locations in the clinic. It also means bringing other people into the therapy session. The size of the audience can be increased. People from the stutterer's world, such as family and friends, can be brought into therapy. The client and the clinician rank such situations from easiest to most difficult, as perceived by the stutterer, who then goes through these situations in sequence. He is to use his FEBs and meet the fluency criterion of 1 or fewer stuttered syllables per minute in each situation for a set period of time before he proceeds to the next, more difficult situation. The clinician continues to reinforce successful use of FEBs. It is important that the stutterer's confidence in using FEBs continues to increase during these activities.

As previously mentioned, the clinician spends half the time in therapy moving the stutterer through this hierarchy and the other half on teaching the stutterer to stutter easily, which we now describe.

Stuttering Easily

Stuttering modification clinicians, particularly Van Riper, have strongly influenced our procedures, as has the work of fluency shaping clinicians. The strategies or physiological movements involved in modifying a moment of stuttering are very similar to FEBs used to modify the overall speech pattern. We attempt to make this clear to clients in the following handout.

STUTTERING EASILY

What do we mean by stuttering easily? First, we mean saying the word without using any of your secondary behaviors, such as postponement, starting, or escape behaviors. Don't use these tricks to help you get started or to help you get out of a word.

Second, we mean you should stutter or say the word in a slow and relaxed manner. This is done by slowly prolonging each syllable of the word. Stutter or say the word in slow motion. Don't be in a hurry to complete it. In other words, you should use your slower rate FEB on the word. Instead of slowing down your whole speech pattern, you are to just slow down on the word that you stutter on or expect to stutter on.

Third, by stuttering easily, we also mean using your other two FEBs, gentle onsets and soft contacts, to say a troublesome word. The word should begin slowly and in as relaxed a manner as possible. Phonation (voice) should be initiated slowly and with as little tension in your larynx (voice box) as possible, that is, use a gentle onset. Movement of the articulators (tongue, lips, and jaw) should also be slow, prolonged, and relaxed. In other words, use soft contacts on consonant sounds. You should also use proprioception to be very aware of the *movement* of your articulators as you work your way through the word.

How does one learn to do this? The first step involves the use of "cancellations." By cancellations, we mean the following. If you stutter and don't make any attempt to use your FEBs, pause for a couple of seconds right after the stutter. Then, say the word again, but this time say the word in a slow, prolonged, relaxed manner. You should use a gentle onset or soft contact at the beginning of the word. Each syllable of the word should be prolonged. Soft contacts should be used on consonant sounds, and you should use proprioception. In other words, you are to say the word again, but this time you are to say it as if you were stuttering easily on it. Don't say it fluently, even if you could, and don't use any of your old tricks. You will practice these cancellations here in the clinic.

The next step in learning to stutter easily involves the use of "pull-outs." This involves catching yourself in a stutter and then pulling yourself out of it. Rather than struggle and hurry out of the word, you should say the rest of the word in a slow, prolonged, relaxed manner. Each remaining syllable should be slowly prolonged (slower rate). Consonant sounds should be produced with a soft contact, and you should be highly aware of the movements of your articulators as you move through the word. These pull-outs will be practiced first in the clinic and then in outside situations around the clinic. You will also use these in your everyday speaking situations.

The last step in learning to stutter easily involves the use of "preparatory sets" (prep sets). When you anticipate stuttering on a word, you should "turn on" your proprioception and prepare to use either a gentle onset or soft contact at the beginning of the word; then each syllable of the word should be slowly prolonged. These prep sets will also be practiced in the clinic and in outside speaking situations. You may need to use these throughout the rest of your life when you expect to stutter on a word.

Once you have learned to use prep sets and pull-outs, you will have another strategy or technique to use if you don't want to use FEBs to modify your overall speech pattern. You can just go ahead and talk spontaneously. If you expect to stutter on a word, you can use a prep set to stutter easily on it. If you unexpectedly get caught in a stutter, you can use a pull-out to come out of it easily.

One word of advice in using these techniques. You should not use them to hide your stuttering. Be honest and open about the fact that you stutter; let your listener know that you are having some difficulty in getting a word out and keep eye contact as you work on your easy stutter. Instead of using these techniques to hide your stuttering, use them to modify your stuttering in the direction of an easier, more relaxed form of stuttering, but let your easy stuttering show.

After the client reads this handout, the clinician makes sure that the client understands that he will now be applying his FEBs only to words on which he either stutters or anticipates stuttering. The clinician then explains and models cancellations. She simulates the client's stuttering on a word and then cancels it by slowly prolonging each sound within the word, using a gentle onset of phonation at the beginning of the word and applying soft articulatory contacts on the word's consonant sounds during this second attempt. She emphasizes that he should be sure to complete the stuttered word the first time he says it; he should not stop part of the way through. She should also point out that the pause between the first and second attempt on the word should be an unhurried pause. During this pause, the stutterer is to calm himself and plan how he will apply his FEBs on the second attempt. The clinician then has him try to use some cancellations as they engage in conversation. At first, it may be difficult for the stutterer to catch himself and cancel stutters. However, with reminders to cancel, feedback regarding his performance, and ample reinforcement from the clinician, most stutterers are soon able to produce some good cancellations while conversing with the clinician. The clinician then tells the stutterer that the goal is to use good cancellations on at least 90% of his stuttered words during conversations in therapy for a session or two. The clinician counts the number of stuttered words and successful cancellations during these sessions. After the stutterer has demonstrated this level of competency in using cancellations, it is time to introduce pull-outs.

The clinician explains to the client that now he is to catch himself while still in the moment of stuttering. Then, he is to slowly prolong the rest of the sounds in the word and use soft contacts on the remaining consonants. The clinician should model pull-outs first, after which the client practices using them. The clinician again informs him that he is to use pull-outs on at least 90% of his stuttered words during conversation for a session or so. She positively reinforces good pull-outs and gives corrective feedback when the client is having difficulty using them.

The final step in learning to stutter easily is preparatory sets, as the client learns to use FEBs on words on which he anticipates stuttering. Many clients may have learned to do this on their own on some words by this time. They approach a feared word by initiating it with a gentle onset or a soft contact, slowly working their way through it by prolonging each sound and using soft contacts on the consonant sounds. If the client is already doing this, the clinician just needs to point out that he is using prep sets and strongly reinforce him for it. If the client has not yet acquired this skill on his own, the clinician will need to explain and model prep sets for him.

As with pull-outs, the client needs practice using prep sets in therapy before he begins to transfer them to the outside speaking world. In this practice, the client should use either a good prep set or a good pull-out on 90% of his stuttered words when conversing with the clinician for a therapy session or two. The clinician reinforces him for their use and gives appropriate corrective feedback as needed. The reason we accept either a prep set or a pull-out is that most clients do not anticipate all their moments of stuttering. Therefore, it is unrealistic to expect the stutterer to use preparatory sets on all of his stutters.

The client is now ready to begin transferring his newly acquired stuttering easily skills to his own speaking environment. To do this, we use the same four hierarchies that were developed for transferring FEBs: (*a*) inside the clinic with the clinician, (*b*) outside the clinic with the clinician, (*c*) everyday speaking situations, and (*d*) the telephone. By now, the stutterer has probably almost completed his inside the clinic with the clinician hierarchy using FEBs. When he does, he completes the same hierarchy again, but this time using stuttering easily skills. Thus, the stutterer goes through the same speaking situations with the clinician in the clinic that he did before, but this time he uses prep sets or pull-outs to modify any moments of stuttering he may have, instead of using FEBs. The criterion for success in each situation is using a good prep set or pull-out on 90% of stutters. The clinician continues to reinforce his stuttering easily during this hierarchy.

Once the client has completed this first hierarchy using both FEBs and stuttering easily skills, it is time to move on to outside the clinic with the clinician hierarchy, involving situations in which the clinician can accompany the client. The clinician and client jointly select and sequence items for this hierarchy. Examples of these situations are asking directions from strangers or obtaining information from store clerks (Fig. 9.3). The client moves through this hierarchy using both FEBs and prep sets or pull-outs—first one, then the other. The client could complete the entire hierarchy using one set of skills, then repeat it using the other set. On the other hand, he could alternate using FEBs and stut-

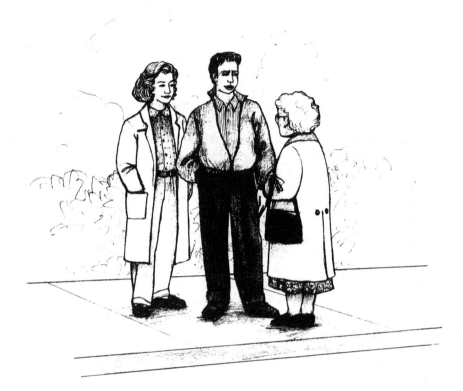

Figure 9.3. Transferring stuttering modification and fluency shaping skills.

tering easily on each step of the hierarchy. It is important, however, that the client begins to generalize both sets of skills from the clinic to outside the clinic situations. Whichever set of skills is being worked on in a given situation, the criterion for success is that both the client and clinician agree that the client has used these skills as well as he did in the clinic. This means that the FEBs or prep sets and pull-outs felt and sounded as good as when he used them in the clinic. This is a subjective evaluation, but realistically it is the type of evaluation the client will use on his own in the future. It is also important that the client be successful in using each set of skills in each situation a number of times so that he gains confidence in his ability to use them. After gaining skill and confidence in using FEBs and prep sets or pull-outs in outside situations with his clinician present, it is time for the client to move on to the next, more difficult hierarchy.

The everyday speaking situation hierarchy involves situations from the client's environment and requires him to complete them on his own. Usually the client ranks, from least to most difficult, 2 to 3 dozen speaking situations that he encounters in a typical week. He may first go through this hierarchy using FEBs, then go through it again using prep sets or pull-outs, or vice versa. He may also choose to use both skills on one step of the hierarchy before going on to the next situation. Most important, the client must begin to generalize his use of both sets of skills to everyday speaking situations. As a general rule, before moving to a more difficult step or situation on the hierarchy, the client should feel that he has successfully used his transfer skills a number of times in the immediately preceding, easier situation. This is important in developing his skill and confidence in using these techniques. During regular therapy sessions, the clinician monitors the client's progress through this hierarchy, praises him when he has successes, encourages him when he has failures, and makes suggestions when he has problems. In time, the client will report to the clinician that his speech is becoming much better in his everyday encounters.

We have also found that most advanced stutterers need a separate hierarchy involving the telephone. The same strategies or principles used in implementing the above hierarchies are applied here as well. In other words, telephone calls, with and without the clinician present, are arranged in a hierarchical order. The client practices both his FEBs and his stuttering easily skills during these calls until the criterion for success is met, and the clinician continues to support and reinforce him during these activities. Soon, the client will report successes in his daily use of the telephone.

By now, the client will be speaking much better in most situations. Although he is not yet out of the woods, he is well on his way. We now move on to the last phase of therapy, increasing and maintaining improvement.

MAINTAINING IMPROVEMENT

The goal of this last phase of therapy is to help the client generalize his improvement, that is, his reduced negative feelings, attitudes, and avoidances and his increased fluency, to all remaining speaking situations and to maintain this improvement following termination of therapy. We introduce the following two procedures during this phase: (*a*) becoming your own clinician and (*b*) establishing long-term fluency goals.

Becoming Your Own Clinician

If the client with advanced stuttering is going to generalize improvement to all speaking situations and maintain this improvement, we believe that he must assume responsibility for his own therapy. We use the following handout to help clients learn how to combat avoidance and continue improving their FEBs.

BECOMING YOUR OWN CLINICIAN

Now that we have covered all the therapy techniques you will need to meet your therapy goals, it is time for you to become your own speech clinician. Although we have helped you improve your fluency and reduce your emotional reactions to stuttering, you will probably still encounter some situations that will give you trouble. Thus, you will need to learn how to handle these situations as well as maintain the fluency you have.

Handling the remaining difficult situations will require you to be honest about where you think you may still stutter and what your fears are. Fear doesn't stand still; if you ignore it, it will grow, but if you pursue it, it will die. So you must be vigilant for words and situations that continue to spark fear in you and make you feel as if you won't be able to handle your stuttering the way you want. For these words and situations, you must be ready to use your techniques, such as openness about your stuttering, voluntary stuttering, and pull-outs and prep sets, to work on these fears. Up to this point, we have been helping you develop and carry out such plans, but now you will be taking more and more responsibility for them.

Working on feared words and situations is not just to make advances. It is also to maintain the level of fluency you have now, because adult stutterers very often relapse or slip back after they leave therapy. Relapse is not inevitable, but neither is it surprising. After all, you have had years of practice at stuttering. In fact, you are an expert. You have avoided words and situations for a long time, and your negative feelings and attitudes about your speech are well learned. Because stuttering is deeply etched in your brain, you may always have some core behaviors, and you will need to cope successfully with them. Therefore, you need to become your own speech clinician. You will have to keep applying—on your own and long after you leave therapy—the techniques you have learned.

What is involved in being your own clinician? You will need to learn to give yourself assignments to overcome remaining difficult speaking situations and new ones that crop up. If you are still avoiding speaking in a certain situation, you will need to design assignments that will eliminate this avoidance. If you are still fearful while talking in some situations, you will need to give yourself assignments to reduce this fear. If you are still stuttering a lot in a given situation, you will need to come up with assignments to improve your fluency in this situation. In the beginning of therapy, we helped you create these assignments, but as you improved, we turned more of the responsibility over to you. We will continue to do this. With additional practice, you will be able to determine your therapy needs and to plan assignments to meet these needs. When you can do this, you will have become your own speech clinician.

We have found the following approach effective in meeting this goal. Every day you need to work at reducing any remaining speech fears and eliminating any remaining avoidances. For example, if you are still fearful while talking in a certain situation, you could give yourself a daily quota of voluntary stuttering in that situation. Every day you also need to work on improving your fluency. If you are still doing a lot of stuttering in a given situation, you could set a daily quota of talking time in that situation during which you use prep sets and pull-outs. These are only examples, but the important thing is that every day you ask yourself which situations are still giving you problems and then give yourself assignments designed to overcome these problems. Let's get started in helping you become your own speech clinician.

By this time, the client is probably getting close to completing his everyday speaking situation hierarchy. The clinician points out to him, however, that completing this hierarchy is not enough. The client needs to become aware of any other situations that are still giving him trouble. The clinician asks him the following kinds of questions. Is he avoiding talking in any situations? Is he still unduly afraid while talking in some situations? Is he unable to successfully use FEBs or prep sets and pull-outs in some situations? If he answers yes to any of these questions, he needs to target these situations in assignments.

If the client is still avoiding some situations, the clinician should remind him of the importance of using feared words and entering feared situations. She should have him reread the handout. She then helps him prepare assignments to overcome these avoidances. The clinician does not assume any more responsibility than is necessary. She asks helpful questions, but she wants him to figure out on his own what he needs to do. As time goes on, she will gradually have the client assuming more and more responsibility for planning his own assignments.

If the client is still unduly apprehensive about talking in some situations, the clinician needs to remind him of the importance of discussing stuttering openly and using voluntary stuttering to reduce these negative feelings. She has him reread the handouts. She helps him create assignments using techniques that will make him more comfortable in these situations. Here again, she does not assume any more responsibility than necessary, guiding the client to becoming his own speech clinician.

If the client is having difficulties using FEBs and prep sets or pull-outs in some situations, the clinician explores with him the nature of his difficulties, helping him determine what types of assignments he needs to have to be successful. Maybe he only needs more practice in some less difficult situations before he can reasonably expect to be successful in these more difficult situations. Perhaps he needs to further reduce his speech fears and the resulting muscular tension in these difficult situations so that his motor control does not break down as readily. We have found that some clients prefer to use FEBs, but others prefer to use preparatory sets and pull-outs. There is no reason why all stutterers need to use both. If the client wants to use only one of these sets of skills, the clinician should accept this. During all of their discussions, the clinician needs to keep in mind that her goal is to help the stutterer become independent of her. So, as she works with a client, she becomes less directing and gradually turns all of the responsibility for his assignments over to him.

Throughout this phase of therapy, the client should be working daily on his outside assignments. During therapy sessions, he discusses his progress with the clinician. During this same period, the clinician is more and more of a consultant, helping the client feel that he can go out and fly on his own.

Establishing Long-term Fluency Goals

Before therapy ends, we believe it is very important for the client to be aware of what he can expect in terms of fluency after termination from therapy. By having realistic goals, we believe he can substantially decrease the possibility of his becoming disappointed and frustrated with his speech. These feelings may lead to relapse. To begin this topic, we share the following handout with the stutterer.

ESTABLISHING LONG-TERM FLUENCY GOALS

You are at the point in therapy at which you need to consider your long-term fluency goals. Before you do this, we need to define some terms we will be using. These are "spontaneous fluency," "controlled fluency," and "acceptable stuttering."

By spontaneous fluency, we mean speech that contains no more than occasional disfluencies and does not contain tension or struggle. This fluency is not maintained by paying attention to or controlling your speech. In other words, you don't use FEBs or prep sets and pull-outs to be fluent. You just talk and pay attention to your ideas. It is the fluency of the normal speaker.

Controlled fluency is similar to spontaneous fluency except that you must attend to or control your speech to maintain relatively normal-sounding fluency. You must use FEBs or prep sets and pull-outs to sound relatively fluent. You sound fluent only because you are working on your speech at the time.

Finally, acceptable stuttering refers to speech that contains noticeable, but mild stuttering that feels comfortable to you. You are not avoiding words or situations. You may or may not need to use FEBs or prep sets and pull-outs to have acceptable stuttering. In other words, sometimes you will have this acceptable stuttering without having to work on or control your speech. At other times, despite your use of FEBs or prep sets and pull-outs, you will still have some mild stuttering.

Now, let's consider long-term fluency goals. A few adults who stutter become spontaneously fluent in all speaking situations on a consistent basis. They become normal speakers. In our experience, however, most adult stutterers do not reach this goal. Instead, they have situations, such as talking to close friends, in which they are spontaneously fluent. In other situations, such as speaking in groups, their stuttering tends to give them trouble. In these troublesome situations, we think it is important for these stutterers—and possibly you—to have the following options.

First, if it *is* important to you to sound fluent in one of these situations, we want you to be able to use either FEBs or prep sets and pull-outs to achieve controlled fluency. We know this is possible in most situations. We also know there will be some situations in which you will not be totally successful. In these situations, we want you to feel comfortable with acceptable stuttering.

Second, if it is *not* important to you to sound fluent in a situation and you do not want to put the effort into using FEBs or prep sets and pull-outs, we would like you to feel comfortable with acceptable stuttering.

These options or goals are both realistic and acceptable. In other words, you don't have to sound perfectly fluent all the time. You don't have to work on your speech constantly. In fact, attempting to sound fluent all the time by using FEBs or prep sets and pull-outs can become burdensome. Where are you now with regard to these fluency goals? Are you satisfied with your present fluency? Where would you like to be in the future with regard to these goals? You should discuss these questions with your clinician and begin to make plans based on your answers.

The clinician makes sure that the client understands the concepts of spontaneous fluency, controlled fluency, and acceptable stuttering. When the clinician is convinced that he understands what is meant by these terms, she explores with him the types of fluency he now has in various, everyday speaking situations. If he is unsure, he gives himself assignments to find out whether or not he is satisfied with the types of fluency he has in these daily speaking situations. If the stutterer is satisfied with his fluency in all situations, then he has met his goals, and the end of therapy is near. If he is not satisfied, then he needs to continue to work along the lines discussed in the previous section, becoming your own clinician, until his goals are met.

We have observed a couple of problems that frequently occur relative to clients' fluency expectations or goals. First, many clients are experiencing a great deal of spontaneous fluency at this point in therapy. They expect and want this spontaneous fluency to last forever without any effort on their part. It can last, but it will require continued work. The client will need to continue to give himself assignments to keep his negative feelings and attitudes at a minimum and his avoidance behaviors eliminated. He will also need to continue to work on his FEBs and prep sets and pull-outs so that he has confidence in his ability to use them when he chooses. Spontaneous fluency will be a by-product of these efforts. The clinician must help the client understand this. If he doesn't understand, he will be disappointed, and possibly panicked, when he begins to lose some of his spontaneous fluency. This may lead to relapse.

The second problem frequently involves clients with more severe advanced stuttering. This client often does not achieve a great deal of spontaneous fluency. If he is going to talk better, he needs to constantly use FEBs or prep sets and pull-outs. Even then, he often achieves only acceptable stuttering, which can be discouraging. It may be too much of a burden for him to constantly monitor and modify his speech. In time, he becomes tired, he gives up doing anything at all. Relapse soon follows. The clinician needs to help this client accept and become comfortable with his acceptable stuttering. She also needs to help him realize the substantial effort he will need to expend to maintain this level of fluency.

Once the client gets to the point at which he feels he is meeting his fluency goals and he has become his own clinician, the frequency of therapy contacts is systematically reduced. We typically fade our contacts to once a week for a month or two, then to once a month for several months, and, finally, to once a semester for 2 years. This gradual transition provides the client with some continued support. If he is doing well, he is reinforced. If he is having a few problems, we can help him find solutions. If he has totally relapsed, he can be reenrolled in therapy. Finally, the day comes to say "goodby." We commend him for all his efforts. We let him know that if he ever needs us again, he should feel free to contact us. If we have done our job well, we will not be hearing from him.

OTHER CLINICIANS

We now discuss the clinical procedures of other clinicians who integrate stuttering modification and fluency shaping therapies for the advanced stutterer. These clinicians do not integrate the two approaches exactly as we do, but you will see that integration of the two approaches can occur in a number of ways.

David Daly

David Daly (1988) has developed a treatment program based on his experience with his own stuttering and the successful therapy he has received. He believes strongly in the power of the client's expectations for success and in the clinician's belief that the stutterer can indeed become fluent. In Daly's program, the groundwork for fluency is achieved through fluency shaping, which is followed by a cognitive therapy program to make long-term success more likely. Daly believes, along with Arnold Lazarus (1971), that "behavioral methods alone are often insufficient to produce durable results."

Daly establishes fluency using three "targets" that are taught through the clinician's models and instructions and then overlearned using highly structured practice in increasingly realistic contexts. The first target is *deliberate phonation,* which is similar to the "phrase continuity" used by Neilson and Andrews (see Chapter 8). However, Daly asks clients to keep phonation going throughout a phrase, even during segments that are normally voiceless, and to use a monotonous drone. At the same time, clients learn to produce speech very slowly. The second target is *normal breath*—essentially a relaxed breathing pattern that ensures adequate air for normal volume without straining. *Easy stretch,* the third and last target, requires clients to use an easy onset of phonation and light articulatory contacts rather than a hard vocal attack and a high level of intraoral air pressure at the beginnings of utterances.

After these targets are learned through extensive drills, provided by Daly in his book, *The Freedom of Fluency* (1988), clients use self-monitoring to maintain the three fluency targets to generalize newly fluent speech. This skill is taught in association with three hand signals (clenched fist, touching the thumb and finger, and pressing a finger on a surface), which clients use to remind themselves to monitor these targets and to gradually fade out self-monitoring once an utterance is underway. Daly follows Shames and Florance's (1980) approach of reinforcing the monitoring of fluency targets by encouraging clients to speak freely, without monitoring, after a certain period of successful self-monitoring has taken place in each speaking situation. This brings clients to a point of being able to speak fluently in most situations. The next phase of Daly's therapy is called *cognitive and self-instructional strategies*. It consists of guided relaxation, mental imagery, and positive self-talk to help clients move through more and more challenging activities to generalize and maintain fluency. Daly provides audiotapes and a reading list for clients to help them continue their cognitive self-therapy.

Hugo Gregory

For the past 20 years, Hugo Gregory (1968, 1979, 1986a) has been integrating stuttering modification and fluency shaping therapies. In his most recent discussion of his therapy for the advanced stutterer, he describes four areas of therapeutic activity: (*a*) changing the attitudes of the stutterer, (*b*) diminishing excessive bodily tension, (*c*) analyzing and modifying speech, and (*d*) building new psychomotor speech patterns and improving speech skills. Although Gregory sees these four areas as being interrelated, he believes changing attitudes and diminishing excessive bodily tension usually precede modifying speech and building new psychomotor speech patterns.

Gregory believes that it is important for the advanced stutterer to change his attitudes about his problem. Thus, he provides the stutterer with an accepting and understanding relationship in which to explore and clarify feelings and attitudes about his problem. These discussions likewise help to reduce the stutterer's negative feelings about his speech. During this period, Gregory also provides the client with information about stuttering. Toward the end of therapy, as the client's speech improves, Gregory helps him to integrate his new fluency into his life patterns.

Gregory thinks that diminishing excessive bodily tension is beneficial for many stutterers. To help them do this, he uses Jacobson's (1938) progressive relaxation techniques. Briefly, this involves having the stutterer systematically tense and relax the muscles in one part of the body at a time until the whole body is relaxed. By going through this process over and over, the stutterer learns to identify the feelings associated with relaxation and to voluntarily relax his muscles. Gregory reports that many stutterers, as they enter a feared speaking situation, are able to consciously reduce bodily tension and to carry this over to the muscles involved in speaking.

Gregory's third area of therapeutic activity is analyzing and modifying speech. At this time, Gregory helps the stutterer to analyze what he does when he stutters by using audio and video recordings. Gregory also helps him to become aware of other aspects of his speech pattern, such as rate, phrasing, and prosody. Following this analysis, Gregory teaches the stutterer to modify his stuttering by relaxing tension, slowing repetitions, and using other similar techniques. Van Riper's cancellations, pull-outs, and preparatory sets are sometimes used. Gregory also teaches the stutterer to use an "easier, more relaxed approach with smooth movements" (ERA-SM) to initiate speech. These relaxed, smooth movements are first practiced in single words, then in phrases, and, finally, in connected speech. Since ERA-SM are used on nonstuttered words, they are much more similar to Neilson and Andrews' fluency skills than to Van Riper's stuttering modification techniques.

The last area that Gregory works on in therapy with the advanced stutterer is building new psychomotor speech patterns. His goal is to make the person who stutters a good speaker. The emphasis is on strengthening normal fluency. Some of the aspects of speech production that are targeted are rate control, loudness, phrasing, and prosody.

In the introduction to this section on the integration of stuttering modification and fluency shaping therapies, we said that we believe it is important to reduce the advanced stutterer's negative feelings and attitudes and eliminate his use of avoidances. We further stated that it is helpful to integrate work on modifying both the stutterer's moments of stuttering and enhancing his fluency skills. It should be clear that Gregory shares many of these beliefs.

Walter Manning

Manning believes that the major handicap of adolescents and adults who stutter is the limitation that stuttering puts on their lives, academically, socially, and occupationally. Consequently, Manning's therapy procedures, which are tailored to each client, are designed to help clients increase the opportunities and choices in their lives. In his book, *Clinical Decision Making in the Diagnosis and Treatment of Fluency Disorders* (1996), Manning describes a therapy approach that usually begins with the client identifying what he does *when* he stutters (core and secondary behaviors) and what he does *because* he stutters (choices motivated by stuttering, such as avoidance of situations). The client then works to modify his behaviors and choices, learning both to feel more comfortable with stuttering in many situations and to modify stuttering to sound more and more like normal speech. After this, the client undergoes fluency shaping to further enhance the smoothness of his speech.

Manning uses fluency shaping from the beginning of treatment with advanced stutterers who may be unable or unwilling to modify their stuttering. Examples are clients who have psychogenic or neurogenic stuttering or those who are mentally retarded. Manning strongly advocates group therapy as a component of treatment to help the client practice speaking skills and deal with emotional issues. He urges stutterers to join support groups after therapy to enhance long-term change.

C. Woodruff Starkweather

In his 1980 article, "A Multiprocess Behavioral Approach to Stuttering Therapy," Starkweather states that he views stuttering as resulting from multiple conditioning processes, namely, operant, classical, avoidance, and vicarious conditioning. Consequently, he takes a multiprocess behavioral approach to its treatment. Specifically, he recommends that treatment for clients with advanced stuttering have the following five goals: (*a*) reversing conditioning processes currently maintaining the disorder, (*b*) reducing or eliminating avoidance behavior, (*c*) modifying stuttering to reduce abnormality, (*d*) rate reduction and monitoring in therapy, and (*e*) rate reduction and monitoring in outside situations.

To achieve the first goal, it is necessary to determine which conditioning processes are currently maintaining the disorder. Starkweather suggests that this becomes apparent from an evaluation. The following two examples, which depict how conditioning processes can maintain the disorder and how conditioning can be reversed, should clarify what Starkweather has in mind in meeting this goal. In one situation, parents may be unintentionally reinforcing an adolescent's stuttering by giving him more attention when he stutters. In this case, the parents need to be advised to discontinue this behavior. In another situation, the spouse of a client may be responding negatively toward his stuttering, thereby increasing his tendency to use avoidance behaviors. If this is so, then the spouse should be counseled to change her responses to those that reflect more acceptance of the disorder.

Starkweather suggests that there are three principles that should guide clinicians in their efforts to reduce or eliminate client's use of avoidance behaviors. The first principle involves reducing fear on which the avoidance behavior is based. Starkweather believes this is fear of stuttering itself or fear of listeners' reactions. To reduce this fear, he recommends many of the identification and desensitization procedures advocated by Van Riper. Among the desensitization procedures, Starkweather believes that pseudostuttering is the most effective. The second principle for reducing avoidance behaviors is motivating the client to approach his fear. A person who stutters needs encouragement to enter feared situations and to stutter openly in them. The third principle for reducing avoidance behaviors is response prevention. The purpose is to keep an individual from using avoidance behaviors and force him to experience his stuttering. Starkweather suggests this can be achieved by using both pseudostuttering and freezing. At the beginning of this section, we said that we believe it is important to reduce negative feelings and attitudes and eliminate avoidances. It is obvious that Starkweather believes this, too.

Starkweather's procedures for modifying stuttering are very similar to Van Riper's. First, the client is taught to vary his stuttering. He deliberately stutters with more tension, and then with less tension. When he has learned to do this, he is introduced to cancellations. In other words, he says a stuttered word again, but stuttering on it the second time with less tension and struggle. Starkweather believes that as the stutterer gets better at using cancellations, he will be able to shift his modification forward in time to catch himself while he is still in a stutter. This is a Van Riper pull-out. Based on his experience, Starkweather suggests that some stutterers will then be able to shift their modification forward in time even more and to ease into anticipated stutters or use a Van Riper preparatory set.

Starkweather's fourth goal is to teach the client to use a form of controlled fluency for situations in which he feels it is important to sound fluent. Based on his experience, Starkweather does not believe it is necessary to use a structured fluency shaping program to do this. Rather, he believes that modeling and instructions help the client achieve a carefully monitored, variably slower rate of speech in the clinical setting. The client learns to vary his speech rate to suit his level of potential fluency, slowing when he feels he may stutter and speeding up when he feels he will be fluent.

Starkweather's last goal is variable rate control and monitoring in all situations. To facilitate the client's ability to use variable rate control, Starkweather recommends the use of hierarchies. Once the client has developed the ability to both modify his stutters and use a variable rate of speech in everyday speaking situations, he is ready to go out on his own.

In 1997, Starkweather and colleague Janet Givens-Ackerman published the book, *Stuttering*, which integrated several new elements into treatment. Their approach is based on a "recovery" philosophy similar to Alcoholics Anonymous, in which the client takes on responsibility for continuous self-therapy in which the clinician is only a guide. The goal is not simply fluent speech, but "freedom of speech, serenity and realizing one's full potential" (p. 150).

Their program is divided into three steps: awareness, acceptance, and change. In awareness, the clinician creates an accepting, safe environment in which the client explores behaviors, thoughts, and emotions associated with stuttering. In so doing, the client reduces denial and avoidance through the process of studying and approaching what has previously seemed scary and mysterious. In addition, by sharing with the clinician as honestly as possible the perceptions of listeners and his feelings about himself and stuttering, the client becomes less defensive, less tense, and therefore able to change.

Acceptance emerges from the way in which the clinician helps the client become aware of his behaviors, thoughts, and feelings. The client changes old patterns of self-condemnation and struggle into calm, disinterested observations of what is happening when he is stuttering. This stage may take much discussion between client and clinician as the client experiments with a different way of responding to stuttering in many different situations.

Change is a process of letting go of the extraneous baggage the stutterer has accumulated as he has learned to struggle, avoid, and defend against speech disruptions. The clinician helps the client learn a variety of strategies to let go. For example, the client may learn to slow down his overall excessive rate in trying to talk when he feels rushed or "stuttery," taking the time he needs to talk. The client may also use a variety of "repair" techniques to modify repetitions, prolongations, or blocks toward looser and more forward-moving, easy stutters. Another domain of change is being more open about stuttering. This includes simply commenting on one's stuttering, discussing it with friends, or letting others know how they can be good listeners by not interrupting or looking away. Being open also includes a willingness to say what one wants to say, even if stuttering occurs, rather than avoiding words or situations. The process of change is gradual and alternates with periods of awareness and acceptance. It also becomes a lifelong process, which is only begun in therapy with a clinician as a guide.

SUMMARY OF INTEGRATION OF APPROACHES

The therapies presented in this chapter represent a variety of integrated approaches. Some are based largely on stuttering modification and use fluency shaping only to refine clients' speech in the later stages of therapy; others use principally fluency shaping, but they deal with thoughts and feelings through additional treatment components, such as positive self-talk and group therapy. Despite these differences, all use both fluency shaping and stuttering modification, and all deal with behaviors, cognitions, and emotions in some way.

STUDY QUESTIONS

1. In integrating stuttering modification and fluency shaping therapies for the advanced stutterer, what position does the author take with regard to the speech behaviors targeted for therapy and the attention given to feelings and attitudes?
2. List the four phases of the author's therapy for the advanced stutterer. What is the goal for each of these phases?
3. Briefly describe the methods involved in the author's "understanding stuttering" phase.
4. List and briefly describe the procedures used in the author's reducing negative feelings and attitudes and eliminating avoidances phase.
5. How does the author integrate stuttering modification and fluency shaping therapies with regard to the speech behaviors targeted in therapy?
6. List and briefly describe the procedures in the author's maintaining fluency phase.
7. Compare the approaches of two "other clinicians" that you think are quite different.
8. Describe how you would structure an integrated approach and what therapy elements you would include.

SUGGESTED READINGS

Ahlbach, J., & Benson, V. (1994). *To say what is ours: The best of 13 years of "letting go."* **San Francisco: National Stuttering Project.**

As its title indicates, this is a compendium of articles written for the National Stuttering Project's newsletter, *Letting Go.* Several dozen authors have contributed essays about their personal experiences with stuttering. This book is full of insights and moving, funny, and honest writing that gives the reader glimpses into the subjective world of those who stutter.

Jezer, M. (1998). *Stuttering: A life bound up in words.* **New York: Basic Books.**

This is a beautifully written and funny autobiography about growing up and learning to cope with a severe stuttering problem. It gives particularly interesting perspectives on various therapies the author has participated in and discusses recent research findings. It provides a deeper understanding of the stutterer's denial of his problem than anything I've ever read.

Manning, W. (1996). *Clinical decision making in the diagnosis and treatment of fluency disorders.* **New York: Delmar Publishers.**

This fine book not only describes diagnosis and treatment of stuttering but gives many clinical insights from the author's own experiences as someone who stutters and who has also helped many persons who stutter. It is one of the few places in which advice on counseling in stuttering therapy can be found, and it provides unique sections on characteristics of the clinician and indicators of progress.

Starkweather, C.W. (1980). A multiprocess behavioral approach to stuttering therapy. *Seminars in Speech, Language and Hearing, 1, 327–337.*

This is an excellent article in which the author applies various learning paradigms to the treatment of the advanced stutterer.

10

Intermediate Stutterer: Stuttering Modification and Fluency Shaping Therapies

The child or adolescent with intermediate-level stuttering may be easier to treat in some ways than the advanced stutterer. This is because typically the intermediate stutterer has not stuttered for so long as the advanced stutterer nor are the learned reactions so well entrenched. On the other hand, the intermediate stutterer may present some management issues that are not a problem with the advanced stutterer. For example, the intermediate stutterer may find it difficult or impossible to use a slower rate or to use voluntary stuttering outside therapy because he wants so much to be like his friends. Another issue is that because he is going through a period of separation from his parents, he may find it difficult to trust an adult clinician. Despite these differences, many of the therapy techniques discussed in the section on advanced stuttering work well with the intermediate stutterer, with some adaptations made for age.

As we describe stuttering modification and fluency shaping approaches for the intermediate stutterer, you will notice that the two approaches are a little more similar for intermediate stuttering than for advanced stuttering. This similarity increases as we move from advanced to intermediate to beginning to borderline stuttering.

Before discussing stuttering modification therapy, fluency shaping therapy, and their integration for the intermediate stutterer, we will review the characteristics of the intermediate stutterer. As discussed, the intermediate stutterer is usually between 6 and 13 years of age and is usually in elementary or junior high school.

In terms of core behaviors, the intermediate stutterer may exhibit part-word or monosyllabic word repetitions that contain excessive tension, vowel prolongations that evidence tension, and blocks. His secondary behaviors may include both escape and starting behaviors and, for the first time, avoidance behaviors. These avoidance behaviors may include word substitutions, circumlocutions (use of a number of words to express a single idea) and avoidance of speaking situations. In terms of the feelings and attitudes associated with stuttering, the intermediate stutterer often feels frustrated and embarrassed and is experiencing fear of stuttering and of listeners' reactions. Finally, he has a definite self-concept as a stutterer. Now, let us turn to the treatment of the intermediate stutterer.

STUTTERING MODIFICATION THERAPY

We have chosen Carl Dell's therapy approach as the major illustration of stuttering modification therapy for the child with intermediate (or what he calls "confirmed") stuttering. This approach focuses strongly on the child's attitudes and feelings about stuttering, while at the same time it helps the child discover that he can stutter in a relaxed way that sounds much like normal speech. The easing of the child's emotions, combined with his ability to modify stuttering often result in near-normal fluency. This same principle can be seen in the other stuttering modification clinicians whose work we describe later.

Carl Dell: Changing Attitudes and Modifying Stutters

CLINICIAN'S BELIEFS

Nature of Stuttering

Dell believes that most stuttering results from a delay in speech motor coordination and suggests that it is similar to such problems as taking longer to develop the gross motor coordinations needed for jumping rope or riding a bike. He believes that many children who begin to stutter are not bothered by their disfluencies and soon outgrow them, but that other children become self-conscious about their difficulty. This leads them to speak with tension and effort. They may be responding to their own discomfort with repetitions and prolongations or to the concerns of parents, relatives, or others. These children are experiencing stuttering as a handicap and need immediate help.

Speech Behaviors Targeted for Therapy

Dell states that children with intermediate stuttering often have a high frequency of stuttering and show signs of tension and struggle in long repetitions with pitch rise or blockages of airflow. They also have negative emotions such as fear or shame and may have developed avoidance behaviors.

The targets of therapy include the child's moments of stuttering—repetitions, prolongations, and blocks—but the child's emotional responses to stuttering are equally important. Consequently, Dell begins therapy slowly and indirectly because children with intermediate stuttering are likely to be embarrassed and ashamed of their stuttering. Too much confrontation before a trusting relationship is established may cause these children to be turned off by therapy.

Fluency Goals

Dell indicates that most of the youngsters he works with at the intermediate level of stuttering will have both controlled fluency and acceptable stuttering when they finish therapy. He believes in dismissing intermediate stutterers from treatment before they are completely fluent, when they are confident that they can control their remaining stuttering. This, he believes, gives them a better chance to become their own therapist in the final stage of therapy, when they become more fluent. Dell keeps his door open, however, for them to return for "booster" sessions of therapy if needed.

Feelings and Attitudes

Dell believes that the child's feelings and attitudes are of major importance. If the child's frustrations and fears are not dealt with, he will react to stuttering with more and more struggle and avoidance, making it more difficult to treat. Dell helps the child change his feelings and attitudes by helping him to confront his stuttering and discover ways of changing it. This is done in a communicative atmosphere in which the clinician shows acceptance of stuttering by voluntarily stuttering herself. This allows the child to feel an equal partnership in therapy and enjoy it.

When working with the child who has intermediate stuttering, Dell achieves many changes in feelings through direct work on stuttering. The success that the child experiences in making stuttering easier goes a long way toward reducing frustration and fear of stuttering.

Maintenance Procedures

Dell believes in discharging the child from therapy before total fluency is achieved to help the child find his own ways of dealing with relapse if it occurs. If he needs to bring children back into therapy after a relapse, he finds them more motivated to work on their speech. Dell believes in nurturing the child's independence and encourages him to feel satisfaction when he is able to reestablish fluency after a momentary setback.

Clinical Methods

Dell's therapy is conducted in a teaching/counseling style in which the clinician teaches and models for the child a new behavior and then informally reinforces the child for using it. The clinician responds spontaneously to the child's responses and reactions within the framework of working on goals but does not follow steps in a formal program. Data are not systematically collected, but the clinician judges the child's progress informally on the basis of his observations and reports by parents, teacher, and the child himself.

CLINICAL PROCEDURES: DIRECT TREATMENT OF THE CHILD

Dell begins direct treatment slowly, testing the readiness of the child to confront his stuttering by putting a few voluntary stutters into his own speech, then commenting on them. If the child does not seem uncomfortable, Dell comments on some of the child's stutters and explores them with him. After the child has developed a trusting relationship with the clinician and appears to feel comfortable with his explorations of stuttering, Dell proceeds with direct therapy, which is divided into eight phases: (*a*) saying words in three ways, (*b*) locating tension, (*c*) cancelling, (*d*) changing stuttering to a milder form, (*e*) inserting easy stuttering into real speech, (*f*) changing hard stutters with pull-outs during real speech, (*g*) building fluency, and (*h*) building independence.

Three Ways of Saying Words

Dell describes and demonstrates for the child three ways of saying words: the regular or fluent way, the hard stuttering way, and the easy stuttering way. The hard way is characterized by typical stuttering and the easy way by an effortless prolongation or repetition. Dell's first step is to have the child identify these three ways of saying words in the clinician's speech in a game in which the child has to identify whether the clinician said a word in the "regular," "hard," or "easy" way.

As the game proceeds, the clinician occasionally asks the child to imitate her hard and easy stutters, allowing her to assess the child's readiness to put voluntary stutters into his own speech. When the child seems ready, the clinician changes the game so that they alternately give each other words to say and instructions to say them hard or easy. Because a major goal of this phase is to help the child learn how to produce easy stuttering, the clinician should develop a variety of ways that portray easy stuttering vividly, such as moving two fingers together slowly (Fig. 10.1) or drawing a gentle curve on a piece of paper.

Throughout this and later phases, the clinician stays alert to the child's spontaneous use of easy stutters when he's talking and praises them. If the therapy sessions that focus on the three ways of saying words are enjoyable and successful for the child, he will complete this phase with feelings of confidence that he can change his speech and will have less fear of stuttering.

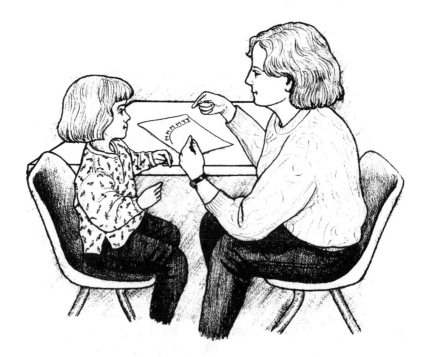

Figure 10.1. Showing a child how to stutter easily by moving two fingers together slowly.

Locating Tension

The next phase, that of locating tension in speech, is designed to help the child confront and explore stuttering as it is happening. Dell begins by doing some voluntary stuttering and asking the child to help him figure out where he is tensing or what he is doing when he is stuttering. He encourages the child to voluntarily stutter in the same way as they explore what is going on, thereby laying the groundwork for the child's exploration of his own stuttering.

The clinician and child experiment with different types of stutters, which cover those that the child shows in his own speech—repetitions and prolongations, as well as labial, lingual, and laryngeal blocks, if appropriate. When the child can identify the types of stutters and places of tension in the clinician's voluntary stutters, he is encouraged to do the same with his own stutters, when the clinician gently points them out in the child's spontaneous speech. Before stopping the child after a stutter, the clinician should explain that such interruptions are needed to work on stuttering, then should help the child confront and briefly explore his stutters during conversations.

Cancellations

After the child has learned to produce easy stutters and has confronted his stutters immediately after they have occurred, he is ready to stop after hard stutters and redo them as easy stutters. This activity is often frustrating, so it is best to use a structured situation for only a few minutes at a time. Dell recommends that a clinician begin this activity by having the child become the teacher and interrupt the clinician when she produces a hard stutter, then teach her how to say the word, not fluently, but with an easier, more relaxed stutter. These cancellations, unlike other ways of modifying stutters, are not used outside the therapy room and are only a means of helping the child begin to change the moment of stuttering as it is happening.

Changing Stuttering to a Milder Form

This phase of transforming his stuttering to an easy stutter begins after the child has mastered cancellations in the previous phase and can redo his hard stuttering as a truly loose and relaxed easy stutter. Now he is ready to change a stutter *as it is happening*, using what Van Riper called "pull-outs." This is begun with the clinician modeling how to make this change during a voluntary stutter, then asking the child to imitate her. Basically, this change is simply a shift from a hard to an easy stutter during a moment of stuttering, and finishing the word without rushing.

Inserting Easy Stuttering Into Real Speech

After the child can use pull-outs during voluntary stuttering, the next step is to have the child put voluntary easy stutters in his speech on words that he doesn't expect to stutter on. These easy stutters are like using a voluntary pull-out at the beginning of a nonfeared word. This gives the child a feel for working on stuttering as he is communicating; it is also a great desensitization activity.

Changing Hard Stutters With Pull-outs During Real Speech

Now Dell is ready to teach the child to change hard stutters into easy stutters while he is talking. Dell notes that this is often a difficult task for the child to learn, but once learned, he is well on the way to recovery. One helpful technique is to touch the child when he gets caught in a real stutter. The child is to hold on to the block voluntarily until Dell lets go, then to release the block, using an easy stutter. Because some children are sensitive about being touched, Dell suggests that clinicians talk with the child before using a touch to signal.

As before, Dell advises the clinician to begin this phase by putting some voluntary stutters in her speech and having the child touch her on the arm for several seconds when she does. She continues to stutter until the child releases his touch, then finishes the word slowly and easily. Roles are then reversed and the clinician gives the child an easy, non-emotional speaking task such as describing a neutral picture. She explains to the child that, when he stutters, she will touch him and that he is to keep stuttering on the same sound in the same way until she releases her touch, and then he is to finish the word slowly and easily.

For example, if the child is stuttering on the /l/ in "like," he is to keep repeating or prolonging the /l/ sound until the clinician takes her hand away; if he is having a silent block on the /b/ in "boy," he should continue the silent block at first, and then slowly change the silent /b/ to a voiced /b/ (even though this may distort the sound). Then, when the clinician's touch is released, the child slowly finishes the word.

After the child can change hard stutters into easy ones in conversational speech using the clinician's touch, he is asked to do so on his own. As he learns to do this successfully, he can begin to set goals, with the clinician's help, for using these techniques in more difficult situations, such as when talking about a complex topic or with a parent. Before transferring this skill to talking with a parent, the child should teach the parent about easy stuttering with the clinician's help. While the parent learns about easy stuttering in the therapy room, the clinician can also teach the parent how to help the child practice at home and especially how to be supportive of changes in the child's speech without being intrusive.

Building Fluency

In the building fluency phase, Dell makes sure that the child has plenty of experiences in which he is fluent every day. At the same time he helps the child work on stuttering by desensitizing him to fluency disrupters and helping him to transfer his more fluent speech into many different everyday situations. Transfer can begin as soon as the child can change hard stutters into easy ones in conversational speech without the clinician's cue. In the context of a game or in role-playing, the child talks and tries to use easy stutters instead of hard ones, while the clinician gradually increases the stress on the child, interrupting the child or looking away while he's talking. If the child begins to have hard stutters instead of easy ones, they stop and discuss what happened and how it might be handled differently.

A hierarchy of more and more stressful therapy or real-life situations are devised by the child and clinician together, and the child enters these situations and uses easy stutters when he stutters as best he can. At the same time, the child is open about his stuttering and comments about it when appropriate.

Building Independence

Finally, in the building independence phase, which begins when both the frequency and severity of stuttering are notably diminished and the child is confident that he can control his stuttering, Dell gradually fades the child from therapy. He does not believe that the child needs to be totally "cured" before he is dropped from therapy. Rather, when the child is doing well, Dell discontinues therapy for a period of time, allowing him to continue on his own and develop the conviction that he, rather than the clinician, is responsible for the change. If the child regresses a bit, Dell brings him in for one or more booster sessions, and often there will be a number of these cycles before the child is finally dismissed.

CLINICAL PROCEDURES: WORKING WITH PARENTS AND TEACHERS

Parents

Dell begins to work with parents during initial interviews when he seeks information about the child and gives parents information about the nature of stuttering. During these initial conversations with parents, some of Dell's other objectives are to create an open, nonjudgmental atmosphere. This is done so that parents can speak freely about their concerns and vent their feelings of frustration about their child's stuttering, and so that Dell can put some of their unspoken feelings into words. These discussions, and informing parents about the nature of stuttering, can also go a long way toward relieving parents of any guilt they may feel about their child's stuttering.

After he has begun to treat the child, Dell invites parents to observe some of their sessions. When the child is changing hard stutters into easy ones, for example, parents may be invited to participate by letting the child teach them how to stutter easily, a situation in which the child is in a position of mastery, compared with the parents, and which is usually very rewarding for both child and parents.

At this time, the child needs to be consulted about including a further role for the parents in his treatment at home. Some children may allow parents to remind them to use easy stuttering; other children may be more comfortable if their parents know what they are working on but are just good listeners. Parents are encouraged to spend a few minutes every day in a quiet time with the child, a time when the parents put aside their agendas and let the child talk about whatever is on his mind.

In addition, Dell asks parents to keep a diary of the times when their child is most disfluent as well as when he is most fluent. In discussions of events surrounding very disfluent times, Dell helps parents to identify and decrease pressures that worsen the child's stuttering. Similarly, he encourages them to find activities and situations that promote the child's fluency and increase these activities. By establishing a continuing partnership with the parents, in which respect and understanding are paramount, Dell is able to help the child while giving the parents an important role in establishing and maintaining the child's fluency.

Teachers

Dell's counseling of classroom teachers involves providing them with information about stuttering, helping them respond more objectively to the child's stuttering in the classroom, and helping them deal more effectively with the difficult issue of the child's oral participation in the class.

Dell believes that an initial meeting with a teacher in a quiet place is very important. In this setting, the teacher can ask questions about the nature of stuttering in general and about the nature of this child's stuttering in particular. By comparing stuttering with other problems that children have, such as making an obvious mistake on a math problem that results in other children laughing, the teacher is better able to see that her response will guide the class and that she needs to ensure that the child who stutters feels confident even though he may have difficulty speaking. In discussions, the clinician can help the teacher discover how she may be most helpful to the child.

When dealing with the issue of how much verbal participation to expect of the child who stutters, Dell believes that this is a topic that the child and teacher can discuss privately and frankly and work out effective strategies for each situation. For example, if the child has to give an oral report, he may prefer to be called on first, so that his fears don't build up. When being called on in class, the child may wish to wait until he feels he is ready and then raise his hand.

In general, Dell finds that helping teachers to understand stuttering is a key to helping children manage their speech in the classroom. With this understanding, teachers can communicate effectively with the child who stutters and, with the help of the clinician, they can work out any difficult situations that arise.

Other Clinicians

To complete our discussion of stuttering modification therapy for the intermediate stutterer, let us now consider what some other stuttering modification clinicians do to treat these children.

OLIVER BLOODSTEIN

Oliver Bloodstein (1975) discusses his treatment for an intermediate or "phase 3" stutterer in his chapter in Eisenson's *Stuttering: A Second Symposium.* He focuses on the child's attitudes and beliefs as well as on his moments of stuttering. Bloodstein targets two components in working on attitudes and beliefs: general speech improvement and personal development. For the first component, the clinician helps the child develop good speaking traits and provides a variety of successful speaking experiences for him so that he can replace previously held beliefs of being a defective speaker with the belief that he can talk well. As the child accumulates more and more successful speaking experiences, he also begins to anticipate an ease of communication rather than difficulty in talking. In working with the child's personal development, the clinician provides a supportive therapeutic relationship and provides successful experiences on many tasks and activities to increase the child's sense of self-worth.

Bloodstein also spends considerable time with the intermediate level stutterer helping him modify his symptoms. The goal of his symptom modification component is to teach the child to reduce the tension and fragmentation in speech by learning to move forward through a stuttered word in a deliberate and unhurried manner.

HAROLD LUPER AND ROBERT MULDER

Many years ago, two superb stuttering clinicians, Harold Luper and Robert Mulder published a book that described stuttering modification therapy in great detail. Although their book, *Stuttering: Therapy for Children* (1964), is out of print, their ideas are still current. Their therapy for the intermediate stutterer (referred to as the "confirmed stutterer" in the book) involves direct treatment of the child and parent counseling. The direct treatment of the child is broken down into five phases.

The first phase has several objectives. During this phase, Luper and Mulder establish a healthy clinical relationship with the child and help him understand that he will need to take an active role in changing his speech behaviors and attitudes. They point out that a cure is not the usual outcome of therapy; rather, a gradual reduction in stuttering and fear of talking is much more typical. To reduce the child's sensitivity to his stuttering, they help him realize that he is a normal individual except for his speech problem.

During the second phase of therapy, Luper and Mulder help the child eliminate unsatisfactory ways of approaching difficult words and situations. First of all, they want him to eliminate avoidances, so they try to instill in the child a willingness to use words he has feared and to talk in difficult situations. In attempting to convince him to be "brave" in facing these difficult tasks, they draw analogies between overcoming fear of talking and other fears the child has overcome, such as fear of going off a diving board. During this phase of treatment, Luper and Mulder also suggest better ways for the child to approach difficult words. They show him how to say such words with reduced tension or "loose contacts," rather than trying to say them with excessive tension.

In the third phase of therapy, Luper and Mulder help the child modify his struggles during moments of stuttering using Van Riper's techniques of cancellations and pull-outs; they provide additional techniques for modifying specific phonemes.

During the fourth phase of therapy, Luper and Mulder help the child reduce any residual word and situation fears. They begin by discussing with him why he is afraid of these words or situations. They believe that by helping the child gain an understanding of his fears it will make it easier for him to alleviate them. They also decondition residual fears using hierarchies of gradually increasing difficulty in which the child experiences his old feared words and situations over and over again under different circumstances until he is no longer afraid of them. Luper and Mulder are careful to ensure that the child has rewarding speaking experiences as he proceeds through these hierarchies.

In the last phase of treatment, Luper and Mulder help the child develop new speech attitudes. They want him to feel free to have a certain amount of "bobbles" in his speech and still find speaking pleasurable.

The thrust of Luper and Mulder's parent counseling is to help parents reduce stress on their child and to help them be good listeners.

WILLIAM MURPHY

Murphy's approach focuses on the speech motor behaviors, attitudes, and feelings of children who stutter, but he places the greatest emphasis on feelings, particularly those of shame. An implicit assumption of his therapy is that stuttering is perpetuated because children are ashamed of it and try to hide or avoid it. Murphy begins by helping the child realize that stuttering is not his fault and that he can learn to change it, but that it is acceptable even if stuttering occurs. Murphy reduces the child's shame about stuttering by having him deliberately stutter (pseudostuttering). This is done gradually, first by having the child catch the clinician stuttering, then by rewarding him for imitating the clinician, and then by rewarding him for being open and playful with pseudostuttering in contests to see who can have the longest, hardest, shortest, loudest, and easiest stutters.

Murphy brings the child's parents into therapy and has the child teach his parents to stutter and grade their efforts.

Another highlight of Murphy's therapy is to help the child deal with teasing. He encourages children to talk about the times when they have been teased and draw pictures of those experiences while they talk. He helps them become more assertive about teasing by having them think of better ways to respond to teasing, then videotaping and replaying a reenactment of the original teasing experience and role playing of the alternative responses to teasing they have planned.

As Murphy helps children diminish their shame, he also teaches them easier ways to stutter, using relaxed pseudostuttering in his speech as a model. The more open and comfortable the child feels with his stuttering, the easier it is for him to stutter in a relaxed and easy way. And as the child finds he can stutter in ways that feel more controlled and less noticeable, he becomes more comfortable and confident about communicating.

JOSEPH SHEEHAN

In Chapter 8, we discuss Joseph Sheehan's therapy for the advanced stutterer, which was based on his view that stuttering is an approach-avoidance conflict. Stuttering occurs whenever a stutterer's tendency to go ahead and talk is equal to his tendency to hold back and avoid talking. Thus, Sheehan's therapy for an advanced stutterer had twin goals: increasing his approach and decreasing his avoidance tendencies. There was an emphasis, however, on reducing avoidance tendencies. This may be a good time to read the description of Sheehan's clinical procedures for the advanced stutterer in Chapter 8. Sheehan recommended similar procedures for the intermediate stutterer, or "older child stutterer."

More specifically, Sheehan (1975) explained to the child that everybody stumbles on some words, but that he had gotten into the habit of struggling or stuttering on words to avoid stumbling on them. Sheehan told the child that, if he would accept the idea that he is going to stumble on some words, then he would not struggle so hard trying not to do it. He would then explain that because the child was going to stumble on some words anyway, it would be best to learn how to say these words smoothly and easily, thereby showing the child that he has a choice in how he stutters. Finally, Sheehan explained that it is unwise to substitute words or avoid certain speaking situations and told the child that it is much better in the long run to go ahead and say what he wants to say.

Sheehan also believed that it is important to counsel parents of all children who stutter about the demand/support ratio in the home. Children who stutter often have too many demands placed on them, and, at the same time, they receive insufficient support. These demands often revolve around such issues as academic performance, music lessons, tidiness, and so on. As part of his therapy for the child who stutters, Sheehan counseled the child's parents to be less demanding and more supportive of their child. Sheehan's capacities and demands perspectives are discussed in Chapter 3.

DEAN WILLIAMS

Dean Williams based his stuttering therapy on the assumption that stuttering was learned behavior, consisting of children's initial responses to mild disfluencies in early childhood, which gradually escalated into tension and struggle. Williams also believed that people who stutter would talk normally if they unlearned all the behaviors that interfered with their speech, such as tensing, breath-holding, and speeding up.

When working with children who had what we call intermediate level stuttering, Williams first taught them about normal speech: how the components of their speech mechanism (such as the tongue, lips, and jaw) work together in normal talking and how they feel in fluent speech. Then he taught them to contrast the feeling of normal talking with the feeling of stuttering. It was very important to Williams for children to understand and accept the idea that stuttering wasn't "something that happened to them" but "something they did," which he established by having them use words that described their stuttering in terms of *what they were doing* when they stuttered. With this understanding, children could better accept responsibility for changing their stuttering.

After the child's initial explorations of normal talking, much of his learning involved examining what he was doing when it was happening. Williams helped the child discover what he was doing to interfere with talking by coaching him to "catch" a moment of stuttering as it was taking place and to "stay there," feeling what he was doing. Once the child could do this, Williams taught him to modify his stuttering as it was happening by letting go of excess tension or allowing air or sound to flow—essentially, changing whatever he was doing to interfere with talking. After he could do this during stutters, Williams taught the child to begin words with a more normal approach, so that he wasn't interfering with talking *in anticipation* of stuttering.

Transfer of more normal talking took place as Williams asked the child to become aware of the feelings he had in speaking situations outside the therapy room. Did he have a feeling that told him he was going to stutter? Did that feeling make him do things to interfere with talking? Thus, Williams helped children discover that they could talk easily even when they anticipated stuttering. As they had more experiences like this—of talking easily even when they felt they might stutter—children changed their feelings and beliefs about their speech and this, in turn, changed their habitual ways of responding to everyday speaking situations and even to stressful situations.

Summary of Stuttering Modification Therapy

All the stuttering modification clinicians we discussed in this section believe that it is important to teach an intermediate stutterer to modify his moments of stuttering. Furthermore, they all believe to some degree that it is important to target the child's feelings about stuttering and attempt to eliminate his use of avoidance behaviors. Thus, with regard to these clinical issues, these clinicians' goals for the intermediate stutterer are similar to those for the advanced stutterer. Of course, their clinical procedures for these two treatment levels are somewhat different because intermediate stutterers are younger and consequently need more support and more concrete explanations of therapy procedures. Finally, all these clinicians believe it is important to counsel parents of intermediate stutterers.

FLUENCY SHAPING THERAPY

To illustrate a fluency shaping approach for the intermediate stutterer, we describe here Bruce Ryan's therapy in detail. Then, we comment briefly on the therapies of a number of other fluency shaping clinicians.

Bruce Ryan: Delayed Auditory Feedback Program

CLINICIAN'S BELIEFS

Nature of Stuttering

Ryan views stuttering as a learned behavior having three components: a speech act, an attitude, and anxiety. The *speech act* consists of words that contain repetitions, prolongations, or struggle. Ryan believes these are operant behaviors. The *attitude component* consists of verbal statements the child makes about himself, which Ryan also believes are operant behaviors. Finally, the *anxiety component* consists of various physiological responses, which may be related to the child's stuttering. Ryan believes these are respondent behaviors. Because speech behaviors are operant behaviors, Ryan believes they can be modified by operant conditioning and programmed instruction procedures. Thus, the focus of his therapy is on increasing fluent speech behaviors and decreasing stuttering behaviors. Furthermore, he believes that concurrent changes are also made in the child's attitude and anxiety components of his problem when speech behaviors are changed.

Speech Behaviors Targeted for Therapy

Ryan organizes treatment into three phases: establishment, transfer, and maintenance. One of several establishment programs he uses is the delayed auditory feedback (DAF) program. He uses DAF with the child who exhibits "severe stuttering." The goal of this program is to establish 5 minutes of fluent conversational speech with the clinician in the therapy room. With the DAF device set on its maximum delay, the child is taught to speak in a slow, prolonged, fluent pattern. This fluent pattern is reinforced, and moments of stuttering are punished. The DAF is then systematically faded, and the child's fluent speech pattern gradually increases in rate, which we describe in more detail in the next section. After the child has attained 5 minutes of fluent conversational speech with the clinician in the therapy room, Ryan systematically transfers the child's fluent speech to his natural environment.

Fluency Goals

Ryan's goals for the intermediate stutterer appear to be either spontaneous fluency or controlled fluency. To pass his criterion test and be dismissed from the program, the child must exhibit no more than 0.5 stuttered words per minute (SW/M). Ryan regards this as "normal-sounding speech."

Feelings and Attitudes

Ryan gives little, if any, attention to changing the child's feelings and attitudes about speech. He believes that, if the child's fluency improves, then any negative feelings or attitudes the child may have will also improve.

Maintenance Procedures

As we previously mentioned, one of Ryan's three phases of treatment is maintenance. The goal is for the child to maintain fluency over a 22-month period. During this period, the child's speech is sampled, and the child, his parents, and his teacher are interviewed about the child's fluency in his everyday environment. If the child regresses, he is recycled through parts of the establishment or transfer phases of the treatment program.

Clinical Methods

Ryan's therapy is based heavily on operant conditioning and programmed instruction principles. This involves a great deal of structure and an emphasis on data collection.

CLINICAL PROCEDURES: DIRECT TREATMENT OF THE CHILD

In his 1984 chapter, "Treatment of Stuttering in School Children," Ryan discusses his treatment procedures for the intermediate stutterer, whom he refers to as the child who exhibits "severe stuttering." This is our primary reference for this section. The reader may wish to refer to Ryan's 1974 book, *Programmed Therapy of Stuttering in Children and Adults*, for additional information. We begin by discussing Ryan's direct treatment of the child during establishment, transfer, and maintenance phases. Then we describe his procedures for counseling the child's parents and classroom teacher.

Establishment

Ryan uses a delayed auditory feedback (DAF) establishment program for the intermediate stutterer (Fig. 10.2). This is also the program he typically uses with an advanced stutterer. The goal is to have the child speaking fluently with the clinician for 5 minutes in the clinical setting. However, before beginning the program, Ryan ensures that the child understands what is expected of him by giving him an overview of the program. He defines stut-

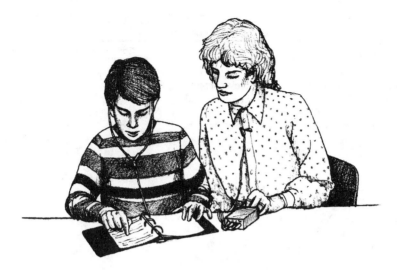

Figure 10.2. Use of delayed auditory feedback (DAF) to establish fluency.

tering for the child—any word that contains a repetition, prolongation, or other struggle behavior—and explains that he will be reinforced for fluent speech and punished for stuttering. The reinforcement involves verbal praise and sometimes tokens. The punishment is a verbal correction. Ryan also administers a pretreatment criterion test, consisting of 5 minutes of reading, monologue, and conversation, which he uses to assess later improvements.

The DAF establishment program is a 26-step program that begins by teaching the child to use a "slow, prolonged, fluent pattern of speech." Training starts with Ryan reading sentences aloud with the child and ends with the child reading aloud in a slow, prolonged, fluent pattern for 5 consecutive minutes. Table 10.1 presents an outline of Ryan's DAF program.

The DAF device is introduced at 250-msec delay, and the child is told to use his slow, prolonged, fluent speech pattern while reading aloud. When he does, his speech pattern is socially reinforced. If the child stutters or speeds up, he is reminded to use slow, prolonged, fluent speech. The child needs to have 5 consecutive minutes of fluent, oral reading at this delay, which means that he needs to meet a criterion of 0 stuttered words per minute (0 SW/M) for 5 consecutive minutes. When he does, DAF is reduced by 50 msec, and the child must now complete another 5 consecutive minutes of fluent, oral reading at the new delay. In this manner, DAF is systematically reduced in 50-msec steps until the child is reading without the aid of the device. During this process, the child is required to have 5 consecutive minutes of fluent, oral reading at each of six delay times (250, 200, 150, 100, 50, and 0 msec) and 5 consecutive minutes of fluent, oral reading without DAF. As delay time is reduced, the child's speaking rate gradually increases. Eventually, the child is reading aloud fluently without the aid of the DAF device at a slightly below normal, oral reading rate.

After the child completes the reading component of the DAF establishment program, he goes on to the monologue and conversation stages of the program. These components replicate the steps used for reading, except that the child now engages in either a monologue or a conversation with the clinician. Everything else, that is, the reinforcement, punishment, 0 SW/M criterion, and so on, remain the same. Ryan reports that most children complete the establishment program speaking fluently at a slightly below-normal speaking rate.

Table 10.1. Outline of Ryan's Delayed Auditory Feedback (DAF) Establishment Program

Antecedent Events	Response	Consequent Event	Criterion
Pattern Training in Reading:			
Instructions to read in a slow, prolonged pattern	Slow, prolonged, fluent reading	"Good"	0 SW/M
Reading:			
Instructions to read. DAF: 250 msec	Slow, prolonged, fluent reading	"Good"	0 SW/M
	Stuttering	"Stop, use your slow, prolonged, fluent pattern"	
Instructions to read. DAF: 200 msec	"	"	"
Instructions to read. DAF: 150 msec	"	"	"
Instructions to read. DAF: 100 msec	"	"	"
Instructions to read. DAF: 50 msec	"	"	"
Instructions to read. DAF: 0 msec	"	"	"
Instructions to read	Fluent reading	"	"
Monologue:			
Repeat the above sequence			
Conversation:			
Repeat the above sequence			

After completing the DAF establishment program, Ryan gives the child a postestablishment criterion test. This consists of 5 minutes of reading, monologue, and conversation. If the child has 0.5 SW/M or less, he goes on to the transfer phase. Otherwise, he is recycled through portions of the establishment program.

Transfer

The goal of Ryan's transfer phase is to transfer the child's fluency from the therapy room to a variety of other settings and other people. He uses a number of hierarchies or sequences of speaking situations, arranged from easy to difficult, in which the child practices his fluent reading and fluent conversation. During these activities, Ryan instructs the child to speak fluently. He continues to reinforce the child's fluency with verbal praise and to remind the child to speak fluently if he stutters. The child must continue to meet the 0 SW/M criterion for specified periods of time to pass each step. The transfer program that Ryan uses with intermediate stutterers involves physical setting, audience size, home, school, telephone, stranger, and all-day hierarchies. These are outlined in Table 10.2.

The first step in the transfer program, the "physical setting" hierarchy, involves the child reading and conversing with Ryan in five different physical settings, arranged in an easy-to-difficult progression, away from the therapy room. The first step is just outside the therapy room door; the last step, just outside the young stutterer's classroom.

The next hierarchy targets "audience size" and begins with one of the stutterer's classmates joining him and Ryan in the therapy room. The stutterer reads and converses with his classmate, and when he meets the criteria, this procedure is repeated with two, then three of his classmates.

The "home" hierarchy is third. Its first step involves a parent joining Ryan and the child in therapy and being trained to carry out the transfer procedures. The parents have been informed previously that they would be involved in these and other treatment activities. (We discuss Ryan's parent counseling procedures in a later section.)

Table 10.2. Outline of Transfer Program

Antecedent Events	Response	Consequent Event	Criterion
Physical Setting:			
5 steps with clinician in different physical settings	One minute of fluent reading	"Good"	0 SW/M
	3 minutes of fluent conversation	"Good"	
	Stuttering	"Stop, speak fluently."	
Audience Size:			
3 steps with 3 classmates in therapy room	"	"	"
Home:			
5 steps with parent in therapy room and at home	"	"	"
School:			
4 steps with clinician in school	"	"	"
Telephone:			
11 steps on the telephone	3 minutes of fluent conversation	"	"
Strangers:			
4 steps with strangers	"	"	"
All Day:			
Up to 16 steps (optional)	Up to 16 hours of fluency	"	"

The first step of the hierarchy is now repeated by the parent and child at home. The remaining steps involve gradual increases in audience size in the home environment by having other family members, and possibly neighbors, join the parent and child as he reads and converses. After successfully completing the home hierarchy, the child is instructed to speak fluently at all times at home, and the parents are instructed to reinforce his fluency.

The fourth hierarchy focuses on the school. The first step consists of the child reading and conversing with Ryan in the classroom. The last and most difficult step is a speech that the child gives to the entire class. After completing this hierarchy, the young stutterer is instructed to speak fluently at all times in the classroom, and the teacher is asked to reinforce his fluency.

The "telephone" hierarchy is an 11-step program. It begins with the child saying, "hello" and "goodbye" into an unplugged telephone. It ends with the child engaging in 3 consecutive minutes of fluent conversation on the telephone with a friend or stranger.

The "stranger" hierarchy begins with the child conversing with people at school, such as the school secretary or principal, and ends with him talking with strangers in local businesses. At each of the four steps in this hierarchy, the child needs to maintain 3 consecutive minutes of fluent conversation.

The final, "all day" hierarchy goes as follows. The child is instructed to speak fluently for increasingly longer periods of time each succeeding day. On the first day, he is to speak fluently for 1 hour. On each subsequent day, 1 hour is added until the child is speaking fluently his entire waking day. The parents and teacher have to monitor and record the child's consecutive hours of fluency.

Ryan reports that, by the end of the transfer phase, the child is usually speaking fluently in all speaking situations and has increased his speaking rate to normal. Ryan gives the child a post-transfer criterion test. If he passes (0.5 SW/M or less), he goes on to the maintenance phase. If not, the child is recycled through portions of the transfer phase.

Maintenance

The goal of Ryan's maintenance phase is for the child to maintain fluent speech in all situations over a 22-month period after completion of the transfer phase. Ryan sees the child and his parents on five separate occasions during this period; these rechecks are scheduled in such a manner as to gradually fade the child from therapy. (See Table 10.3 for an outline of this maintenance program.) During each recheck, Ryan administers the criterion test to the child and questions him and his parents about his fluency at home and at school. If the child has 0.5 SW/M or less on the criterion test and if he is reported to be doing well in all other situations as well, Ryan schedules the next recheck. If the child's speech has regressed, he is recycled through portions of the treatment program, depending on the severity of the regression. After the child has demonstrated and the parents have reported fluent speech for 22 months, Ryan dismisses the child from treatment.

CLINICAL PROCEDURES: PARENT COUNSELING

Ryan begins working with the parents before beginning the DAF program with the child. He explains the DAF program and the overall treatment plan to them. He wants the parents to understand what their child will be doing in therapy and what they can expect in terms of improvement in his speech. Ryan also tries to enlist the parents' cooperation for the "home practice" program and the "home" and "all day" hierarchies of the transfer phase. The home practice program involves the parents helping the child practice being fluent while engaging in reading, monologue, and conversation at home. After the child completes the reading portion of the program, he is ready to begin to practice reading at home. At this point, Ryan brings the parents into therapy to teach them how to identify stuttered words and how to carry out treatment procedures at home. They then help the child practice reading 5 minutes daily. After the child completes the monologue portion, home practice is modified to include 2 minutes of reading and 5 minutes of monologue. Later, when the child has completed the conversation mode, the home practice is again modified to include 2 minutes of reading, 2 minutes of monologue, and 5 minutes of conversation. This routine continues daily until the child begins the home hierarchy of the transfer program, which we discussed earlier in the home portion section of the transfer program.

CLINICAL PROCEDURES: CLASSROOM TEACHER COUNSELING

Before the child's treatment begins, Ryan explains the overall treatment plan to the classroom teacher and enlists her aid in the "school" hierarchy of the transfer phase. He explains that she may observe improvements in the child's speech at any time during the treatment program.

Table 10.3. Outline of Maintenance Program

Antecedent Events	Response	Consequent Event	Criterion
2 weeks	5 minutes of reading, monologue, and conversation	—	0.5 SW/M or less
1 month	"	"	"
3 months	"	"	"
6 months	"	"	"
12 months	"	"	"

Other Clinicians

We conclude our discussion of fluency shaping therapy for the intermediate stutterer with a brief description of the clinical procedures used by other fluency shaping clinicians.

JANIS COSTELLO

In our description of fluency shaping with the beginning stutterer (Chapter 12), we describe Janis Costello's extended length of utterance (ELU) program. The reader may wish to consult this section to learn the details of Costello's basic program for all children who stutter. Costello notes that if this basic program produces "less-than-satisfactory" results with a child, she considers using "additives" with the basic program, including rate control, gentle onset, linguistic simplification, and attitude modification. Because these additional techniques may be more necessary for the intermediate than for the beginning stutterer, we describe them here.

Rate control is the first additive Costello considers using with her ELU program. This is especially true if assessment data indicate the child speaks too rapidly. Costello believes it is not necessary to use DAF to control the child's speaking rate. She prefers to simply instruct the child to talk slower during the ELU program. She reinforces only those responses that are both fluent and within a given speaking rate limit. Costello may also occasionally model the desired rate for the child. As the child progresses through the ELU program, speaking rate is allowed to increase gradually, as long as fluency is maintained, until a normal speaking rate is attained.

The next additive that Costello considers using is gentle onset of phonation. She believes this is most appropriate for the child who exhibits hard blocks. She instructs the child to use gentle onsets during the ELU program. As the child moves through the program, his use of gentle onsets is faded out.

Costello's third additive is linguistic simplification. She considers using this strategy, along with her ELU program, only when the child has documented deficiencies in such areas as word retrieval or the use of age-appropriate syntactic rules.

The last additive that Costello uses is attitude modification. By and large, Costello believes that most children who stutter do not have attitudinal problems because of their stuttering. She recommends that unless there is reason to suspect that the child has a serious attitude problem, it is best to use just the basic ELU program.

ASHLEY CRAIG

Although many of Ashley Craig's early publications dealt with advanced stuttering, he has also developed treatments for young adolescents who are presumably intermediate stutterers. In a relatively recent article (Craig et al., 1996), he describes a treatment approach for 9- to 14-year-old children who stutter, involving group therapy and carefully assessed procedures for establishment, generalization, and maintenance of fluency.

Craig and his coworkers developed and tested three different programs for establishing fluency: intensive smooth speech, home-based smooth speech, and intensive electromyographic (EMG) feedback. In *smooth speech treatment,* individuals are trained to initially speak at a slow rate, with prolonged syllables, light articulatory contacts, continuous airflow, and relaxed breathing. Then speech rate is increased until it approximates natural-sounding speech. This is achieved by means of a programmed approach similar to Neilson and Andrews' treatment, described in Chapter 8. The intensive version of smooth speech treatment is conducted in a therapy setting for 6½ hours per day over the course of a week.

Fluency is established in group sessions in which the children read aloud, tell jokes and stories, perform plays, and give speeches. The *home-based version* of smooth speech treatment is focused on developing a parent-child therapeutic relationship in which the parent and child both learn and practice smooth speech (as previously described) in a group of other parent-child pairs 1 day (6½ hours) per week for 4 weeks and practice at home in between sessions. *EMG feedback* treatment trains children to lower the tension in facial muscles before beginning an utterance, first with EMG feedback and then without, in a clinical setting.

All three treatments for stuttering use highly structured, behavior modification procedures with an emphasis on operant conditioning for both establishment and transfer of fluency. Transfer activities for all treatments involve speaking assignments outside the clinic, such as making telephone calls to acquaintances and talking to strangers. Maintenance sessions, at 1-month and 3-month intervals, are designed to help the children continue to use the fluency skills they learned during treatment. Sessions involve assessment and retraining of these skills and assessment of tape recordings of speech brought in by the children.

In their evaluation of these programs, Craig and coworkers found that all three treatments were successful in establishing and maintaining fluency for 70% of the children. The home-based smooth speech and EMG feedback treatments were slightly superior when the criterion was less than 2% syllables stuttered in the 1-year follow-up.

CHARLES AND SARA RUNYAN

The Runyans' therapeutic program (1986, 1993) is organized around three sets of "rules" or treatment components. First, there are two "universal rules," which are used with all children who stutter and may be the only rules needed for treating very young stutterers. Then, for children who do not eliminate all stuttering using the universal rules, two "primary rules," which have a physiological orientation, are taught. Finally, there are "secondary rules," which are applied when needed for children who have hard articulatory contacts, stoppages of speech, or extra body movements that are not eliminated by the universal and primary rules.

The two universal rules, which are taught together, are (1) speak slowly and (2) say one word at a time. The first universal rule has the child speak at a slow, but normal rate. It is taught using various games incorporating turtles and racehorses or a metronome set at 60 beats per minute and through the clinician's model of a relaxed, slow speaking rate. The Runyans caution that the more normal the rate and style of the child's speech, the easier it will be for him to generalize fluency. They also point out that it may not be just a slow rate that is important, but the overall calming effect of talking more slowly.

The second universal rule—to say a word only once—is taught along with the first universal rule. This rule is used to help the child who has many whole- or part-word repetitions. The Runyans may teach this principle with two toy trains—one with all the same cars and one with all different cars, or they may play games that compare walking on alternate feet (speaking without repetitions) with hopping on the same foot (repetitions). They also help the child understand repetitions by having him count the repetitions in the clinician's and his parents' speech. Finally, the Runyans use a raised index finger as a signal whenever the child produces a part-word or whole-word repetition any time during therapy session.

Children who do not become normally fluent using the two universal rules are taught two primary rules: (1) use speech breathing; and (2) start voicing gently. The first rule helps children who "lock up" their vocal folds or take a quick breath just before they be-

gin speaking. These children are taught to take a normal breath and exhale slowly, beginning their speech soon after they start exhalation. To teach this rule, the Runyans use
a drawing of the inhalation-exhalation cycle, placing a mark where speech should begin.
The child is asked to trace this breathing curve as he inhales, exhales, and begins to speak.

Tactile feedback may be used in teaching this rule by having the child place one hand
just below the sternum and feel the chest wall move in and out while breathing. Negative and positive practice (e.g., deliberately stopping breathing and tensely closing the
glottis, contrasted with keeping the vocal folds relaxed) is added for those children who
hold their breath when stuttering.

The other primary rule, starting the voice smoothly at the beginning of an utterance,
is taught by making the child more aware of his "voice box," contrasting gentle and hard
onset of phonation, and using single-syllable words beginning with vowels to practice
gentle onset. The Runyans caution that children should not be taught a breathy onset and
that they must continue to use normal intensity as they learn the gentle onset concept.

Three secondary rules are used in addition to the universal and primary rules whenever
they are needed in treatment: (1) use light articulatory contacts; (2) keep the articulators
moving; and (3) use only the "speech helpers" to talk. The appropriate secondary rule is
taught immediately whenever the child exhibits what the Runyans call a "secondary behavior," essentially squeezing, or cessation of movement of the articulators, or extra body
movements during stuttering. After the child is aware of the secondary rule and can speak
fluently and without struggle behavior, the therapeutic program is continued.

Children are taught the first secondary rule by comparing the difference between hard
articulatory contacts and light contacts and by experiencing, in animated exaggeration in
front of a mirror, how hard contacts can completely stop their speech production. The
child is asked to note the difference between hard contacts during stuttering and light
contacts during fluency. The child is then helped to change from hard to easy contacts in
conversational speech as the clinician squeezes his arm in proportion to the articulatory
tension perceived in the child's speech as they talk.

The second rule—to keep the articulators moving—was originally designed to eliminate prolongations, but the Runyans found that it combines well with light articulatory
contacts to help the child learn an overall flow of speech. They use such props as "turtle
tracks" or "lily pads" to help the child learn to move from one syllable to the next smoothly
and lightly. They use five-syllable phrases at this stage of training and have the child say
them as he steps from one track or pad to the next. After each phrase, the child pauses,
then uses proper speech breathing combined with a gentle onset to begin the next phrase.

The Runyans also teach the child to keep his articulators moving by having him touch
the table top, sequentially with his thumb and four fingers, producing a five-syllable
phrase as he does it.

The final secondary rule—use only the speech helpers to talk—is designed to eliminate extraneous body movements, which some children develop as part of their stuttering pattern. The Runyans use a mirror and an accepting, playful attitude to work side by
side with the child to highlight unnecessary body movements and help the child speak
without them.

After the child has learned the rules necessary to be fluent in the clinic, the Runyans
use loosely structured play situations with conversational speech designed to make therapy enjoyable and to provide opportunities for the child to practice fluency rules and generalize fluency to other activities. The clinician's sense of humor and spontaneity are key
elements. When needed, the Runyans use hand signals to remind the child of fluency
rules. For example, they may move a hand downward to signal a slower speaking rate or
hold up a giant rubber finger to remind the child to say a word only once. Generalization

to spontaneous speech in the therapy setting often happens suddenly and is closely related to the child's ability to monitor his own and his parents' speech production.

To help children carry over therapeutic principles from the clinic setting to home and school, the Runyans use small objects, such as refrigerator magnets and stickers, video games, and the telephone. These items are used to remind children of their fluency rules so that they will use them in a variety of home and school situations, thereby extending their fluency outside the therapy sessions. For example, the Runyans have found that some children are highly motivated to practice fluency rules at home using video games that were first used in the clinic as opportunities to practice fluency in conversational speech.

Another technique to help with carryover and maintenance is to telephone the child at home to remind him of his rules. There are numerous calls at first when the child is just beginning to transfer his new speaking skills, but fewer as time goes on and fluency is better established in the child's daily life.

The Runyans' guiding principles for therapy with children are (1) therapy must be fun; (2) establish fluency with as little deviation from normal speech as possible; and (3) once fluency is established, use every possible method to keep the child's fluency rules at a conscious level. The Runyans note that if the child has an articulation or language problem in addition to stuttering, they do fluency therapy simultaneously with their work on the other problem.

GEORGE SHAMES AND CHERI FLORANCE

We describe George Shames and Cheri Florance's (1980) "stutter-free speech" programs for the adult stutterer in Chapter 8 and briefly review it here before discussing what they suggest for the intermediate stutterer.

As mentioned earlier, the adult program is divided into five phases: (*a*) volitional control, (*b*) self-reinforcement, (*c*) transfer, (*d*) training in unmonitored speech, and (*e*) follow-up. The children's program, devised for children from approximately 3 to 8 years of age, is similar except for the omission of phase 4—training in unmonitored speech. Shames and Florance indicate that phase 4 is not necessary with children, because they begin to use unmonitored, stutter-free speech or spontaneous fluency by themselves. Another difference in the two programs is the major involvement of parents in the transfer phase of the child program.

So what do Shames and Florance do with intermediate stutterers, who are usually between 6 and 13 years of age? They suggest that an adolescent, intermediate stutterer who is demonstrating a need to be independent from his parents will probably do better in the adult program, whereas a younger, intermediate stutterer will probably do better in the children's program. They admit that it is difficult at times to determine when the child is too old for the child program. As the child moves through the volitional control and self-reinforcement phases of the program, Shames and Florance believe the clinician will get to know the child well enough to determine which path to take in the remaining phases of the program.

RONALD WEBSTER

We discuss Ronald Webster's "precision fluency shaping program" in Chapter 8 when we cover the treatment of the advanced stutterer. The goal of this program is to teach the advanced stutterer to use certain fluency-generating target behaviors. When a stutterer uses these target behaviors, he will be fluent. The two behaviors that are most important are slightly increased syllable duration and gentle voice onset. For a review of these target behaviors and Webster's entire program, you can turn to our previous discussion of it in Chapter 8.

With children between 5 and 12 years of age, Webster (1979) modifies his precision fluency shaping program by simplifying instructions and adapting therapy materials that are appropriate to the child's language abilities. He stresses the importance of giving the child a great deal of positive feedback when he is working on target behaviors. He also requires that one of the child's parents attend a number of therapy sessions to learn how to provide support for the child as he is acquiring the use of target behaviors. Webster reports that children in this age range readily develop the use of fluency-generating target behaviors.

Summary of Fluency Shaping Therapy

All the fluency shaping clinicians discussed in this section use procedures that first establish fluency in the clinical setting, then generalize it to the intermediate stutterer's everyday speaking environment. In all cases, their procedures are the same or modifications of the procedures they use with either beginning or advanced stutterers.

COMPARISON OF THE TWO APPROACHES

At the beginning of this chapter, we suggested that stuttering modification and fluency shaping therapies for the intermediate stutterer are more similar than they are for the advanced stutterer but less similar than for the beginning stutterer. Let us compare these two therapeutic approaches for the intermediate stutterer on the following clinical issues: (*a*) speech behaviors targeted for therapy, (*b*) fluency goals, (*c*) attention given to feelings and attitudes, (*d*) maintenance procedures, and (*e*) clinical methods. Table 10.4 provides an overview of the similarities and differences between these two approaches for the intermediate stutterer.

With regard to speech behaviors targeted for therapy, all the stuttering modification clinicians we reviewed teach the intermediate stutterer to modify his moments of stut-

Table 10.4. Similarities and Differences Between Stuttering Modification and Fluency Shaping Therapies for the Intermediate Stutterer

Clinical Issue	Therapy Approach	
	Stuttering Modification Therapy	Fluency Shaping Therapy
Speech behaviors targeted for therapy	Moments of stuttering	Fluent responses or fluency skills
Fluency goals	Spontaneous fluency, controlled fluency, or acceptable stuttering	Spontaneous fluency or controlled fluency
Feeling and attitudes	Some attention given to reducing negative feelings and attitudes	No attention given to reducing negative feelings and attitudes
Maintenance procedures	Minimal emphasis given to maintenance procedures	Minimal emphasis given to maintenance procedures
Clinical methods	Therapy often characterized by loosely structured interaction—play activity	Therapy often characterized by tightly structured interaction or programmed instruction
	Little emphasis on collection of objective data	Considerable emphasis on collection of objective data

tering. All the fluency shaping clinicians target fluent responses or train fluency skills. Thus, these two therapy approaches differ substantially with regard to this issue, much as they did for the advanced stutterer.

On the second issue, fluency goals, both stuttering modification and fluency shaping clinicians have spontaneous fluency and controlled fluency as their goals for the intermediate stutterer. Stuttering modification clinicians, however, include acceptable stuttering as a realistic goal, whereas fluency shaping clinicians do not.

Stuttering modification and fluency shaping clinicians differ with regard to the attention they give to reducing the negative feelings and attitudes of an intermediate stutterer. They do not differ as much on this issue as they do in the case of the advanced stutterer. With the advanced stutterer, stuttering modification clinicians pay considerable attention to reducing negative feelings and attitudes, but with an intermediate stutterer, these clinicians seem to pay somewhat less attention to changing such feelings and attitudes. Fluency shaping clinicians do not target feelings and attitudes with either the advanced or the intermediate stutterer.

Regarding maintenance procedures, stuttering modification and fluency shaping therapies are similar. Both give minimal attention to the issue.

Stuttering modification and fluency shaping therapies usually differ with regard to clinical methods, just as in the treatment of advanced stuttering. Stuttering modification therapy is usually characterized by loosely structured interactions between clinician and child. Fluency shaping therapy, on the other hand, is usually characterized by a programmed instruction approach. Furthermore, stuttering modification therapy usually places little emphasis on data collection, but fluency shaping therapy puts considerable emphasis on it.

In summary, stuttering modification and fluency shaping therapies for the intermediate stutterer are more similar than they are for the advanced stutterer. However, they are less similar here than they are for the beginning stutterer. The greatest difference, excluding clinical methods, is in the speech behaviors targeted for therapy and, to a lesser degree, the attention they give to reducing negative feelings and attitudes.

STUDY QUESTIONS

1. What are Dell's "three ways of saying words?" Describe how he teaches the child to distinguish one from the other.

2. Suggest a new way you might teach a child to understand what "easy stuttering" is. For example, devise a gesture or a metaphor or an activity the child could do to help him grasp this concept.

3. Explain how two of Dell's clinical procedures with a child might involve the left hemisphere emotions described in Chapter 4.

4. As Dell works on changing stuttering, he often uses physical touch to signal the child. Why might this be more effective than other kinds of signals? How do you feel about the use of physical touch?

5. Describe Dell's philosophy of terminating therapy; comment on it.

6. What are Ryan's goals for the intermediate stutterer during each of the following three phases of treatment: (a) establishment phase, (b) transfer phase, and (c) maintenance phase?

7. Describe Ryan's delayed auditory feedback (DAF) program for the intermediate stutterer.

8. Briefly describe Ryan's transfer procedures for the intermediate stutterer.

9. Compare Dell's and Ryan's ways of involving parents in therapy.

10. Compare stuttering modification and fluency shaping therapies for the intermediate stutterer on the following five clinical issues: (*a*) speech behaviors targeted for therapy, (*b*) fluency goals, (*c*) attention given to feelings and attitudes, (*d*) maintenance procedures, and (*e*) clinical methods.

SUGGESTED READINGS

Craig, A., Hancock, K., Chang, E., et al. (1996). A controlled clinical trial for stuttering in persons aged 9 to 14 years. *Journal of Speech and Hearing Research, 39,* 808–826.
This article describes three different treatment approaches for intermediate stuttering and assesses the effectiveness of each.

Dell, C. (1993), Treating school-age stutterers. In R. Curlee (Ed.), *Stuttering and related disorders of fluency.* **New York: Thieme Medical Publishers.**
This is an updated and realistic account of the therapy Dell developed in his work with Van Riper.

Dell, C. (1979). *Treating the school age stutterer: A guide for clinicians.* **Memphis: Stuttering Foundation of America.**
This bargain-priced booklet contains a wealth of clinical information about stuttering modification with the school-age child, as well as helpful advice on working with parents and teachers.

Manning, W. (1996). *Clinical decision making in the diagnosis and treatment of fluency disorders.* **New York: Delmar Publishers.**
Chapter 5, Treatment of Young Children, contains excellent information on both fluency shaping and stuttering modification approaches with children between 2 and 12 years old.

Ryan, B.P. (1974). *Programmed therapy of stuttering in children and adults.* **Springfield, IL: Charles C Thomas; and Ryan, B.P. (1984).**
This book contains a highly detailed description of several operant approaches developed by Ryan and his wife.

Ryan, B.P. (1984). Treatment of stuttering in school children. In W.H. Perkins (Ed.), *Stuttering disorders* (pp. 95–105). **New York: Thieme-Stratton.**
In this brief chapter, Ryan describes his fluency shaping procedures for the school-age child.

Van Riper, C. (1973). Treatment of the young confirmed stutterer. In *The treatment of stuttering* (pp. 426–451). **Englewood Cliffs, NJ: Prentice-Hall.**
In this chapter, Van Riper provides a comprehensive discussion of a classic stuttering modification approach to the treatment of the intermediate stutterer.

II

Intermediate Stutterer: Integration of Approaches

As we move from the advanced level of stuttering to the intermediate level, fluency shaping and stuttering modification therapies become a little more similar. Therefore, integrating them becomes easier. Stuttering modification therapies do not focus on working with deep-seated beliefs and years of emotional conditioning. Fluency shaping therapies do not involve working so hard on overlearning and generalizing each component of slow, smooth speech. Often the intermediate stutterer is able to use just the slowing or the gentle onsets to establish and generalize fluency.

Before we begin discussing the integration of these two approaches, let's review the characteristics of the intermediate stutterer.

The child with intermediate-level stuttering is usually an elementary or junior high school student between 6 and 13 years of age. He exhibits part-word and monosyllabic whole-word repetitions and vowel prolongations that contain excessive tension. However, for many of these children, blocks, typically with considerable tension and struggle, are the most evident sign of stuttering. This child may use escape devices, such as body movements or brief verbalizations (e.g., "uh"), to break free of stutters. He may use various avoidance strategies such as starters, word substitutions, circumlocutions, and evasion of difficult speaking situations. He experiences the frustration and embarrassment of earlier stages and the fear of stuttering and of many speaking situations. Finally, he has a definite concept of himself as a stutterer. Let us now turn to the integration of stuttering modification and fluency shaping therapies for this child.

As noted in the last chapter, the greatest difference (excluding clinical methods) between stuttering modification and fluency shaping therapies for the intermediate stutterer is the speech behaviors targeted for therapy. To a lesser degree, these two approaches also differ with regard to the attention they give to reducing negative feelings and attitudes. Therefore, in our integration of these two approaches, we concentrate on these two aspects of therapy. As will become apparent, our direct treatment of the intermediate stutterer contains elements of both stuttering modification and fluency shaping therapies, with parent counseling and classroom teacher counseling more strongly influenced by stuttering modification therapy.

We first discuss our own approach to integrating stuttering modification and fluency shaping therapies for the intermediate stutterer, then describe the clinical procedures of other clinicians who integrate these two approaches at this treatment level.

OUR APPROACH

Clinician's Beliefs

NATURE OF STUTTERING

As discussed previously, we believe that predisposing physiological factors related to the neural organization of speech and a vulnerable temperament interact with developmental and environmental factors to produce or exacerbate the core behaviors of repetitions and prolongations. The child responds to these disfluencies with increased tension in an effort to inhibit them. This increases the severity of struggle behavior. Furthermore, as the young stutterer attempts to cope with these core behaviors, he develops a variety of escape and starting devices. We believe these behaviors are operantly reinforced. Then, in the early elementary school years, frustration and embarrassment are associated with the stuttering, and fear begins to develop. These negative emotions generalize through classical conditioning to more and more words and speaking situations. Finally, the child begins to avoid these feared words and situations. These avoidance behaviors are reinforced through avoidance conditioning. With the onset of avoidance behaviors, the child has become an intermediate stutterer. By this time, stuttering has also become a part of his self-concept.

Because the tension response, escape and avoidance behaviors, and negative feelings and attitudes are learned, we believe they can be unlearned or modified. Furthermore, since these learned components are not as well established in the intermediate stutterer as they are in the advanced stutterer, they are easier to change. The context for change must be an accepting, supportive environment that focuses on the child as a person, rather than just on his stuttering.

Many intermediate stutterers feel that they have failed in previous therapy and have disappointed their parents and teachers because they did not become fluent. Thus, we must help these children feel accepted with their current level of stuttering, as well as help them to experience mastery and success with their speech.

If we can provide the intermediate stutterer with a sufficient number of fluent and emotionally positive speaking experiences in therapy, fluency and the positive feelings associated with speaking will generalize to other environments. We use operant and classical conditioning principles to achieve this. Furthermore, because predisposing physiological factors may contribute to the core behaviors or physiological disruptions in the speech of many intermediate stutterers, we believe it is also important to help them cope more effectively with these disruptions in their speech. These twin goals of positive speaking experiences and coping with the remaining stuttering can be achieved using a combination of fluency shaping and stuttering modification. In implementing these goals with an intermediate stutterer, we need to keep in mind that the client is younger than the advanced stutterer. This will influence the selection of our clinical procedures.

Finally, we believe it is important to reduce developmental and environmental influences that may be contributing to the child's stuttering. We do this by counseling the child's parents and classroom teachers, helping them to create an environment that accepts the child and facilitates change. In addition, we help the child communicate more easily with his parents and teachers about how they can best help him deal with his stuttering.

SPEECH BEHAVIORS TARGETED FOR THERAPY

We believe it is beneficial to combine fluency shaping and stuttering modification strategies for the intermediate stutterer. In terms of fluency shaping procedures, we occasionally use a delayed auditory feedback (DAF) program (as described for Ryan's approach in Chapter 10). However, we prefer to teach fluency enhancing behaviors (FEBs) without DAF, using the approach we describe in Chapter 9 on integrated therapy for the advanced stutterer. The latter approach often enhances the child's confidence so that he can regain fluency by himself if he relapses, without having to return to a DAF device. Using modeling and instruction, we teach the child to speak fluently with a slower rate, gentle onsets, soft contacts, and proprioception. Once fluency is achieved in the therapy room, we help the child transfer it to other situations.

Our stuttering modification component for the intermediate stutterer is similar to that used for the advanced stutterer. We usually find that our efforts to help the child pay off more quickly because his fear of stuttering is less intense. In the first stage, understanding stuttering, a great deal of desensitization occurs while we are helping the child to understand, confront, and accept his stuttering. All of this also contributes to reducing the tension in his stutters. The second stage, modification, is facilitated by work on FEBs, which focuses largely on using FEBs to change hard stutters into easier ones.

FLUENCY GOALS

Which fluency goals are realistic for the intermediate stutterer? Some intermediate stutterers may become normal or spontaneously fluent speakers. This is more likely for the younger than for the older intermediate stutterer. Typically, the intermediate stutterer will need to use controlled fluency to sound normal. This is often a difficult task for a youngster to do on a consistent basis. Although he may use controlled fluency in some situations, a child this age often does not have the motivation or self-discipline to control his fluency throughout his daily talking. Thus, we believe that a realistic fluency goal for many intermediate stutterers is acceptable stuttering, that is, fluency characterized by mild or very mild stuttering.

FEELINGS AND ATTITUDES

How much attention should be given to the intermediate stutterer's feelings and attitudes about his speech? Whenever a child is experiencing frustration and embarrassment and is beginning to experience some fear related to speech, as is usually the case for intermediate stutterers, we believe it is important to reduce these negative feelings. Furthermore, because these children are beginning to avoid certain words and avoid speaking in certain situations, it is important to eliminate or reduce these avoidances also. Even though negative feelings and avoidance behaviors are not as pronounced or as well established in the intermediate as in the advanced stutterer, we believe that, for effective treatment to occur, these aspects of the problem must be given some attention in therapy.

In selecting clinical procedures to reduce the intermediate stutterer's negative feelings about speaking and to eliminate or reduce avoidance behaviors, it is important to keep in mind that this client is younger than the advanced stutterer. Therefore, the clinical procedures discussed in Chapter 9 for the advanced stutterer would not be appropriate for this younger client. Different or modified procedures are needed.

MAINTENANCE PROCEDURES

The typical intermediate stutterer may need some help in maintaining improvement. He will certainly not need the extensive help required by advanced stutterers, but he may need more than the minimal help required by beginning stutterers.

To help an intermediate stutterer maintain improvement, we believe it is very important to reevaluate his fluency periodically. During these reevaluations, we obtain samples of his speech and discuss with him what his speech is like in everyday speaking situations. We also interview his parents and classroom teachers about his fluency. If we find there has been some regression, we reenroll the child in therapy for 1 or 2 months. Our experience indicates that some of these children may have one or two mild regressions before their fluency finally stabilizes. In time, the child's regressions and our reevaluations become farther apart. The day then comes to dismiss the child from treatment. We have found that these procedures are usually adequate for helping intermediate stutterers maintain improved fluency.

CLINICAL METHODS

The clinical methods we use for the intermediate stutterer—our structure of therapy and our data collection procedures—are influenced by both stuttering modification and fluency shaping therapies. In terms of the structure of therapy, we may use a loosely structured type of interaction between the clinician and the child. Typically, with the younger intermediate stutterer, we use a game-orientated approach. With the older intermediate stutterer, we use a teaching/counseling type of interaction. Both types of interactions are loosely structured. Occasionally, we may decide to use a highly structured, programmed instruction approach with both the younger and the older intermediate stutterer. The type of interaction that we decide to use depends on the outcome of some trial therapy.

In terms of data collection, we believe it is important to measure the child's stuttering and rate of speech before, during, and after the treatment program. If we use a game-orientated or teaching/counseling type of approach, we will take a probe or sample of the child's speech at the end of each therapy session. If we use a programmed instruction approach, we will measure all the child's responses during each therapy session.

Clinical Procedures: Direct Treatment of the Child

We have been combining or integrating aspects of stuttering modification and fluency shaping therapies for intermediate stutterers for a number of years.[1] Based on our current beliefs, we include the following components in their treatment: (*a*) understanding stuttering, (*b*) using fluency enhancing skills and modifying the moments of stuttering, (*c*) reducing negative feelings and attitudes and eliminating avoidances, and (*d*) maintaining improvement. As you may recall, these same components are included in our treatment of the advanced stutterer, but the procedures we use are different. The procedures are designed for a younger client whose stuttering is not as fully developed. Let us now consider the specific clinical procedures used in our direct work with this child.

UNDERSTANDING STUTTERING

In this phase of treatment, we have a number of goals. First, we help the child to explore and understand his moments of stuttering. Second, we provide an explanation for his stuttering at an appropriate level. Third, we give the child an overview of what he will be doing in therapy. We discuss each of these goals separately, but in actual practice, our efforts to achieve these goals are often interwoven into the same therapy sessions.

Exploring Moments of Stuttering

When we first meet the child, we believe it is most important to establish good rapport with him. During the first several therapy sessions, we spend considerable time getting to know the child. We show our interest in him and in what he has to say. We let him know through our attention to what he says that we really want to understand him. We also convey acceptance of his stuttering through our interest and curiosity and our willingness to stutter ourselves as we explore his stuttering with him. This relationship continues to develop as we work with the child throughout therapy. We do this while we are teaching him to use FEBs and to modify his moments of stuttering and are helping him reduce his negative feelings and attitudes and eliminate his avoidance behaviors. We convey our acceptance of his stuttering as it is now, and we demonstrate our belief in his ability to improve his speech by our enthusiasm for the changes he makes in his stuttering and his feelings about speech. We believe that an accepting, supporting relationship is necessary if the child's speech fears are going to become deconditioned. We also believe such rapport is mandatory if a child is going to take our advice and attempt to change his manner of speaking and to risk giving up his avoidance behaviors.

After we get to know a child and he feels at ease with us, we bring up the topic of stuttering with him. Our aim is to help him become interested in his stuttering, rather than denying it and hoping it will go away. Because talking about stuttering is often uncomfortable for a child, we begin our discussion when we are playing a game, drawing, or doing something else the child enjoys. Thus, we can alternate between confronting a difficult issue and retreating, when the child appears to be anxious, to an island of safety. To

---

[1] The reader is referred to Guitar, B., & Peters, T.J. (1980). The elementary school child who stutters. In B. Guitar & T.J. Peters, *Stuttering: An integration of contemporary therapies.* (pp. 51–62). Memphis: Speech Foundation of America for an earlier version of integrating stuttering modification and fluency shaping therapies with the intermediate stutterer.

begin, we simply comment on the child's stuttering in an accepting manner. We may say something like "Hey, you really eased out of that one pretty well," or "That was a tough one, huh?" We take note of how he responds—whether he appears uncomfortable or whether he acknowledges his stuttering, even subtly and nonverbally—when we comment on it. This first approach to stuttering may go quite easily if we have won the child's trust and if he is not excessively embarrassed by his stuttering. However, many children at the intermediate level feel helpless, frustrated, and ashamed about their stuttering. Most can be helped to face their stuttering if we proceed slowly.

For a particularly sensitive child, we begin by providing him with a feeling of mastery over something else, such as a board game, drawing, or "shooting hoops" in the therapy room. We then alternate between exploring the stuttering and giving him relief through other activities of his choice. As we explore the child's stuttering with him, we not only comment on it, but we also ask him to describe what he's doing when he stutters. For example, we might say, "Okay, there was an interesting one. What did you do when you stuttered on that word?" Then we help him feel and identify what he actually does when he stutters. For many children, this focus on the stuttering behavior can change their emotion from shame and helpless confusion to a more hopeful and objective outlook.

At some point during the early exploration of a child's stuttering, we teach him about "speech helpers"—the lungs, larynx, and articulators—and their involvement in speech production. For the more sensitive child, we start with instruction about how speech helpers work during fluent speech and later explore what the child does with his speech helpers when he stutters. For children who are less emotional about their stuttering, we incorporate instruction about speech helpers into exploration of what they are doing when they stutter.

Once the child is able to tolerate discussing his stuttering for a few minutes, we move on to activities that focus more consistently on stuttering. We begin by having the child try to "catch us" stuttering. We throw in a few mild disfluencies and ask him to let us know by signaling whenever he notices a stutter in our speech. We reward him when he is successful and sometimes talk about what we did when we got stuck. This lets him know that we are unafraid of stuttering. This in turn provides a model of talking objectively about stuttering. Most clinicians can do this legitimately even though they do not really stutter. Most children know that the stutters are voluntary and usually aren't bothered that they are not real. After several minutes of putting stutters in our speech, we might ask the child to signal us when *he* stutters. If he misses many of them, we comment on a few that he has missed.

Our primary purpose at this stage is to continue to make stuttering something that we can talk about. This decreases some of the fear, frustration, and shame associated with stuttering. We continue to question the child about his stutters, and we maintain an interested, accepting style of inquiry. What did he do when he stuttered? Where was it tight? Could he show us again what it sounded like? Again, we continually assess how much confrontation a child can tolerate, and we intersperse it with activities the child enjoys.

In addition to helping the child explore his core stuttering behaviors, we help him become aware of secondary symptoms, such as starters, postponements, and word and situation avoidances. We approach these as we approach the core behaviors—with interest and acceptance, not criticism. We usually begin this process by mentioning some examples of starters, postponements, and avoidance behaviors that we have seen in other children. We tell the child about children we know who use "well" or "um" before difficult words, who don't talk in class because they're afraid they might stutter, or who substitute easy words for hard ones. By sharing examples such as these with the child and asking him if he has tried any of them, we make it easier for him to be open with us about the secondary behaviors he uses—or at least those he is aware of. If a child has difficulty identifying or discussing secondary behaviors, we put it aside for now. He may be more able to explore these behaviors after he has learned some coping skills.

In addition to identifying strategies that the child uses to hide or avoid his stuttering, we also explore feelings underlying his need to use them. Many of these children are unwilling, perhaps unable, to discuss in much detail their feelings of embarrassment or fear associated with stuttering. We do not push a child on this point but do let him know that these sorts of feelings are understandable and natural. We encourage his expression of such feelings, reinforce any comments of this nature, and continue to show our acceptance. We use several approaches to help the child express, and thereby diminish, feelings about stuttering. We often comment on experiences and feelings other children have when they stutter, such as the angry and sad feelings that result from being teased, being told by adults to slow down, having words finished for them, and being interrupted.

We also find that some children express their feelings more freely through drawings. Thus, we often draw together for a while, then ask the child to draw a picture of how it feels when he gets stuck on a word. In explaining his drawing, the child is often able to express how he feels. Therefore, we use drawing throughout therapy to help the child deal with old feelings of hurt and new feelings that are encountered during various stages of therapy. Our experience has been that children's feelings often affect their fluency. The more practice they get in expressing their feelings, the less those feelings interfere with talking.

By now, the child has shared with us his moments of stuttering and the strategies he uses to hide them. Moreover, he has found us to be understanding and accepting listeners. Some deconditioning of speech fears has already occurred, and the child has also learned some of the terms we will be using in the remaining phases of therapy. Thus, some basic groundwork for the following phases of treatment has been laid.

Explaining Stuttering

We believe it is important for an intermediate stutterer to be given some explanation for his stuttering. He knows he stutters. He knows he has been stuttering, probably for a number of years. He needs to have an explanation for why he talks differently from his friends. So, what do we say to this child?

Choosing words that are appropriate for the child's age and comprehension level, we let him know that stuttering is not his fault and that much of it is learned and can be unlearned. For example, we may say that he stutters because his "speech machine" has a tendency to be more disfluent or bumpy than that of his peers. We may even suggest that he was born this way but that he can still change it. We do not want him to believe that he caused his speech problem or to feel guilty about his stuttering. We are careful to explain that his tendency to be disfluent has nothing to do with his intelligence or personality, that it is related only to his ability or lack of ability, to say words smoothly.

We point out that many children have problems in other areas. For example, some children have problems in learning to read, and some children have a hard time at sports. We go on to explain that this tendency to be disfluent accounts only for his individual moments of stuttering, what we call the *core behaviors*. Other parts, the most bothersome parts, are learned. He can change them. One tool we sometimes use to help teach intermediate stutterers about stuttering is the videotape, *Do You Stutter? Straight Talk for Teens*, available from the Stuttering Foundation of America (Guitar & Conture, 1996).

In helping a child to better understand his stuttering, we believe it is beneficial for him to know that a lot of children stutter, that he is not the only person in the world who stut-ters. Often the child may not know any other children who stutter. He may believe that he is one of only a very few who have this problem. So, we tell him that about 1 in 100 children stutter. We tell him that there are over 2 million people in the United States who share this problem with him. We believe this sort of information helps a child to feel less unique and less isolated because of his stuttering.

Giving an Overview of Therapy

Finally, we believe that it is important for the intermediate stutterer in the early stages of therapy to have an overview of later stages of his treatment program. We explain that we will help him learn to talk more fluently and to stutter more easily on any remaining moments of stuttering. To help the child understand how he will do this, we model FEBs and stuttering modification techniques. We also tell him that we will help him to become more comfortable with his stuttering and to overcome his habit of using tricks to hide it. Finally, we explain that it is going to take time and effort, but by working together, we can lick this problem.

USING FLUENCY ENHANCING BEHAVIORS AND MODIFYING THE MOMENTS OF STUTTERING

When we discussed the treatment of the advanced stutterer in Chapter 9, we preceded the "reducing negative feelings and attitudes and eliminating avoidances" phase of ther-apy with the "using fluency enhancing behaviors and modifying the moments of stutter-ing" phase. We commented that we found it beneficial to reverse this order with some advanced stutterers, especially those who found it difficult to confront their speech fears. Because of their younger ages, we believe this applies also to most intermediate stutter-ers. Thus, with intermediate stutterers we typically have the "using fluency enhancing be-haviors and modifying the moments of stuttering" phase precede the "reducing negative feelings and attitudes and eliminating avoidances" phase. We have found that interme-diate stutterers usually deal with their speech fears and avoidance behaviors much more easily after they have increased their fluency.

Teaching Fluency Enhancing Behaviors

To increase the intermediate stutterer's fluency, we begin by teaching him to use FEBs, using one of two options. The first follows procedures such as those Bruce Ryan uses with intermediate-level stutterers as described in Chapter 10. A DAF device is used to teach the child to slow his rate of speech and to talk in a smooth, continuous fashion. This de-vice is needed just to establish FEBs. Once FEBs are established, these behaviors can be combined with stuttering modification strategies (as described in the text that follows).

The second fluency shaping option in our integrated approach is to teach FEBs with-out using DAF, through direct instructions and models of slow speech, gentle onsets, light contacts, and proprioception, just as we did with the advanced stutterer in Chapter 9. You may wish to reread this section to ensure a full understanding of FEB components. With an intermediate stutterer, we begin with single words, teaching slow speech by modeling slow productions of words, initiated by a variety of sounds, and eliciting the child's slow, fluent imitations. Our models also use gentle onsets and light contacts. For the first few words, however, we emphasize only their slowness.

After the child is able to produce words slowly, we model and elicit imitations of gen-tle onsets. We first use words that begin with vowels, later those that begin with consonants. We then do the same for light contacts. We use words that begin with plosives, fricatives, and affricates before trying words with these sounds in medial and final positions. Finally, we teach proprioception (awareness of movement) first by demonstrating it in arm movements, then in speech movements, emphasizing the child's awareness of his lip, tongue, and jaw movements. Although it is not always easy to judge accurately whether a child is using proprioception, we look for slightly exaggerated, slow movements to verify that he is trying to feel the movements of his articulators.

After a child can produce single words fluently using all four FEBs, we move to the next level of difficulty—saying sentences fluently using FEBs. The child is again given a model for a sentence and asked to imitate it. Our models are produced with slow rate, gentle onsets, light contacts, and proprioception, but we now add the concept of continuous breath groups. First, the child is taught to produce only two or three syllables at a very slow rate before taking a breath. For example, if you were to model the phrase, "My name is Jim," you should take 4 to 5 seconds to produce "My name," take a breath, then produce " . . . is Jim," taking another 4 seconds. We call these phrases *continuous* breath groups because a phrase is produced as one continuous word within each breath group. Thus, "my" is linked with "name" in "My name.." without a pause between them; so are "is" and "Jim" in the second phrase.

We work with the child at this level until we believe that he has learned how to produce sentences consistently and fluently and has used all the attributes just described. This may take several sessions, but learning FEBs well, especially when talking at a very slow rate, is critical to future success. The next level is to have the child in structured conversation for 1, 2, 3, 4, and finally 5 consecutive minutes of the child's talking at approximately 40 syllables per minute, verified with a stopwatch and calculator as described in Chapter 7. We begin by having the child describe a series of pictures or talk about various objects in the room for 1 minute. To pass each step (1 minute, 2 minutes, and so on), the child must be entirely fluent and use all the FEBs. We continue this progression until the child is able to speak for 5 minutes (interspersed with our comments and questions) without disfluencies while using FEBs. If the child stutters at any time, we stop and discuss what happened and explore various options such as gearing down to a very slow rate before saying a difficult word to prevent future stutters. At this point, rather than speed up speech rate, as Ryan does in his traditional fluency shaping approach for the intermediate stutterer, we use the slow rate of speech with other FEBs to modify moments of stuttering.

Modifying the Moments of Stuttering

In this phase of treatment, we use the FEBs that the child has just learned to teach him to modify his stutters from "hard" to "easy." The first goal is for him to learn how to "downshift" when he catches himself in a stutter, that is, making the transition from feeling "jammed up" by easing into saying the rest of the word slowly and easily, using proprioceptive cues. The second goal is for the child to learn to anticipate stutters and to downshift into a slower rate of speech and to use a gentle onset, light articulatory contacts, and proprioception as he begins the anticipated word.

We begin working on the first goal by using voluntary stutters, first in our own speech, then by having the child use them. We make extensive use of voluntary stutters in this phase to teach the necessary motor skills in a relatively nonemotional situation. By overlearning these skills in a calm situation, the child has a better chance of succeeding with real stutters, which are often accompanied by negative emotions, such as fear and shame. After we teach the child to make downshifted voluntary stutters on words using plenty of models in our speech, we set quotas for numbers of downshifted stutters in our conversation during various games the child chooses to play. After the child can do this with his voluntary stutters, we encourage him to hunt for real stutters. When he catches a real stutter, we coach him to hang onto it, maintaining its posture and production, then downshifting slowly out of it. When the child can do this, we reward his efforts highly.

Many children with intermediate stuttering begin to downshift automatically when they anticipate a stutter. But if a child does not do this on his own, we use voluntary stuttering to teach the skill. We do this by modeling how to use FEBs to say a word that might be stuttered with our own voluntary stutters and by teaching him to use voluntary stutters to practice the skill. Interspersed with downshifting practice, we refresh the child's memory of speaking slightly slowly while using the other FEBs in conversational speech. We make sure that we give the child the experience of slow, fluent speech in every session. Then we use voluntary downshifts again, in our speech and his, to practice moving from stutters, or anticipated stutters, into brief periods of "FEB speech." Although our voluntary downshifts, both before and during a stutter, may be somewhat exaggerated at first, we emphasize to the child that once this skill is mastered, the downshifts can be done without sounding weird, giving plenty of examples in our speech of smooth, brief downshifts.

Typically, transfer of downshifting begins by setting up a hierarchy with the child of easy-to-difficult situations in which we can use voluntary downshifts together. We carry out the tasks on this hierarchy together, and we use small rewards when each task is completed. At the same time, we are getting information from the child's parents about his progress at home. At the appropriate level of difficulty in the hierarchy, we bring the child's parents into therapy and have him teach them about downshifting and then develop a plan to have him use both voluntary and real downshifts at home. One or both parents (depending on the child's preference) help him keep a log of the number of downshifts he makes each day.

For some children, involving parents as therapy helpers is not effective. They prefer not to have their parents function in this way, but merely be supportive listeners. In these cases, we use telephone calls and have the child tape-record himself when transferring downshifting into speech at home.

By now, the child is speaking with little difficulty in many situations, but some situations are probably still giving him problems. As we continue with these transfer procedures, we turn more of our attention toward reducing the child's negative feelings about his speech and toward eliminating any avoidance behaviors.

REDUCING NEGATIVE FEELINGS AND ATTITUDES AND ELIMINATING AVOIDANCES

In addition to being an understanding and accepting listener for the child, we have four goals during this phase of treatment. First, we help the child cope with any teasing. In fact, if this has been a significant problem, we would have responded to it earlier. Second, we desensitize the child to any remaining fluency disrupters. Third, we help the child eliminate the use of avoidance behaviors, including both word and situation avoidances. Fourth, we help the child to be open about his stuttering. Each of these goals is dealt with in turn.

Coping With Teasing

We believe it is important to minimize any teasing that a child may be receiving because of his stuttering. We address this issue in more detail when we discuss parent and classroom teacher counseling. Regardless of how hard parents, teachers, clinicians, and friends may try to eliminate teasing, we doubt that it is possible to eliminate all of it. Thus, we try to give a child some defenses against the teasing he is likely to receive.

We agree with Van Riper that the best defense against teasing is acceptance, if a child is emotionally mature enough to feel and express acceptance. For example, if a child can say, "I know I stutter, but I'm working on it," or some similar statement, this will disarm most teasers. Nobody likes to tease someone who does not appear to be bothered. Running away, on the other hand, just reinforces teasing. Nevertheless, we have found it is difficult for a child in this age range to calmly accept and admit his stuttering to tormentors. When we have been successful at it, we have done the following things.

First, we discuss the importance of calmly and openly admitting to teasers that we stutter, rather than saying nothing. We explain how this type of response usually discourages teasers. We then explore with the child the sort of statement he can imagine himself making. The words he uses must be words with which he feels comfortable. Next, we initiate role playing with the child. As we play the role of the teaser, the child's task is to respond calmly to our heckling. He practices saying the type of statement he has chosen to use to counteract the teasing. We role-play this many times, until the child feels comfortable with his response and can see himself doing this in a real-life situation. Finally, the day comes when he tries out this new behavior. We hope it works. If it does not, we are there to give support and encouragement.

Some children are especially sensitive to teasing and need our patience and understanding as they work to develop effective responses. These children may have more inhibited temperaments. Their first reaction to a threatening situation is to withdraw or avoid. Hence, these children need practice in asserting themselves. In our role playing, we experiment with a variety of ways in which the child can feel they confronted the teaser. For some children, it might be teasing back; for others, it might be reporting the teaser to a teacher or principal.

Desensitizing the Child to Fluency Disrupters

At this point in therapy, as noted earlier, the child is probably speaking rather well in many situations. Furthermore, many of the child's fluency disrupters have been eliminated or substantially reduced as a result of parent counseling. However, some fluency disrupters, because of their nature, cannot be totally eliminated from a child's life. The child needs to learn to cope with them. For example, one young intermediate stutterer with whom we worked became angry and cried whenever he lost a competitive game. When this happened, he also lost control of his speech, and his stuttering increased. We thought it was important to desensitize this child to losing. After all, everybody loses sometime in their lives. Other stutterers have different fluency disrupters, and we try to desensitize them to these, too.

As an example of desensitization, we briefly describe here the procedures we used with the young intermediate stutterer who hated to lose. This boy had completed the fluency hierarchy and was speaking fluently in therapy. We told him that we were going to play games and were going to play our hardest and try to beat him. We told him further that he was to use his FEBs and be fluent, even if he were losing the game. We reinforced his fluency and reminded him to use his FEBs to downshift whenever he was not fluent. In the beginning, we lost more than we won, and his fluency remained good. Gradually, we began to win more and more. His fluency began to drop. When we reminded him to use his FEBs and he did, his fluency returned. Eventually, we were winning most of the time, but he was remaining fluent. He had learned to maintain his fluency, even though he was losing, and had also learned to become a better loser!

Eliminating Avoidances

We believe it is critical for an intermediate stutterer to eliminate or substantially reduce his use of avoidances. We begin by helping the child to understand that the more he runs away from saying a specific word or from talking in a given situation, the more afraid of that word or situation he will become. We explain that in the long run it is better for him to say what he wants to say, even if he is afraid and even if he stutters. We go on to explain that, by confronting his fears, he can overcome them.

For most children, it helps to use analogies. We help them to think about other fears that they have overcome or about people they know, such as younger brothers or sisters, who are still afraid of something, such as the dark, bugs, or swimming in deep water. By analyzing how people get over their fears and by describing the rewards of facing fears and conquering them, we are often able to motivate children to tackle their fears of difficult words and situations.

If a child does not recall overcoming some other fear in his life, we make up a hypothetical situation. For example, we may talk about overcoming being afraid of jumping off the high diving board at the local swimming pool (Fig. 11.1). We suggest to the child that, if he wanted to overcome his fear of the high board, it would be best for him to start by just jumping off the side of the pool. When he could imagine being comfortable with this, he could imagine jumping off the low board. After becoming comfortable with the low board, he would be ready to take on the medium-high board. Eventually, he would reach the high diving board. After jumping off the high diving board a number of times, he would find himself no longer afraid of it. Therefore, there would be no reason for him to avoid the high diving board any more either. We then explain to the child that we will use this same easy-to-hard strategy, or hierarchies, to help him overcome his speech fears and avoidances.

It is usually easier to help a child overcome his fear and avoidance of words than of situations. This is because we can provide the child with more support in confronting word

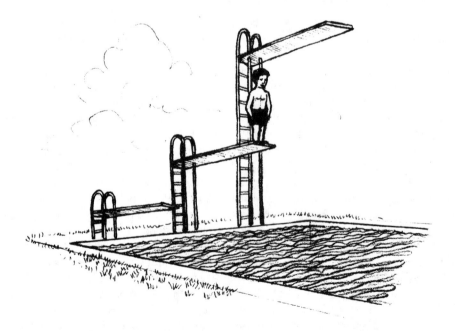

Figure 11.1. Using an easy to hard hierarchy to overcome fear and avoidance.

fears in the therapy room than we can provide when he confronts his situation fears in his daily life. We can also use feared words over and over again within the therapy situation. For example, we recall a young intermediate stutterer who consistently substituted "me" for "I." This was not symptomatic of a language disorder, and his parents reported that he had used "I" appropriately for a number of years before he began using this substitution. With this child, we began to practice saying "I" in unison with him while we both used a slow, easy stutter on the word. We strongly reinforced his efforts. Next, we used "I" many, many times in carrier phrases while playing games, with both of us using easy stutters when saying "I." Gradually, the child regained his confidence in saying "I." Within a week or two, his avoidance of "I" was eliminated in the therapy situation, and his parents reported that he was again using this pronoun appropriately at home.

Now, how do we help a child overcome his fear and avoidance of speaking situations? To the degree that we can in therapy, we devise a series of speaking situations that gradually lead up to and approximate the feared situation. For example, suppose a child was afraid to speak aloud in the classroom. In this case, with the child's consent, we would invite one or two of the child's classmates into therapy. We would play the role of the classroom teacher and have this small group of two or three children ask and answer questions. When the child began to feel comfortable doing this, we would expand the group to three or four classmates. Next, it might be helpful for the child and the rest of us to go to his classroom during a noon hour or a recess. After explaining our goal and therapy procedures to the classroom teacher, we would have the child sit at his desk and have his teacher ask questions about his lessons. These activities are about as far as we can go in simulating this child's feared situation. The child needs to take the last step by himself. He has been successful in a number of situations that approximate his feared situation, and his classroom teacher is now sensitized to his problem and understands his therapy. The chances are that, after some initial ambivalence, he will overcome his reluctance to talk in class.

Being Open About Stuttering. One of the best ways to combat fear, embarrassment, and the physical tension that these emotions often elicit is to be open about stuttering: to talk about it casually with friends, to refer to it in humorous ways when it happens, and to educate people about it. Children differ widely in their readiness to be open about their stuttering. However, once most of them feel some sense of mastery over what has made them feel helpless in the past, they are much more able to let people know about their stuttering. If the child stutters in class, we rehearse casual comments that he can make about his stuttering when he is giving an oral report or answering a question in class. He might say, for example, "My report is about how maple syrup is produced. Before I begin, I just want to say that I'll probably stutter sometimes while I'm talking, but don't let it bother you. I'm learning to deal with it." Or, the child might say, "It makes it easier for me if you can keep pretty good eye contact with me when I get stuck in a stutter." Basically, it is not so much the content that is important as the fact that the child has acknowledged his stuttering. He feels good that he acknowledged it, and his audience is more comfortable than if he stutters and tries to hide it.

A child may also benefit from developing a repertoire of casual comments to make about his stuttering if he gets particularly hung up on a word while talking to friends, relatives, or strangers. He might learn to say, "Wow! I really got hung up there," or, "I'm really running into a lot of blocks; I better slow down a bit." In our experience, the most effective comments are those that the child comes up with spontaneously, when he feels comfortable with his stuttering. These are unforced, often funny remarks that put the child and his listeners at ease.

Teaching other children and his teachers about stuttering can be a powerful tool in combatting the shame and embarrassment that often accompany a school child's stuttering. Although this can be done with small groups of students brought into the therapy room or in meetings with the child and his teachers, our experience has been that, eventually, sharing information about stuttering in front of the entire class is extremely effective for many children. When and if a child is ready to do this, we rehearse a presentation that informs the class about stuttering in general and the child's own stuttering in particular. A question-and-answer period is a crucial part of the presentation because it gives the child's classmates a chance to express their curiosity about stuttering. It also gives the child an opportunity to feel his expertise about the very behavior that previously made him feel so helpless.

Here is an example of how this may work. A second grader who was very sensitive about his stuttering was also rather proud of a brief segment on local access television that showed him working on his stuttering. He was willing to show a videotape of this segment in class and answer questions about his stuttering. The following year, we accompanied him to class for a full-scale presentation about stuttering. The presentation included posters he had made, demonstrations of therapy techniques, and a question-and-answer segment. A year after this program, the child had a particularly rocky beginning to the school year, but he was still willing to do another presentation with us. This time he used more videotaped clips of himself talking (because he was more reluctant to talk at length) and talked to the class about some of the "ups and downs" of his progress with stuttering.

MAINTAINING IMPROVEMENT

By this point in therapy, a child is usually speaking well in most situations. He is having a great deal of spontaneous fluency in many situations and either controlled fluency or acceptable stuttering in others. His speech fears and avoidances have been eliminated or significantly reduced. We do not dismiss the child from therapy at this point. Rather, we gradually phase him out of therapy. We see him for therapy on a weekly basis for a month or so, then on a twice-monthly basis for a month or so. If all continues to go well, we see him for a series of reevaluations over the next 2 years. At first, these reevaluations are monthly, then bimonthly, and, finally, once per semester.

During these reevaluations, we obtain samples of the child's speech and oral reading and talk with him about how he has been talking in everyday speaking situations. We also interview his parents and classroom teacher about his speech at home and school. If we find that the child's fluency has regressed or if he has begun to use avoidance behaviors again, we reenroll him in therapy. Our experience shows that a number of children may have one or two mild regressions before their fluency stabilizes. Such regressions are often associated with the beginning of a school year or with transfers from one school to another or with other disrupting factors.

When we bring a child back into therapy, it is usually for only a month or two. During these "booster" sessions, he may need to have his fluency enhancing or stuttering modification skills tuned up. He may need a brief refresher course on the importance of not avoiding, or he may just need an opportunity to talk to an understanding listener about his stuttering. In time, these regressions and our reevaluations become farther apart. Finally, the day arrives when we dismiss the child from treatment.

Clinical Procedures: Parent Counseling

We have five goals in mind when counseling parents of an intermediate stutterer: (*a*) explaining the treatment program and the parents' role in it, (*b*) explaining the possible causes of stuttering, (*c*) identifying and reducing fluency disrupters, (*d*) identifying and increasing fluency enhancing situations, and (e) eliminating teasing. We discuss each of these goals in turn.

EXPLAINING THE TREATMENT PROGRAM AND THE PARENTS' ROLE IN IT

First, we discuss the stages of our therapy program with the child's parents, letting them know how we hope to take the mystery out of stuttering for the child by exploring with him what he does when he stutters. We also tell them about our goal of teaching the child to stutter in easier ways rather than trying to eliminate the stuttering. Second, we tell them that therapy may take time, perhaps from 1 to 3 years and, in some cases, even longer. Third, we inform them that communicating with their child about his stuttering is important. They should communicate their acceptance of his stuttering and acknowledge their understanding that it is often difficult for the child to work on it.

EXPLAINING THE POSSIBLE CAUSES OF STUTTERING

We believe it is very important for the parents of an intermediate stutterer to be given an explanation of the possible causes of stuttering. We explain our interpretations of the current theoretical and research literature with them. In some cases, parents have no information about the causes of stuttering. Since we want them to participate in their child's treatment, they need to understand the rationale for our treatment program. Many parents feel guilty about the stuttering because of some outdated or inaccurate information they may have. They may have been exposed to a theory that is no longer valid, or they may have been given some erroneous information by a well-meaning, but misinformed, friend or relative. Such parents then blame themselves for some supposed misdeed on their part. They need good, current information about the nature of stuttering. Often, just supplying this information relieves them of their guilt. The following materials have been helpful supplements to our parent counseling: Eugene Cooper's (1979) pamphlet, *Understanding Stuttering: Information for Parents,* and the Speech Foundation of America's booklets (Conture & Fraser, 1989), *Stuttering and Your Child: Questions and Answers,* and (Guitar & Conture, undated), *If You Think Your Child Is Stuttering.* The video, *Do You Stutter? Straight Talk for Teens* (Guitar & Conture, 1996), is also helpful for parents.

What do we tell the parents about the possible causes of the disorder? Using language that is appropriate to their level of understanding, we provide the type of information that was discussed in Section I of this book. We tell them that we believe that predisposing physiological factors interact with developmental and environmental influences to produce or exacerbate a child's initial repetitions and prolongations. The child responds to these disfluencies with increased tension in an effort to inhibit them. In time, the child also learns a variety of escape and, possibly, starting behaviors to cope with these repetitions and prolongations. We go on to suggest that the predisposing physiological factors are most likely neurological in nature and are related to a child's deficits in the area of speech production. We suggest that the child may have problems in the timing of fine motor movements required for fluent speech. We also note that in many cases the predisposing physiological factors are probably genetic in origin. Thus, there are many possible sources for this speech difficulty.

We explore, with the parents' assistance, the developmental and environmental influences that may be interacting with the child's predisposing physiological factors to affect the child's stuttering. These are reviewed in Chapter 3. In some cases, we may not identify any developmental or environmental factors that seem to be contributing to the problem. However, when we do identify one or more possible factors, we attempt to lessen their influence. Our experience suggests that, in most cases, the solution to reducing the impact of these developmental and environmental influences is fairly straightforward. In a few cases, when it may be more difficult, we have suggested that counseling by a private psychotherapist or mental health agency may be helpful.

We also need to talk with parents of an intermediate stutterer about avoidance behaviors. We need to describe these behaviors to the parents and explain how these word and situation avoidances are behaviors their child has learned to use in coping with the embarrassment and fear of talking. We also need to explain how, in therapy, we will be helping the child eliminate his use of these avoidance behaviors.

IDENTIFYING AND REDUCING FLUENCY DISRUPTERS

As we explain in later chapters, environmental influences are often critical factors for managing beginning and borderline level stuttering. Intermediate-level stuttering is more complex and requires direct treatment of a child's behaviors and attitudes, but environmental factors are important for this level of stuttering as well. An intermediate stutterer's home environment may involve stresses that can be substantially alleviated if the clinician can join forces with an interested, motivated family. We begin by asking the family to observe when the child's stuttering is greatest and when it is least. With this information, we brainstorm with them various ways to reduce potential stresses and to observe the effect on the child's stuttering. For example, some children stutter a lot when there is competition for attention at the dinner table or when several children arrive home from school at the same time, all wanting to talk to their parents. In other cases, changes in a family routine may spark an increase in stuttering. Whatever the sources of stress, we encourage the parents and other family members to take the lead in identifying them and in planning ways of reducing stress. Even in cases in which stress may come from relatively abstract sources, such as a family's attitude that stuttering is shameful, the family is unlikely to change unless they feel that they and their points of view are respected and understood by the clinician. In an accepting environment, a trusting relationship can be developed, and a family may be open to seeing the child and his stuttering in new ways.

IDENTIFYING AND INCREASING FLUENCY ENHANCING SITUATIONS

During the process of identifying the times when the child stutters more frequently, families also discover there are times when a child is extremely fluent. These may be specific situations or just days or weeks when the child is particularly fluent. Whatever the case, families can find ways of increasing factors that promote fluency and letting the child have plenty of opportunities to talk when he is fluent. For example, children may be especially fluent when they are talking to parents at bedtime, providing parents with the opportunity to comment on this "smooth speech" and to let the child know that they can imagine how good it feels to talk easily. We are also interested in helping parents find ways of increasing fluency enhancing situations and of reinforcing fluency without implying that the times when a child stutters are bad. We can accomplish this by having the family empathize with the child that fluency is great, but that stuttering just can't be helped sometimes.

ELIMINATING TEASING

If any of the intermediate stutterer's siblings are teasing him about his stuttering, his parents need to stop it. We have found the best way to do this is to have parents have a serious talk with the teasing sibling. They need to explain that teasing makes the stuttering worse and must be discontinued. Usually, this is sufficient. If it is not, we have found it effective for us to talk to the sibling about the importance of not teasing a young stutterer. Having an adult other than a parent talk seriously about this matter often carries more weight with the teaser.

Clinical Procedures: Classroom Teacher Counseling

We believe it is very important to have the intermediate stutterer's classroom teacher involved in the child's treatment program (Fig. 11.2). After all, the teacher spends as much, if not more, time with the child than any other adult. We have four goals in mind when we are working with a classroom teacher: (*a*) explaining the treatment program and the teacher's role in it, (*b*) talking with the child about his stuttering, (*c*) coping with oral participation, and (*d*) eliminating teasing.

EXPLAINING THE TREATMENT PROGRAM AND THE TEACHER'S ROLE IN IT

We believe it is beneficial for classroom teachers to have an overview of the child's treatment program. We discuss how we are helping the child increase his fluency and modify his stutters and how we are attempting to help the child become more comfortable with his stuttering and eliminate his speech avoidance behaviors. We want the teacher to understand the rationale behind our procedures. Therefore, we are careful to answer any questions the teacher may have, believing that helping the teacher understand our goals will have at least two benefits. (1) The teacher will have a better understanding of how to

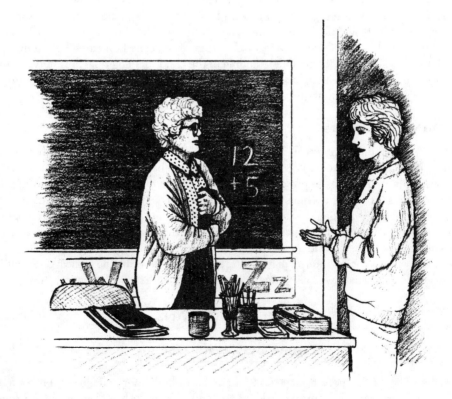

Figure 11.2. It is important to have the classroom teacher involved in the child's treatment.

interact with the child. (2) The teacher will be better able to give us feedback regarding the child's fluency in the classroom.

We also explain the teacher's role in the child's therapy. We discuss why and how we would like the teacher to implement the last three goals, how to talk with the child about his stuttering, how to help him cope with oral participation, and how to eliminate any teasing he may be receiving. We discuss each of these in the following text.

TALKING WITH THE CHILD ABOUT HIS STUTTERING

A friend recalls going all the way through school, from kindergarten through high school, without any teacher ever mentioning his stuttering. He stuttered severely year after year, and everyone knew he stuttered, but nobody ever acknowledged it. He described this silence as very painful.

We believe, along with Van Riper, that it is better for a classroom teacher to sit down with an intermediate stutterer and talk calmly with him about his stuttering, letting him know that she or he is aware of his stuttering and would like to help him in any way possible. The classroom teacher should tell the stutter that she will not interrupt or hurry him when he is talking. Just this acknowledgment and acceptance of the child's stuttering by the teacher will make the child feel more comfortable in the classroom.

COPING WITH ORAL PARTICIPATION

The teacher should also talk with the child about his oral participation in class. Again, like Van Riper, we believe it is important for an intermediate stutterer to participate orally in class. It is also important for the child to feel comfortable in participating. The teacher should seek the child's input on this matter. Possibly some classroom procedure, such as calling on students in alphabetical order, is creating apprehension for the stutterer and could be modified. Possibly the child would prefer to be called on early, before his apprehension builds up. With an understanding of the child's feelings and flexibility in procedures, most teachers can help an intermediate stutterer become much more comfortable in his oral classroom participation.

ELIMINATING TEASING

It is not unusual for stutterers in elementary or junior high school to be teased about stuttering. If a classroom teacher becomes aware of teasing, he or she should attempt to stop it. As we indicated during our previous discussion of parent counseling, we believe the best way to do this is to have a serious talk with the teaser. The teacher needs to explain that the child's teasing is making the stutterer's speech worse and that he needs to discontinue it immediately. The teacher should make it clear that this behavior will not be tolerated.

This concludes the description of our integration of stuttering modification and fluency shaping therapies for the intermediate stutterer. We now describe the clinical procedures of some other clinicians who also integrate procedures from these two approaches.

OTHER CLINICIANS

Eugene and Crystal Cooper

A hallmark of the Coopers' therapy (1995) is that they help intermediate stutterers (or at least those in their adolescent years) define their goal not as perfect fluency, but as a feeling of fluency control. Using four stages of treatment, they work on attitudes, feelings, and behaviors related to stuttering so that the adolescents they work with feel able to modify their speech in any situation, even though they may stutter to some degree.

In the first stage of therapy, "structuring," the adolescent and clinician develop a plan of therapy together and identify the attitudes, feelings, and behaviors that seem to make up the stuttering problem. Then, in the "targeting" stage, the clinician assists the teen in confronting his stuttering behaviors and attitudes. The child and the clinician develop a clinical relationship that values the free expression of feelings. The "adjusting" stage focuses on learning new attitudes and new behaviors to decrease the maladaptive aspects of stuttering. A variety of "fluency initiating gestures" are used to increase the adolescent's feeling of fluency control in the therapy room. In the final stage of therapy, the "regulating stage," the intermediate stutterer learns techniques of self-management, such as realistic perception and self-reinforcement, and learns to transfer his use of fluency initiating gestures to everyday situations at school and at home.

Hugo Gregory and June Campbell

Hugo Gregory and June Campbell (Gregory, 1984b, 1986a; Gregory & Campbell, 1988) refer to the intermediate stutterer as the "more confirmed school-aged stutterer." In terms of the speech behaviors targeted in therapy, they begin by using a less specific approach and move to a more specific approach only if needed.

In their less specific approach, Gregory and Campbell do not attempt to modify moments of stuttering. Rather, they model an "easy, relaxed approach with smooth movements" (ERA-SM) for the child, a technique they also use with advanced stutterers. ERA-SM involves a slower rate of speech and smooth transitions from sound to sound and from word to word. These changes occur at the beginning of a word or phrase, but not during the entire sentence. Thus, Gregory and Campbell are teaching the use of fluency enhancing skills at the beginning of an utterance. They also integrate work on ERA-SM with general body relaxation and emphasize that feelings of general body relaxation are being carried over into the movements involved in speech. In teaching ERA-SM, Gregory and Campbell take the child through a progression of tasks that begins with one-word responses and ends with longer, more complex responses. In going through this hierarchy, they use the following types of activities to elicit speech from the child: choral reading, reading alone, answering questions, describing pictures, and engaging in conversation.

If a child still has residual stutters associated with certain sounds or words, Gregory and Campbell use their more specific approach, which involves teaching the child to modify individual moments of stuttering. To do this, they feign a stutter for the child and ask him to imitate them. They then model a modification of this stutter and ask the child to imitate the modification. This may involve slowing down a repetition or easing the tension on a prolongation. Next, Gregory and Campbell model the child's typical stutter and have the child imitate and experiment with ways to modify it. Eventually, this modification evolves into an easy, relaxed approach with smooth movements.

Gregory and Campbell also believe it is important to deal with an intermediate stutterer's feelings and attitudes about his speech. By being supportive and understanding listeners, they encourage the child to explore areas of concern he may have about his problem and recommend that discussions with the child be concrete and related to specific events. In addition, Gregory and Campbell may teach the child to use voluntary disfluency if he is overly sensitive about his speech. This involves putting normal disfluencies, such as revisions and insertions, into his speech. They want the child to realize that some disfluency is a normal part of talking.

In terms of transferring the new speech patterns into the child's environment, Gregory and Campbell teach the child's parents to model ERA-SM in their speech and to reinforce their child's use of it at home. They also work with the child's classroom teacher so that he or she understands the child's therapy and can be supportive of it. Finally, to help the child maintain improvement, they recommend that the child have monthly rechecks for 12 to 18 months after intensive therapy.

Peter Ramig and Ellen Bennett

Both clinicians have published a number of articles and chapters detailing their therapy approach to school-age or intermediate-level stutterers (Ramig & Bennett, 1995; 1997). The first of these publications describes the process of stuttering treatment like that of building a house. The first stage is "laying the foundation." In this stage, the child learns about the nature of stuttering and about the processes of normal speech. The child learns to name the parts of the speech mechanism and what each part does. The second stage is "installing the plumbing." In this stage, the child explores what happens when he stutters in terms of where the plumbing "clogs up" and what it feels like to release the clog by reducing the tension at the points where the child is interfering with the smooth flow of speech. The third stage is "building rooms and walls." In this stage, the child and the clinician build rooms that meet the child's special needs, addressing such things as teasing, being open about stuttering, voluntary stuttering, modifying moments of stuttering, relaxation, positive self-talk, and handling time pressures. In this stage, the possibilities of relapse are also discussed in terms of the repairs that may need to be made to the house from time to time. The final stage is "the roof of fluency." In this stage, the child increases fluency through fluency shaping techniques (slowing, gentle onsets, light contacts) or through stuttering modification techniques of cancellations, pull-outs, and preparatory sets and openness about stuttering. The child is also provided with a "tool box" of techniques to make the repairs and do the upkeep on fluency that will be needed after formal therapy is completed.

Lena Rustin, Frances Cook, and Rob Spence

Rustin, Cook, and Spence have been conducting stuttering treatment for many years at the Michael Palin Centre for Stuttering Children in London. Their program for the intermediate stutterer, described in *The Management of Stuttering in Adolescence* (1995), is focused not only on fluency but also on general communication skills and family therapy. Although they use group therapy in an intensive format, they suggest that their approach can also be carried out on an individual basis in a nonintensive format (see Rustin & Cook, 1995, for details).

The program developed by Rustin, Cook, and Spence has six essential, interdependent components. The first is "fluency control." The client learns about normal speech and the characteristics of his own stuttering and is then taught to use FEBs such as slower rate, easy onsets, and soft contacts. The second component is "relaxation." This is learned both as a concept of self-management and as a specific technique for handling stress and tension. The third component, "social skills," is taught through the use of exercises, modeling, and role playing. The fourth and fifth components, "problem solving" and "negotiation," extend social skills and help the child to deal with speech difficulties. The sixth and final component, "environmental factors," refers primarily to the family's involvement, extending throughout the course of treatment. This component also includes the school environment and the youngster's friends, although these aspects are treated at the end of the intensive program.

Treatment components are carefully tailored to each client, and many are worked on simultaneously and complement each other. For example, fluency control is practiced as the client is learning various social skills. Family involvement means adolescents can work on their speech in the social context of family life via clinic homework assignments. Assignments given in problem solving and negotiation encourage them to develop ways in which working on stuttering at home and in school can be rewarding. Preliminary follow-up data for 11 adolescents in this program (Rustin, personal communication, 1997) indicate that fluency and other communication skills were significantly improved 6 months after treatment ended. More complete outcome results are being prepared for publication.

Meryl Wall and Florence Myers

Meryl Wall and Florence Myers (1984, 1995) believe stuttering results from a lack of synergism among psycholinguistic, physiological, and psychosocial factors in children and that all three factors need to be taken into account in a treatment program. In their therapy, Wall and Myers control the length and semantic-syntactic complexity of the child's utterances. They typically begin by eliciting one- or two-word utterances, then gradually build to conversation, requiring the child to be fluent at one level of linguistic difficulty before moving on to the next. During these activities, Wall and Myers provide the child with an "easy speech" model to facilitate fluency. This model is characterized by a slow-normal rate, relaxed articulation, gentle voice onset, and slightly reduced volume. If the child still stutters on some words, they teach the child to modify these stutters, using such traditional tools as Van Riper's loose contacts, pull-outs, and cancellations. When necessary, they work on the child's respiratory, phonatory, and articulatory control as well. They also share information about the child's stuttering with his parents and help them to reduce fluency disrupters in the home.

In addition to these direct treatment procedures, Wall and Myers work with other components of stuttering that are influenced by psychosocial aspects of the problem—the child's feelings and attitudes. First, they state that this child "knows" he stutters and that it is important to openly deal with this in therapy. They suggest that not acknowledging the child's stuttering is insensitive and believe the child will be relieved by this openness.

Second, Wall and Myers believe it is important to deal with the intermediate stutterer's word and situation fears and avoidances. They begin work on fears and avoidances after the child has increased his fluency and has gained some control over his blocks. In dealing with situational avoidances, Wall and Myers use hierarchies. For example, if a child is afraid of reading aloud in front of the class, they role-play this situation with him in therapy. They have the child practice pull-outs while standing and reading to them in therapy. Then they have some other children come to therapy sessions, and they have the child practice pull-outs while standing and reading to the other children. Finally, with the cooperation of the classroom teacher, they have the child use pull-outs while reading aloud to the entire class.

Third, Wall and Myers believe it is important to work on the intermediate stutterer's response to teasing. They deal with this through discussion and role playing with the child. They take turns being the teaser and the teased. They help the child explore alternate ways of responding to being teased and help him gain insight into the motives of teasers. Eventually, they want the child to learn to respond calmly with an appropriate statement that defuses the teaser.

SUMMARY OF INTEGRATION OF APPROACHES

In this chapter, a variety of methods of integrating stuttering modification and fluency shaping for the intermediate stutterer have been described. All these approaches teach the child to maintain fluency and manage moments of stuttering. All give some attention to attitudes and feelings.

Our own approach begins with a tactful confrontation of stuttering to decrease some of the negative emotions associated with stuttering, then teaches slow rate, gentle onset, light contacts, and proprioception to enhance fluency and manage stuttering. The young client then uses voluntary stuttering to practice management skills and subsequently works on fear and avoidance by being open about stuttering, becoming desensitized to fluency disrupters, and learning to deal with teasing.

The other clinicians whose therapies are described in this chapter use many of these same techniques. All of them teach fluency enhancing skills in a hierarchy from words to sentences to conversation in the clinic and then to everyday situations outside the clinic. Most of them foster a change in attitude about speech and stuttering, not only to provide positive expectations for fluency but also to help clients accept any residual stuttering so they will deal with it rather than avoid it. Several of these clinicians use relaxation techniques to enhance fluency. Many also prepare the child to deal with teasing. One of these approaches includes teaching communication skills. Thus, we see that the core of these programs is very similar but several clinicians have added innovations.

STUDY QUESTIONS

1. List the four phases of our treatment for the intermediate stutterer. What is the goal for each of these phases?
2. List and briefly describe the clinical procedures involved in our understanding stuttering phase.
3. How do we decide which fluency shaping procedure to use in the "using fluency enhancing behaviors and modifying the moments of stuttering" phase?
4. What procedures do we use to transfer fluency out of the clinical setting in the "using fluency enhancing behaviors and modifying the moments of stuttering" phase?
5. List and briefly describe the clinical procedures involved in our phase for reducing negative feelings and attitudes and eliminating avoidances.
6. Briefly describe the clinical procedures involved in our fluency maintenance phase.
7. Describe how we counsel parents of the intermediate stutterer.
8. Describe our counseling techniques with the classroom teacher.
9. Considering the Coopers' therapy procedures, what do you think they mean by their goal of a feeling of fluency control rather than perfect fluency?
10. How do Gregory and Campbell integrate their ERA-SM technique into stuttering modification?
11. Why are the activities in Ramig and Bennett's "laying the foundation" stage of therapy critical for accomplishing the activities in the "installing the plumbing" stage?
12. Describe how treatment components in Rustin, Cook, and Spence's program are often interactive or carried out simultaneously.
13. What are three ways in which Wall and Myers work on psychosocial factors with the child who has intermediate-level stuttering?

SUGGESTED READINGS

Fosnot, S. (Ed.). (1995). Clinical forum. *Language, Speech, and Hearing Services in Schools, 26(2).*

The Clinical Forum in this issue is devoted to stuttering in school-age children. It contains many excellent treatment approaches for the intermediate stutterer in the school setting.

Turnbaugh, K.R., & Guitar, B.E. (1981). Short-term intensive stuttering treatment in a public school setting. *Language, Speech, and Hearing Services in Schools, 12,* 107–114.

This article describes an integrated treatment program for an intermediate stutterer in which the "reducing negative feelings and attitudes and eliminating avoidances" phase precedes the "using fluency enhancing skills and modifying the moments of stuttering" phase. This is the reverse of the sequence discussed in this chapter.

Wall, M.J., & Myers, F.L. (1995). Therapy for the child stutterer. In M.J. Wall & F.L. Myers (Eds.), *Clinical management of childhood stuttering.* (pp. 179–227). Baltimore: University Park Press.

We recommended this excellent chapter at the end of Chapter 10 also. We recommend it again as an example of how the clinician can integrate stuttering modification and fluency shaping procedures with the intermediate stutterer.

12

Beginning Stutterer: Stuttering Modification and Fluency Shaping Therapies

In the earlier treatment chapters on advanced and intermediate stuttering, we describe fluency shaping and stuttering modification therapies as being divergent in their approaches. They differ in the speech behaviors they target for change, fluency goals, attention given to feelings and attitudes, maintenance procedures, and clinical methods. In this chapter on the beginning stutterer, we describe how these two approaches begin to converge.

Before presenting the details of these two approaches, let us briefly review the characteristics of the beginning stutterer. Children at this treatment level are usually between 2 and 8 years of age and thus are either preschool or early elementary school children.

Their core stuttering behaviors are often part-word or monosyllabic word repetitions, which are produced rapidly and with irregular rhythm, and prolongations, which may have pitch rises. Excessive tension is often present in these stutterers. As tension increases, repetitions and prolongations turn into blocks. Secondary behaviors may include escape behaviors and possibly some starting behaviors. This child may have a self-concept as someone who has trouble talking. However, he has little, or only occasional, concern about it. He may also be experiencing frustration because of his stuttering. These children often respond well to therapy using either approach. Let us begin with stuttering modification.

STUTTERING MODIFICATION THERAPY

Charles Van Riper called his approach to beginning stuttering "prevention."[1] He believed that early intervention could prevent a child's stuttering from becoming chronic. Although he was not in favor of direct work on the child's stuttering, he believed in working directly with the child, as well as with the family. We present his ideas in the following text. We also present the ideas of several other stuttering modification clinicians.

Charles Van Riper: Facilitating Fluency and Desensitizing to Fluency Disrupters

CLINICIAN'S BELIEFS

Nature of Stuttering

As previously noted, the late Charles Van Riper (1982) viewed stuttering as a disorder of timing. He believed that when a child stutters, there is a disruption in the proper timing and sequencing of the muscle movements involved in producing a word. When this happens, the child exhibits a core behavior—that is, a repetition or prolongation. Van Riper suggested that the mistiming could be due to an organic predisposition, to a faulty feedback system, or to communicative and emotional stress. He further suggested that the child's motor speech system is less mature and less stable than that of an adult's. Therefore, it is more subject to disruption by stress, especially *communicative stress*. These stresses include such fluency disrupters as losing listener attention, being frequently interrupted, speaking under time pressures, or attempting to imitate speech and language models that are too advanced.

   The focus of Van Riper's therapy for the beginning stutterer is on facilitating the acquisition of normal fluency and on increasing the child's tolerance for communicative stress. To achieve these goals, Van Riper worked directly with the child, while he also counseled the child's parents.

Speech Behaviors Targeted for Therapy

At this treatment level, Van Riper did not teach the child to modify moments of stuttering. Rather, his goal was to create a "basal level of fluency" in the clinical setting.[2] Van Riper accomplished this by manipulating clinical conditions so that the child could speak fluently. By providing a simple fluency model, engaging in certain fluency facilitating activities, and reinforcing fluency, Van Riper established a basal level of fluency in the clinic. Then, by gradually introducing fluency disrupters while the child was experienc-

---

[1] Van Riper described his "prevention" approach in such a way that it can be used with both borderline and beginning stutterers. Here we highlight the aspects of Van Riper's "prevention" that are appropriate for beginning stuttering and that have inspired so many other clinicians' work with this age group.

[2] The reference for Van Riper's point of view on this and remaining clinical issues is Van Riper, C. (1973). *The treatment of stuttering.* Englewood Cliffs, NJ: Prentice-Hall.

ing this basal fluency, Van Riper steadily increased the child's tolerance for these communicative stresses.

Fluency Goals

Van Riper's goals for a child with beginning stuttering were, quite simply, spontaneous fluency in all speaking situations.

Feelings and Attitudes

As you may recall, a child at this treatment level is not highly concerned about his stuttering. He may be momentarily surprised or frustrated when he repeats or prolongs a syllable for several seconds without being able to complete the word. If this happens too often, he may begin to feel wary of speech. He may add effort to force words out. Van Riper's aim was to prevent this escalation in stuttering development by making speech fun, thus counteracting any negative associations the child may have made with talking. More is said about this when we discuss Van Riper's "making speech pleasant" procedure later in this chapter.

We also believe that in some cases Van Riper's "desensitizing the child to fluency disrupters" procedure involved responding to the child's feelings and attitudes about his speech. For example, when Van Riper desensitized the child to speaking under emotionally disruptive conditions, we believe he was to some degree dealing with the child's feelings.

Maintenance Procedures

Van Riper did not discuss maintenance procedures for the child with beginning stuttering. This fact, together with his belief that the prognosis for this child to achieve normal or spontaneous fluency is excellent, leads us to conclude that Van Riper did not feel formal maintenance procedures are necessary. He believed that fluency will be maintained by the positive experiences the child has had in therapy and the changes that have occurred in the child's environment.

Clinical Methods

In terms of the structure of therapy, Van Riper's interactions with the beginning stutterer took place during play activity. Even though he had definite goals for a therapy session, each session was loosely structured, as will become apparent when we discuss his procedures in the next section. Van Riper did not address the collection of data in his discussion of therapy procedures.

CLINICAL PROCEDURES: DIRECT TREATMENT OF THE CHILD

The reference for material in this section is Chapter 14, "Treatment of the Beginning Stutterer: Prevention," in Van Riper's (1973) *The Treatment of Stuttering*. We describe his therapy in sufficient detail to allow the reader to understand his basic procedures. However, the above chapter includes additional information.

As mentioned earlier, Van Riper's therapy for the beginning stutterer involves a two-pronged attack on the problem: (*a*) direct treatment of the child and (*b*) counseling and training parents. We discuss his direct treatment of the child first.

In working with the beginning stutterer, Van Riper stressed the importance of building a relationship in which the child feels accepted and supported. As Van Riper was developing this relationship, he was working on the following goals: (*a*) making speech pleasant, (*b*) creating suitable fluency models, (*c*) integrating and facilitating fluency, (*d*) reinforcing fluency, (*e*) desensitizing the child to fluency disrupters, (*f*) counterconditioning integrative responses to fluency disrupters, and (*g*) preventing stuttering from becoming a stimulus for struggle and avoidance.

Before discussing the clinical procedures used to achieve these goals, we should point out that Van Riper expected parents to be involved in therapy. At first they observed him working with the child, then they participated with him, and finally, they worked with the child while he observed. By doing this, he trained them in a fluency-facilitating interaction style that they then used on their own at home.

Making Speech Pleasant

Not every beginning stutterer will need help in this area. Only when the child is exhibiting signs of frustration or concern about his speech did Van Riper plan activities aimed at reducing negative feelings. If the child was reluctant to talk and play, he used a series of steps to make the child comfortable. He brought out two boxes of toys: one for the child and one for himself. They sat on the floor and began to take the toys out of their respective boxes. At this point, they were engaged in "solo play," in which each is involved only with his own toys and play activities. At first, Van Riper was silent and put no demands on the child to speak. After a while, Van Riper began to vocalize as he played, perhaps making animal or car noises as he played with his toys. Soon, he may have begun to use one-word commentaries about what he was doing as he played, but was still careful not to put demands on the child to talk. If things continued to go well, Van Riper moved into "tangential play," in which his toys occasionally bumped into the child's or he and the child interacted intermittently. Van Riper then began to use short phrases and sentences as he commented on their activities.

Gradually, play became more and more "cooperative play," and little by little the child began to verbalize (Fig. 12.1). This may have taken a number of sessions, but in time, the child was talking more and more. Once this stage was reached, Van Riper began to engage the child in a variety of games and activities with the goal of having a good time and

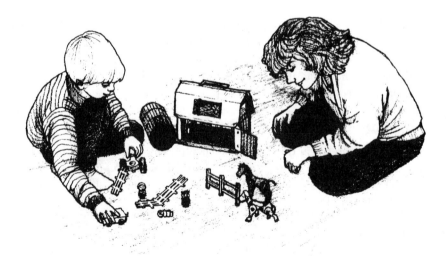

Figure 12.1. Making speech fun.

a by-product of having fun talking. He had the parents observe and then participate in these activities, with the intention of having them carry out similar activities at home.

Creating Suitable Fluency Models

Van Riper believed that when a child attempts to use speech and language patterns that are too difficult for him to produce, he becomes disfluent. Thus, while interacting with the child in play activities, he provided the child with simple speech and language models. In early sessions, he used single words. Later, he used simple phrases, and still later, he used short, simple sentences as he talked with the child. Van Riper used a normal speech rate, with many pauses and silent periods mixed in.[3] He believed it is very important for the child's acquisition of normal fluency to be bombarded by unhurried, simple speech and language patterns. Van Riper also expected the parents to follow this model after they had heard him use it and had tried it themselves under his guidance.

Integrating and Facilitating Fluency

Van Riper believed that the beginning stutterer's motor speech system is prone to breakdown or disfluency. Consequently, it was important to provide a young stutterer with activities that will integrate and stabilize his motor speech fluency. To do this, Van Riper used rhythm or timing techniques. These techniques are not to be used by themselves to make the beginning stutterer fluent but can be embedded in games to provide the young stutterer with fluent speaking experiences. Van Riper told the child to talk this way only when they were playing their speech games together. A typical game may be playing "Indian." Both Van Riper and the child clapped their hands against their mouths as they spoke. At first, each clapping movement was accompanied by a syllable, later a word, and eventually a short phrase or sentence. Other activities might involve the use of puppets, who need to echo or repeat everything that is said to them. Again, Van Riper began by having the child repeat words, then phrases, and finally short sentences. Using these and similar games, Van Riper provided the beginning stutterer with experiences that facilitate fluency.

Reinforcing Fluency

Van Riper's goal here was to reinforce a child's fluency without making the child aware of why he is being reinforced. One way he did this was to show great interest or enthusiasm in a child's fluent communication but only ordinary acceptance of the child's stuttered speech. Another way to achieve this goal was to play games like "Say the Magic Word." During this game, the child would name what he saw out a window or in a picture book. When he said the magic word, a bell was rung and the child won a reward, like a peanut or a sip of soda. Van Riper did not have a specific magic word in mind; instead, he reinforced the child's fluent words, and he chose one of the fluent words as the magic word. In these ways, Van Riper reinforced fluency without the child being made aware of why he was being reinforced.

Desensitizing the Child to Fluency Disrupters

By this time, Van Riper had developed a warm, friendly relationship with the child, and the child felt comfortable talking with him. Van Riper had also learned how to create a

---

[3] This is very much like television's "Mr. Rogers," who talks at a relatively normal rate (we have clocked him at about 165 syllables per minute), but pauses frequently.

basal level of fluency—a few minutes of fluent, continuous speech on the part of the child—by providing simple fluency models, engaging in rhythmic activities, and reinforcing fluency. Van Riper was now ready to begin desensitizing the child to the fluency disrupters or conditions that had been identified by the parents and himself as being particularly important in disrupting this child's fluency. We discuss some of the common fluency disrupters later when we discuss Van Riper's parent counseling. For an example we assume that Van Riper wanted to desensitize the child to being interrupted.

First, Van Riper would interact with the child until a basal level of fluency was achieved. Then, gradually he would begin to interrupt the child, but only occasionally in the beginning. If the child's fluency did not break down, he would interrupt him a bit more frequently. Van Riper continued to do this until just before the child began to stutter. How did Van Riper know when this was about to occur? It varies with the child, but usually a child's speech becomes less spontaneous and free-flowing and may sound somewhat halting and jerky. Once this point is reached, Van Riper stopped interrupting the child and allowed the child's basal fluency to return. After letting the child experience his basal fluency for a few minutes, Van Riper repeated the above cycle. Thus, gradually and systematically he again interrupted the child until just before he began to stutter, then returned the child to his basal fluency level for a few minutes.

In the beginning of this desensitization process, Van Riper went through only two such cycles during a therapy session. Later, as the child became able to handle more and more interruptions, he would be able to tolerate several more such cycles during a session. Using similar strategies and procedures, Van Riper would desensitize a beginning stutterer to the major fluency disrupters that he and the child's parents identified. Van Riper believed that these desensitization procedures also increase a child's tolerance for fluency disrupters in home and school environments, thereby increasing his fluency in these situations.

Counterconditioning Integrative Responses to Fluency Disrupters

Now we turn to Van Riper's procedures for counterconditioning integrative (i.e., fluency facilitating) responses to fluency disrupters. His goal was to have the child establish new, competing, integrative responses to situations that disrupt his fluency. Suppose a young stutterer responded to direct questions with increased stuttering, like most beginning stutterers. How would Van Riper countercondition an integrative response to this fluency disrupter?

One way was to play "can't catch me." In this game, Van Riper produced a jar of peanuts and told the child that one of them would get a peanut whenever the other one asked a question. However, the person who got a peanut had to put it back in the jar if he began to answer the question before he ate the peanut. Van Riper saw to it that he lost a lot of his peanuts by answering too soon and that the child was asked a lot of questions and won a lot of peanuts. Thus, at least two kinds of learning were occurring here. First, the child was learning that answering questions is a pleasant experience. Second, the child was learning to respond to questions slowly and was not giving in to time pressure. Both facilitate fluency. Through games such as this, Van Riper counterconditioned more adaptive and integrative responses to a child's usual fluency disrupters.

Preventing Stuttering From Becoming a Stimulus for Struggle and Avoidance

Van Riper believed it is very important to keep a child from reacting to his moments of stuttering with frustration and concern. He thought that once a child began to do this, he would soon respond to moments of stuttering with struggle and avoidance behaviors. If this could be prevented, Van Riper believed that the chances were very good that stuttering would disappear. Much of the work in meeting this goal is done by the parents, and we return to this topic when we describe parent counseling in the next section. For now, we discuss what therapeutic technique Van Riper used with the child directly.

It is common for a beginning stutterer's stuttering to come and go, and Van Riper liked to see the child more frequently during periods of increased stuttering. At such times, Van Riper wanted to create as many fluency experiences for the child as possible, and Van Riper felt it was especially important for the child to have these fluent experiences during these periods of increased stuttering.

Another technique Van Riper used to reduce the stimulus value (i.e., negative influence) of a child's moments of stuttering was "restimulation." After those stutters to which the child responded with apparent frustration or concern—and after the child completed his utterance—Van Riper casually repeated or paraphrased what the child said, without the disfluencies. By calmly restimulating the child with the stuttered word said normally, Van Riper hoped that the child's memory of the unpleasant experience was reduced and soon forgotten.

This completes the list of goals and procedures that Van Riper employed in his direct treatment of the child. We now turn to the ways in which he helped parents use these procedures at home.

CLINICAL PROCEDURES: PARENT COUNSELING

The second component of Van Riper's treatment for the child with beginning stuttering is parent counseling. Van Riper believed that it is very important to provide the child with an environment that is conducive to fluency, and this requires working with the significant people in the child's life.

Van Riper (1973) was careful in how he approached the parents. For example, on page 418 he commented:

> Far too often the clinical counseling of parents consists of advice alone. In our experience we have not found that giving them a barrage of do's and don'ts changes the child's situation except for the worse. They only make the parents feel more guilty.

Instead, Van Riper tried to form a permissive and supportive relationship with the parents, freeing them from the burden of guilt and energizing them to make changes in their child's environment.

In early sessions, Van Riper attempted to achieve a number of objectives: he obtained information about the child and the family, provided the parents with some basic information about the nature of stuttering, and informed them about his overall plan of treatment. He also gave parents absolution for any past mistakes they may have made in their handling of the child's stuttering. He was much more concerned with the present and the future than the past. He always encouraged parents to observe and participate in their child's therapy sessions. This was important because Van Riper wanted them to try out some of the procedures he used in direct therapy with the child, while he observed them and gave them guidance. For instance, it was especially desirable to have the parents provide the child with unhurried, simple speech and language models when they interacted with him throughout the day.

The main thrust of Van Riper's parent counseling was to help parents increase the conditions that facilitate the child's fluency and decrease those that disrupt it. If parents are to do this, they first need to identify each of these conditions. Van Riper shared some ideas about which conditions may facilitate and which may disrupt fluency. He then asked parents to observe their child in daily activities to determine which conditions are associated with increased fluency and which with increased stuttering. Through discussions of their observations, Van Riper helped parents discover for themselves that fluency and stuttering have predictable patterns and that parents can influence them.

Finally, Van Riper suggested ways the parents could help prevent the child from becoming more aware of his stuttering, thereby helping to prevent his stutters from becoming stimuli for struggle and avoidance reactions. One way was for the parents to arrange activities in such a way that there is little need for the child to talk on days when he is having a lot of stuttering and to create many opportunities for the child to talk on days when he is more fluent. In addition, Van Riper gave the parents ideas for handling those times when their child was having frequent moments of stuttering. He recommended that they attempt to distract the child from his speech at these difficult times. If this was not possible, he suggested that they reassure him and use the restimulation technique they had observed in therapy.

It may appear as if Van Riper's treatment of children with beginning stuttering is long and complex. However, he indicated that neither is the case. Van Riper said that he was often successful after only brief periods of therapy or by working on only a few of his goals. In short, Van Riper reported that he had been very successful using these procedures with beginning stutterers.

Other Clinicians

Let us now take a brief look at the treatment procedures used with beginning stutterers by other clinicians who have been associated with the stuttering modification approach. By being aware of these clinicians' contributions, you will gain a broader appreciation of stuttering modification therapy for the beginning stutterer.

OLIVER BLOODSTEIN

Oliver Bloodstein (1975) discusses his therapy for the beginning stutterer, or what he calls the "phase 2" stutterer, in a chapter that also discusses his viewpoint of stuttering as an anticipatory struggle reaction (see Suggested Readings). In line with this anticipatory struggle theory, which we described in Chapter 3, Bloodstein's primary objective is to combat the beginning stutterer's concept of himself as a defective speaker. The essence of Bloodstein's anticipatory struggle theory is that stuttering is caused by the child's development of the belief that speaking is difficult and that he is a defective speaker or communicator. This attitude grows out of a background in which the child experiences frequent or severe communicative failures and pressures. Bloodstein wants to reverse this belief on the part of the child. Consequently, his therapy for the beginning stutterer focuses on (a) general speech improvement designed to establish a self-image as an effective speaker, (b) general personal development, (c) subtle and appropriate use of suggestion, and (d) parent counseling.

In working on the first goal, to improve the child's self-confidence as a communicator, Bloodstein targets all areas of communication except fluency. For example, a treatment program may involve improving the child's voice and diction or improving his conversational skills. Bloodstein's focus on general personal development is aimed at increasing the child's sense of personal worth by helping him develop new interests and abilities, minimizing his old liabilities, and enhancing his image with his friends and classmates. With regard to the third therapy emphasis, Bloodstein conjectures that almost any form of suggestion that the child is doing well in therapy will be effective in improving his confidence in his speaking ability and will thereby improve his fluency.

Bloodstein's approach to therapy for the beginning stutterer was inspired by the success of many clinicians working in New York in the 1950s who used "chewing therapy,"[4] a form of fluency shaping that gave children a method for speaking fluently. This method, which was imbued with the conviction that the child would succeed, seemed to give beginning stutterers confidence in their general speaking ability and many opportunities to experience fluency.

Bloodstein's goals when counseling parents of beginning stutterers are to remove environmental pressures and reinforce the child's anticipation of fluency. In removing environmental pressures, Bloodstein insists that parents remove all speech pressures on the child. He also suggests that, when pertinent, they be less restrictive in their child-rearing practices. Bloodstein recommends that, in reinforcing their child's anticipation of fluency, parents provide more situations in which their child is fluent and eliminate those in which he is disfluent.

Like Van Riper, Bloodstein believes that the prognosis for the beginning stutterer is excellent. Also like Van Riper, his therapy is characterized by a low level of structure and little emphasis on data collection.

EDWARD CONTURE

Conture's therapy is a form of stuttering modification. His clinical methods are loosely structured, and he does not use programmed instruction.

Conture begins therapy by using an analogy between the speech mechanism and a garden hose. He compares the larynx or voice box with the faucet at the house, the throat and tongue with the hose, and the lips with the nozzle at the end of the hose. He and the child then practice stopping the water or air at various points. Next, he introduces the notion of "air stoppers" in the child's speech. Once the child understands that he is stopping air at various points in his speech mechanism when he stutters, Conture explains that the tightness or pressure he feels when he stutters is like the pressure in a garden hose when he squeezes it and stops the water. He then explains that the child can change his feelings of tightness by doing things differently with his speech mechanism.

At this point, Conture introduces another analogy. He explains that speech requires movement from one sound to the next, much like the frog jumping from one lily pad to the next when it crosses a stream. If a frog jumps up and down on a lily pad (repetition) or stays too long on one pad (prolongation), it will get wet and will not get across the stream. Similarly, if the child wishes to say a word, he needs to keep moving from sound to sound and not stop too long on any one of them. Conture then helps the child learn to use "smooth, easy movements" as he says words.

Conture believes that it is very important for parents to be kept informed regarding their child's therapy and to understand what is happening. He also believes that it is important to provide them with information about stuttering and to relieve any guilt about their child's speech problem.

CARL DELL

Carl Dell (1979) was trained by Van Riper to become a stuttering specialist in the public schools, after which he worked for several years in the schools in Grand Rapids, Michigan. Based on this training with Van Riper and his experiences in schools, Dell wrote

---

[4] This approach was pioneered by the Viennese therapist Emil Froeschels (1943), who emigrated to New York in the 1940s and taught stutterers to move their mouths when speaking as if they were chewing.

Treating the School Age Stutterer: A Guide for Clinicians. Dell describes his therapy procedures for the beginning stutterer, or what he calls the "mild stutterer," in a chapter in that booklet. His therapy is discussed under the following headings: (*a*) gradual but direct confrontation, (*b*) making stuttering more voluntary, (*c*) exploring the emotional nature of the child, (*d*) exploring struggle and tension, and (*e*) reducing the severity of repetitions and prolongations. Dell implements therapy goals in low-structured, play interactions with the child and places little emphasis on data collection.

In gradual but direct confrontation, Dell inserts pseudostuttering into his own speech and comments about it. This allows him to begin to talk with the child about stuttering in an objective and relaxed manner. When appropriate, Dell also encourages the child to engage in some pseudostuttering with him.

Once the child is doing some pseudostuttering, Dell has him try different types of pseudostuttering. In doing this, the child learns that stuttering is not completely involuntary, that he has some control over it.

In exploring the emotional nature of the child, Dell attempts to provide an emotional climate in which the child feels comfortable talking about his stuttering and related matters. Although Dell may probe from time to time, he never forces the child to talk about any topic that he does not want to talk about.

A fourth focus of Dell's therapy is helping the child learn to identify what he does when he stutters. Dell wants the child to identify the sites of tension and to feel the difference between speaking with just the right amount of tension and not squeezing too hard.

The final goal involves teaching the child to reduce the severity of his moments of stuttering by reducing the number of repetitions per stutter and shortening the length of prolongations. From his experience with beginning stutterers, Dell believes that once the beginning stutterer learns what he is doing when he stutters and learns that he has a choice in how he says the word, he will choose the easier way to say it.

In addition to working directly with the child, Dell also works with parents. He attempts to alleviate any guilt they may have about their child's stuttering, provides them with information about stuttering, and gives them suggestions on how to help facilitate their child's therapy at home. Based on his experience with this treatment approach, Dell is optimistic about the outcome of therapy with beginning stutterers.

HAROLD LUPER AND ROBERT MULDER

Harold Luper and Robert Mulder developed a treatment program for children whom they describe as "transitional stutterers." Their description matches ours of children who have beginning-level stuttering. Luper and Mulder believe it is realistic to have spontaneous or normal fluency as a goal with the beginning stutterer. Their treatment may involve only parent counseling, without any direct contact with the child. If a child is seen directly, their procedures may or may not involve modifying the child's moments of stuttering. Their therapy is loosely structured, not programmed instruction. As a general rule, Luper and Mulder prefer to start with less direct procedures, such as parent counseling, before beginning more direct procedures with the child.

In terms of parent counseling, Luper and Mulder provide parents with information about speech and language development and about stuttering and its development and encourage them to implement a variety of "do's" and "don'ts" with their child. Do's include providing good fluency models for the child, looking at the child when he talks, and showing interest in what he has to say. Common don'ts are calling negative attention to the child's stuttering, putting undue pressure on the child for good speech, and interrupting the child.

If the decision is made to involve the child directly in treatment, but not work on modifying moments of stuttering, Luper and Mulder recommend the following procedures: desensitizing the child to fluency disrupters in a way similar to Van Riper's approach; providing the child with ample and successful opportunities to talk freely in therapy; allowing the child, if he chooses, to talk about his speech problem; and providing opportunities for the child to speak fluently, such as speaking in rhythm or choral reading.

If the decision is made to help the child modify moments of stuttering, Luper and Mulder model "loose contacts" and producing difficult or hard words while emphasizing relaxation and smooth movements of the speech mechanism.

Summary of Stuttering Modification Therapy

Although all stuttering modification clinicians emphasize teaching advanced stutterers to modify moments of stuttering, this is less true for the beginning stutterer. Van Riper focuses on facilitating a child's fluency by providing an environment that enhances fluency and by encouraging the child to ignore his stuttering. Dell works on a child's feelings about stuttering before working on symptom modification. When negative feelings have subsided, he has the child modify stutters by making them looser and more normal-sounding. Dell and Bloodstein borrow from fluency shaping approaches by also focusing on the child's feelings of fluency and sense of competence as a speaker. Luper and Mulder recommend teaching a child to use loose contacts to modify moments of stuttering only if less direct procedures are unsuccessful. In contrast, Conture emphasizes modifying moments of stuttering by teaching the child to stutter in an easier, looser fashion.

FLUENCY SHAPING THERAPY

At the beginning of this chapter, we suggest that in the treatment of the beginning stutterer, the differences between stuttering modification and fluency shaping therapies become less and their similarities become greater. Before we compare these two therapy approaches at this treatment level, however, we need to present a representative example of fluency shaping therapy for the beginning stutterer. We have selected Mark Onslow as a fluency shaping clinician because of his data-based publications about his approach. His treatment of beginning stuttering illustrates two principles of fluency shaping with a young child who stutters: The clinician and parents are direct in calling the child's attention to his fluency and stuttering, and they make sure that the child enjoys therapy and doesn't feel embarrassed or ashamed of stuttering. Although generally representative of fluency shaping clinicians, Onslow is unique in beginning his treatment with a child's natural conversational speech, having the parent reward fluency and punish stuttering.

Mark Onslow: The Lidcombe Program

CLINICIAN'S BELIEFS

Nature of Stuttering

Onslow acknowledges that research on the nature of stuttering is incomplete, but suggests that there is evidence that stuttering is a disorder related to speech motor control. Furthermore, he believes that genetic, environmental, and learning factors may work together to create the various behaviors of stuttering.

Speech Behaviors Targeted for Therapy

Parents are trained to give positive reinforcement to their child for fluent speech and to correct the child's stuttered speech, using a positive and encouraging tone of voice. In addition, parents positively reinforce the child's corrections of his stutters. Thus, both fluency and stuttering are targets of treatment.

Fluency Goals

Onslow believes that stutter-free speech is attainable by those children between 2 and 5 years of age, whose stuttering has recently begun. His clinical data indicate that his procedures result in less than 1% of syllables stuttered. This is well within the range of normal fluency for this age group, if this 1% of residual stuttering consists of brief repetitions and prolongations.

Feelings and Attitudes

In his book, *Behavioral Management of Stuttering* (1996), Onslow acknowledges that feelings and attitudes are important in the treatment of stuttering, but he does not advocate their specific treatment. Instead he emphasizes the importance of positive, constructive, and supportive parent behaviors when they respond to the child's fluency or stuttering. Describing their treatment, Onslow and his coworkers (1994) say that "parents were trained to correct stuttered speech in a positive and nonpunitive manner" and "the parental RCS [response contingent stimulation] was conducted in an atmosphere of support and positiveness." This suggests that Onslow believes that the child's feelings and attitudes about his speech can influence the outcome of treatment.

Maintenance Procedures

In Onslow's program, maintenance is simply the systematic and gradual fading of clinic assessments. Criteria for progressing through his maintenance component consist of minimal stuttering in the clinic, on audiotapes of the child's speech outside the clinic, and low overall severity ratings by the parents.

Clinical Methods

Onslow's program is a structured approach that can be tailored to the needs of individual children and their families. Parents are taught how to systematically reinforce fluency and punish stuttering before they use these contingencies in the child's natural environment. Careful data are kept, to ensure that parents are reliably identifying stuttering and properly presenting contingencies and to chart the child's progress through treatment and maintenance.

CLINICAL PROCEDURES

The procedures described, taken from the two journal articles and Onslow's book listed earlier, are still evolving. The version presented here includes weekly clinic visits by the parent and child for parent guidance, sessions delivered at home by parents, contingent responses to the child's fluency and stuttering throughout each day, and the maintenance program of clinic assessments. The sequence of therapy is (*a*) parent training, (*b*) treatment during sessions, (*c*) treatment on-line, and (*d*) maintenance.

Parent Training

In the first clinic session, the parents and clinician decide on the length and frequency of the treatment sessions that parents will deliver at home. For many children, a 5-minute session administered each day is sufficient at the start. Onslow points out that a gradual onset of treatment is desirable for children who have been stuttering for some time without receiving intervention.

Parents are trained to praise and reward the child when he is fluent and gently correct him when he stutters.[5] Onslow recommends that parents use five positive contingencies for each negative one, to ensure that the child will feel good about these procedures. Parents are first coached through a treatment session in the clinic. Then they tape-record themselves conducting a treatment session at home and review it with the clinician to ensure that they are responding accurately to the child's fluency and stuttering and that the child is enjoying treatment. If all is well, parents then administer treatment sessions at home, once a day, or more frequently if the child's stuttering is severe.

On-line treatment begins gradually, after home treatment sessions are going smoothly. In on-line treatment, parents give contingent reinforcements and corrections to the child in natural conversations at home and in outside speaking situations. Parents use praise and tangible rewards when the child is fluent and intermittently call attention to the child's stuttering and ask him to say the word again fluently. For example, when a child is fluent, a parent might say, "Gee, that was really smooth speech" or "You said that without any stutters. Nice." When a child stutters the parent might say, "Oops, you were a little bumpy there" or "I think that was a stutter on the word 'I,' wasn't it?" At first, contingencies in natural conversations are used sparingly. Then gradually as the child's stuttering diminishes, contingencies are applied more frequently. The parents make regular visits to the clinician to ensure that this program is providing the child with a positive experience. As treatment progresses, clinic sessions fade out and only on-line feedback is used.

Maintenance begins when the clinician is satisfied that the child has only minimal stuttering in most situations. The criteria are that the child shows 1% or fewer syllables stuttered during clinic measurement, shows fewer than two stutters per minute in an outside speaking situation, and has an average rating below 2 on a 10-point scale on which parents assess stuttering severity in a variety of different situations. These criteria are flexible and may be adapted to the individual child.

The maintenance program consists of simply having the child come to the clinic for formal assessments of fluency. Clinic contact is gradually faded from once every few weeks to once every few months over a period of 2 years. If a child fails on any of the fluency criteria at any time, he begins the maintenance program all over again. Throughout the maintenance program, parents continue to use contingencies for the child's stuttering in natural conversations, but formal home treatment sessions are discontinued.

Other Clinicians

MARTIN ADAMS

Martin Adams has been a productive researcher and clinician for many years. In his 1980 article, "The young stutterer: Diagnosis, treatment and assessment of progress, he sug-

---

[5] Onslow has found that children 2 to 3 years of age respond best to verbal contingencies only, but children 4 years and older may need such tangible reinforcers as stickers or stamps. Contingencies are adjusted to suit the individual child.

gests that beginning stutterers may come from two different etiological backgrounds. One consists of a motor-impaired group with problems starting or sustaining phonation. The other consists of a language-impaired group with problems encoding language. It is interesting that Adams recommends a similar treatment program for both groups. His therapy for both groups includes speech rate reduction by prolonging sounds and the principles embedded in Ryan's gradual increase in length and complexity of utterance (GILCU) program (discussed later in this chapter). Adams believes these two strategies are helpful for both groups, but for different reasons.

Like many fluency shaping clinicians, Adams is a strong supporter of operant conditioning principles in the treatment of stuttering. For example, in his 1980 article, he emphasizes four aspects of reinforcement that warrant a clinician's careful attention. First, he stresses the fact that a reinforcer needs to be something the child "really wants." Second, he suggests that the clinician should also tell the child "why" he is being reinforced. Third, he emphasizes the importance of providing reinforcement as soon as possible after the correct response. Fourth, he discusses the effects that various schedules of reinforcement have on the rate and permanence of learning.

In this article, Adams also provides helpful suggestions for transfer and maintenance activities. For example, he recommends that clinicians obtain from the child's parents a "hierarchy of speech-related stimuli" to use in transferring fluency from the clinic to the child's environment. Items on this hierarchy should be consistently associated with stuttering on the part of the child. Adams concludes this article with a discussion of the importance of measuring treatment effects.

JANIS COSTELLO

Janis Costello is a leading advocate of operant conditioning and programmed instruction procedures in the treatment of the beginning stutterer. Costello refers to her "basic" program as the extended length of utterance (ELU) program, which is similar to Ryan's GILCU program. A detailed description of her ELU program is provided in *Treatment of Stuttering in Early Childhood: Methods and Issues* (1983). We describe it briefly in this section. Costello uses "additives" to her basic program if progress is not satisfactory. These are described in Chapter 10, where we discuss her approach for the intermediate stutterer.

Costello's ELU program begins with the child producing fluent responses that consist of single monosyllabic words. After 20 graduated steps, it ends with the child conversing fluently for 5 minutes in the therapy setting. Throughout the program, Costello reinforces the child's fluent responses both socially and with tokens that are periodically redeemed for backup reinforcers. She also punishes or gives the child feedback for his stuttered responses. Costello observes and charts each response, using predetermined criteria to decide when to move a child from one step to the next.

If, after the child completes the ELU program, he has not spontaneously generalized fluency to his natural environment, Costello engages the child in activities similar to those Ryan uses in his transfer phase. In other words, she brings people from the child's natural environment into the therapy setting, and she also accompanies the child into his real world.

Like most of the other authors discussed so far in this chapter, Costello is optimistic about the chances of improving the fluency of the beginning stutterer.

REBEKAH PINDZOLA

Pindzola's approach, as described in her book, *SIP: Stuttering Intervention Program* (1983), consists of four segments: evaluation, involving the parents, enhancing fluency (treatment), and public school commitments. We omit the evaluation segment and describe the essentials of her treatment, which comprise the remaining three parts.

Pindzola's treatment begins with her involvement of the parents in an evaluation interview. In this first parent counseling session, Pindzola gathers information about the child and his problem and gets the parents involved in discovering the nature of their child's stuttering and how they can help their child. In later sessions, she helps parents study how they respond to their child's stuttering and discusses such topics as discipline, sibling relationships, and other important aspects of the home environment. Parents are involved in treatment first as observers of therapy, then as models of the fluency enhancing style of speech that the child is learning with the clinician.

In her direct treatment of the child, Pindzola relies on three principal procedures: (*a*) reinforcement and punishment to increase fluency and decrease stuttering; (*b*) stretched, soft, and smooth speech; and (*c*) a hierarchy of language complexity, going from short and simple utterances to complex ones. She begins by teaching the child how to produce stretched, slow speech on monosyllables. When the child is able to use this style of speaking, Pindzola has the child move up to combined monosyllables and add a soft speaking voice.

Throughout treatment, the child uses stretched, slow speech only on the first syllable of a sentence or following a pause, not during the entire utterance. A softer voice is used throughout all speech but is even softer on the first syllable of an utterance. When this is mastered, Pindzola moves the child to polysyllable words and adds a smooth talking component that involves blending all the words within a breath group. The child then uses these three fluency enhancing speech production behaviors together as he progresses through a linguistic hierarchy from single phrases to longer utterances to spontaneous speech.

Reinforcement is given immediately when the child uses proper speech patterns and is fluent, as he progresses. Punishment, in the form of corrective feedback and retrials, is used when the child stutters. In her book, Pindzola provides examples of the kinds of activities that can be used with the child at each level.

Another element in Pindzola's treatment package focuses on how to involve the child's school. She provides materials and ideas that can be used to plan an individual education program for the child as well as materials and suggestions for the child's teachers.

BRUCE RYAN AND BARBARA VAN KIRK RYAN

Bruce Ryan and his wife Barbara Van Kirk Ryan pioneered fluency shaping therapy for children in the 1960s and 1970s. One of their earliest treatment programs was the gradual increase in length and complexity of utterance, or GILCU. It is still in use, and Ryan continues to publish data on its effectiveness (Ryan & Van Kirk, 1974). This program consists of establishment, transfer, and maintenance phases and is based on operant principles of reward for fluency and punishment for stuttering. Each step within a phase is carefully controlled so that the child is given specific instructions, makes a specific response, and receives a specific consequence. The aim is to ensure that a child successfully progresses from one step to a slightly harder one with complete fluency.

In the first phase of therapy, the clinician establishes fluent speech in the child in each of three modes—reading, monologue, and conversation—progressing in 18 steps from uttering one word fluently to two words fluently, and so on, to 5 minutes of fluency. Very young children, who do not read, participate in modified monologue and conversational modes. After each fluent response, the clinician says "good" and gives the child a token, which is later redeemed for a tangible reward. If the child stutters on a response, the clinician immediately says, "Stop, speak fluently," and the step is redone. If the child has repeated difficulty on a step, the clinician then uses a "branching step" in which the desired response is modeled (e.g., a three-word phrase said fluently), and the child imitates it. As the child becomes successful in imitating the clinician's model, modeling is gradually faded, and the normal sequence of the program is resumed.

After the child completes the establishment phase of the GILCU program, he must pass a criterion test of 5 minutes each of reading, monologue, and conversation (or monologue and conversation for nonreaders) with no more than two stuttered words in a 2-minute period. Once past this stage, the child goes through a transfer phase, conducted like the establishment program, in which complete fluency is required at each step before progressing to the next.

Transfer occurs in four areas: physical setting, audience size, home environment, and school environment. Each is achieved through a sequence of small, manageable steps. After completing the entire transfer phase, the child is again assessed in criterion tests of reading, monologue, and conversation with no more than one stutter in 2 minutes of speaking. When the child passes this criterion test, he can begin the maintenance phase of treatment. This is simply a 22-month period during which the child is given periodic rechecks at longer and longer intervals, so that contact with the clinician is faded gradually. Performance at school and performance at home are also evaluated by teacher and parent reports. If the child is having trouble in any area, he is recycled through that particular transfer program before returning to a maintenance schedule.

Ryan involves the parents fully in therapy from the beginning of the program. The parents are trained to identify stuttering and to carry out the treatment program at home. Once the child completes the reading part of the GILCU program (or monologue, for nonreaders), he begins practice at home with his parents. This is continued through with the monologue and conversation sections and continues as the home transfer phase is carried out.

Like other therapies for stuttering, the GILCU approach is most efficient when it can be completed on a regular schedule. Ryan points out that when this approach used in a clinic setting with the child attending sessions consistently, progress can be swift and satisfying. When the GILCU approach is used in school, vacation periods and other schedule interruptions can stretch treatment out for a longer period of time.

GEORGE SHAMES AND CHERI FLORANCE

In Chapter 8, we describe George Shames and Cheri Florance's "stutter-free speech" program for the adult or advanced stutterer. We indicate that they divide their adult therapy program into five phases: (*a*) volitional control, (*b*) self-reinforcement, (*c*) transfer, (*d*) training in unmonitored speech, and (*e*) follow-up. Their child's or beginning stutterer's program is similar to their adult program, except that it omits phase 4, training in unmonitored speech. Shames and Florance report that children begin using unmonitored stutter-free speech or spontaneous fluency by themselves. The child's program is also accompanied by a parent-training program.

The goal of the first phase of therapy is met if the child gains volitional control over his speech. Shames and Florance use delayed auditory feedback (DAF) to help the child learn two important skills—control of rate and continuous phonation. They begin with DAF set at its maximum delay and instruct the child how to use rate control and continuous phonation to produce slow, prolonged, stutter-free speech. Gradually, they increase the child's speaking rate by systematically reducing delay times of DAF. By the end of this phase, the child is producing stutter-free speech at a near-normal rate while still on DAF. Data are recorded, and token reinforcement is used throughout this phase.

As in the adult program, the goal of the self-reinforcement phase is to teach the young stutterer to monitor, evaluate, and reinforce himself for using stutter-free speech while off DAF. As the child is systematically withdrawn from DAF, reinforcement is gradually shifted from the clinician to the child. In the adult program, self-reinforcement is the opportunity for the stutterer to use brief units of unmonitored speech. In the child's program, self-reinforcement is a token.

The child's parents become involved in the transfer phase. They meet with the child and the clinician to plan a home transfer program. This involves designing transfer situations and a reinforcement system. At first, these transfer situations involve activities similar to those used in therapy. Later, the parents, clinician, and child plan and develop contracts to expand the child's use of his stutter-free speech into other speaking situations. Token reinforcement continues to be used in early stages of the transfer phase, but it is gradually replaced with social reinforcement.

After the completion of the transfer phase, the child is enrolled in a 5-year follow-up program.

RICHARD SHINE

Richard Shine is another clinician who advocates a fluency shaping approach for the beginning stutterer. He refers to his therapy as "systematic fluency training" and throughout this program, he uses operant conditioning and programmed instruction principles (Shine, 1988). The following seven phases are included: (*a*) picture selection for monosyllabic words, (*b*) determining a fluent speaking mode—whispered or prolonged, (*c*) establishing an easy speaking voice, (*d*) environmental program, (*e*) picture identification, storybook, picture matching, and surprise box, (*f*) transfer, and (*g*) maintenance.

During the first phase, Shine selects, from a large number of pictures, 69 pictures of things that the child can readily identify and say fluently.

The goal of the second phase is to train the child to speak totally fluently. This involves teaching the child to speak in a whisper. The clinician provides models of counting, then of sentences to train the child. The child must speak fluently for 2 minutes, using four-to six-word sentences to pass this step. In the few cases in which a child is not able to whisper fluently, Shine suggests using prolonged speech.

During the third phase, Shine teaches the child to use a more normal-sounding voice than is used with whispering or prolonged speech. This is called an "easy speaking voice" and consists primarily of loose articulatory contacts, slower rate, and easy onsets of phonation, but intonation, loudness, and vocal quality are essentially normal.

In the fourth phase, a parent, or someone having regular contact with the child, is taught how to work with the child at specified times during the week. This enables the child to receive training that parallels his therapy with the clinician at a different site, so that transfer can begin.

The fifth phase consists of a variety of activities in which the child uses first his easy speaking voice, then his new speaking voice, which is even more normal-sounding than the easy voice. Throughout this phase, the child gradually progresses from simple speaking tasks to more complex, natural ones, speaking almost entirely fluently. Parents work on these same goals in the environmental program.

In the transfer phase, the clinician and parent work together to help the child transfer his fluency to all of his natural speaking environments. After the child has completed the transfer phase and is gradually faded from regular treatment sessions, he is reevaluated periodically to ensure that fluency is maintained.

Summary of Fluency Shaping Therapy

The clinicians reviewed in this section all work directly with the child's speech, using operant conditioning principles first to change stuttering into fluent speech in a structured treatment situation, then to transfer fluency to more natural contexts. Onslow's approach differs from the other clinicians in his use of parents as clinicians who reinforce fluency and punish stuttering during parent-child conversations. Onslow does not attempt to alter the child's natural speech rate or length of utterances, whereas the other clinicians establish fluency using a variety of speech changes. Costello and Ryan elicit short and simple responses from the child. Adams, Pindzola, and Shames and Florance use modeling or DAF to slow the child's utterances. Shine instructs the child to first whisper, then use slow, prolonged speech.

All these clinicians shape the child's altered speech pattern into normal-sounding fluency before helping the child to transfer it to everyday situations.

COMPARISON OF THE TWO APPROACHES

At the outset of this chapter, we suggested that most of the differences between stuttering modification and fluency shaping therapies diminish as we move from the treatment of advanced and intermediate stutterers to the treatment of a beginning stutterer. This trend is readily apparent as we compare stuttering modification and fluency therapies for the beginning stutterer on the following five issues: (*a*) speech behaviors targeted for therapy, (*b*) fluency goals, (*c*) attention to feelings and attitudes, (*d*) maintenance procedures, and (*e*) clinical methods. Table 12.1 provides an overview of the similarities and differences between these two therapy approaches for the beginning stutterer.

With regard to the speech behaviors targeted for therapy, much of Van Riper's stuttering modification therapy and Onslow's fluency shaping therapy target a child's fluent responses. Van Riper uses various stimuli and reinforcers to increase fluency, as does Onslow, but Onslow also corrects stuttering. Not all stuttering modification clinicians try to facilitate fluency as part of their approach. Luper and Mulder, for example, and Conture work mainly on helping a child stutter more easily.

Table 12.1. Similarities and Differences Between Stuttering Modification and Fluency Shaping Therapy for the Beginning Stutterer

Clinical Issue	Therapy Approach	
	Stuttering Modification Therapy	Fluency Shaping Therapy
Speech behaviors targeted for therapy	Moments of stuttering or fluent responses	Fluent responses or moments of stuttering
Fluency goals	Spontaneous fluency	Spontaneous fluency or controlled fluency
Feelings and attitudes	Some approaches focus on negative attitudes; others don't	No attention given to changing negative feelings and attitudes
Maintenance procedures	Little emphasis on maintenance procedures	Some emphasis on maintenance procedures or periodic rechecks
Clinical methods	Therapy often characterized by loosely structured interaction—play activity	Therapy often characterized by tightly structured interaction or programmed instruction
	Little emphasis on collection of objective data	Considerable emphasis on collection of objective data

By and large, both stuttering modification and fluency shaping clinicians agree that spontaneous fluency is a realistic goal for the beginning stutterer. They also agree that the probability of this occurring is very high.

Some stuttering modification clinicians feel that some beginning stutterers may have begun to develop negative feelings and attitudes about their speech. Van Riper and Dell, for instance, suggest that significant frustration may be present in these children and may lead to more tension and struggle. Van Riper tries to keep the child's attention away from his stuttering to prevent any increase in negative feelings. On the other hand, Dell encourages the release of feelings to help the child. Bloodstein counteracts negative feelings by giving the child positive speaking experiences. Conture attends to feelings indirectly by helping the beginning stutterer learn an easier form of stuttering. Fluency shaping clinicians, such as Onslow and Ryan, also endeavor to affect feelings only indirectly, by teaching the child more fluent responses. Overall, in approaches to feelings and attitudes, the fluency shaping clinicians are more similar than are the stuttering modification clinicians.

On the fourth issue, maintenance procedures, the two approaches differ somewhat in their concern. Beginning stutterers seldom regress, so stuttering modification clinicians do not emphasize maintenance procedures. Fluency shaping clinicians, on the other hand, incorporate maintenance phases into their programs, even though they consist primarily of periodic reassessments.

On the final issue, clinical methods, the two approaches continue to be dissimilar in their treatments for beginning stutterers. The interactions between the clinician and the child in stuttering modification therapy is loosely structured, often involving play activities. Fluency shaping therapy, on the other hand, is highly structured, often characterized by programmed instruction. The two approaches also differ with regard to data collection. Stuttering modification therapy places little importance on the collection of objective data, but fluency shaping therapy places considerable emphasis on it.

In summary, stuttering modification therapy and fluency shaping therapy have some similarities in their treatment of beginning stutterers. Specifically, they often do not differ significantly in terms of the speech behaviors targeted for therapy, fluency goals, or maintenance procedures. They may differ, depending on the clinician, in their attention to and approach to feelings and attitudes. Moreover, they differ consistently in how they structure therapy and in the collection of data. Thus, as is apparent in the next chapter, the task of integrating these two approaches for the beginning stutterer is not difficult.

STUDY QUESTIONS

1. Describe the following clinical procedures that Van Riper uses to create a basal level of fluency: (a) creating suitable fluency models, (b) integrating and facilitating fluency, and (c) reinforcing fluency.
2. Describe how Van Riper desensitizes the beginning stutterer to fluency disrupters.
3. Describe Van Riper's counseling with parents of a beginning stutterer.
4. Onslow's approach begins by training parents to reward their child's fluency and correct his stuttering; several examples are given in the text. Suggest a variety of other things a parent might say to their child to reward fluency. Suggest other ways in which a parent might correct the child's stuttering.

5. Onslow suggests that a child's feelings and attitudes are important. How do his treatment procedures reflect this?

6. Discuss how Onslow involves parents in treatment. Compare this with other fluency shaping clinicians' involvement of parents.

7. Compare Onslow's sequence of treating the beginning stutterer with Ryan's fluency shaping hierarchy in this chapter.

8. Describe the ways in which Van Riper's approach to the beginning stutterer is like fluency shaping.

9. Compare stuttering modification therapy and fluency shaping therapy for the beginning stutterer on the following five clinical issues: (a) speech behaviors targeted for therapy, (b) fluency goals, (c) attention to feelings and attitudes, (d) maintenance procedures, and (e) clinical methods.

10. Find the clinicians you think represent the most extreme differences between fluency shaping and stuttering modification among the "other clinicians" for the two approaches and describe their differences.

SUGGESTED READINGS

Adams, M.R. (1980). The young stutterer: Diagnosis, treatment and assessment of progress. *Seminars in Speech, Language, and Hearing, 1*, 289–299.
This is a brief overview of Adam's approach to beginning and intermediate stuttering.

Bloodstein, O. (1975). Stuttering as tension and fragmentation. In J. Eisenson (Ed.), *Stuttering: A second symposium.* New York: Harper & Row.

Bloodstein, O. (1993). The treatment of early stuttering. In *Stuttering: The search for a cause and cure.* Boston: Allyn & Bacon.
These readings give an overview of Bloodstein's insightful and unique approach to treating beginning stutterers.

Conture, E.G. (1990). *Stuttering,* 2nd ed. Englewood Cliffs, NJ: Prentice-Hall.
In this book, Edward Conture presents his therapy for a beginning stutterer under the heading of "children who clearly stutter and parents who are (un) concerned."

Costello, J.M. (1980). Operant conditioning and the treatment of stuttering. *Seminars in Speech, Language, and Hearing, 1*, 311–325.

Costello, J.M. (1983). Current behavioral treatments for children. In D. Prins & R.J. Ingham (Eds.), *Treatment of stuttering in early childhood: Methods and issues.* San Diego: College-Hill Press.
These are accounts of Costello's approach. Written versions of her therapy do not fully convey her enthusiasm as a clinician, which is evident on videotapes of her therapy.

Dell, C. (1979). *Treating the school age stutterer: A guide for clinicians.* Memphis: Speech Foundation of America.

Dell, C. (1993). Treating school-age stutterers. In R. Curlee (Ed.), *Stuttering and related disorders of fluency.* New York: Thieme Medical Publishers.
These are interesting reports written by a masterful clinician.

Luper, H.L., & Mulder, R.L. (1964). *Stuttering: Therapy for children.* Englewood Cliffs, NJ: Prentice-Hall. [Note: Although this book is out of print, many university libraries still have copies.]

This account of therapy is very relevant today despite that fact that it was written more than 30 years ago.

Onslow, M. (1996). *Behavioral management of stuttering.* San Diego: Singular Publishing Group.

Onslow, M., Andrews, C., & Lincoln, M.A. (1994). Control/experimental trial of an operant treatment for early stuttering. *Journal of Speech and Hearing Research, 37,* 1244–1259.

Onslow, M., Costa, L., & Rue, S. (1990). Direct early intervention with stuttering: Some preliminary data. *Journal of Speech and Hearing Disorders, 55,* 405–416.

Because Onslow is constantly updating his procedures, the reader should also see any more recent publications written by Onslow.

Pindzola, R. (1987). *SIP: Stuttering intervention program.* Austin: Pro-Ed.

This program is especially good for younger stutterers.

Ryan, B.P. (1974). *Programmed therapy of stuttering in children and adults.* Springfield, IL: Charles C Thomas.

Ryan, B.P. (1979). Stuttering therapy in a framework of operant conditioning and programmed learning. In H.H. Gregory (Ed.), *Controversies about stuttering therapy.* (pp. 129–173). Baltimore: University Park Press.

Ryan, B.P. (1986). Postscript: Operant therapy for children. In G.H. Shames & H. Rubin (Eds.), *Stuttering: Then and now.* (pp. 431–443). Columbus, OH: Charles E. Merrill.

Ryan is a pioneer and purist in the operant approach to stuttering therapy.

Shames, G.H., & Florance, C.L. (1980). *Stutter-free speech: A goal for therapy.* Columbus, OH: Charles E. Merrill.

This is a detailed description of an operant approach with the authors' innovative supplements to a traditional fluency shaping approach.

Shine, R.E. (1988). *Systematic fluency training for young children,* 3rd ed. Austin: Pro-Ed.

This kit provides all the material to carry out Shine's approach.

Van Riper, C. (1973). Treatment of the beginning stutterer: Prevention. In *The treatment of stuttering.* Englewood Cliffs, NJ: Prentice-Hall.

This is a detailed report, written in Van Riper's unique style, of his pioneering therapy for beginning stutterers. The section on parent counseling applies to parents of children who stutter.

13

Beginning Stutterer: Integration of Approaches

As pointed out in the last chapter, stuttering modification and fluency shaping therapies do not differ substantially in their treatment goals for the beginning stutterer. Thus, integration of these two approaches at this level is relatively easy and straightforward. Our direct treatment of the child is strongly influenced by fluency shaping therapy, although stuttering modification components are included, whereas our parent counseling is most strongly influenced by stuttering modification therapy.

Before beginning the discussion of the integration of stuttering modification and fluency shaping therapies for the child with beginning-level stuttering, let us review the characteristics of a beginning stutterer.

The child is usually between 2 and 8 years of age. Core stuttering behaviors are usually part-word repetitions that are produced rapidly and with irregular rhythm. Some prolongations may be present. Many of these core behaviors contain excessive tension, and the child may also exhibit blocks. Secondary behaviors are typically escape devices, such as eye blinks and head nods, although mild avoidance maneuvers, such as starting sentences with extra sounds, like "uh," may be observed. These struggles with speech are often frustrating so the child may have a self-concept as someone who has trouble talking, but usually he is not concerned about this.

Let us now discuss the integration of the two major therapy approaches with the beginning stutterer.

OUR APPROACH

Clinician's Beliefs

NATURE OF STUTTERING

Even though we have discussed our views on the six clinical issues before, here we summarize our beliefs as they pertain to the beginning stutterer. We believe that predisposing physiological factors interact with developmental and environmental influences to produce or exacerbate repetitions and prolongations. The young stutterer usually feels frustration and responds to these early disfluencies with increased tension in an effort to free himself from them. Furthermore, as the child attempts to cope with these core behaviors, he may develop a variety of escape and possibly starting behaviors that are instrumentally reinforced. Through classical conditioning, certain speech situations may begin to elicit tension responses, which may lead to more severe, tense stutters. Even though the beginning stutterer is aware of his stuttering, he has little or only occasional concern about it.

Like Oliver Bloodstein (1975), we believe that if we can provide a beginning stutterer with a sufficient number of positive, fluent speaking experiences during treatment, this fluency will generalize to more and more speaking situations. We describe how to do this in the following text with a hierarchy for establishing and transferring fluency. Increased fluency reduces the opportunities the child has to respond to any remaining disfluencies with tension, frustration, or escape and starting behaviors and allows time for the child's physiological system to mature and for normal fluency patterns to become stabilized.

We also believe that it is important to reduce, through parent counseling, any developmental or environmental influences that may be contributing to the child's stuttering.

SPEECH BEHAVIORS TARGETED FOR THERAPY

Which speech behaviors do we target for the beginning stutterer? Like fluency shaping clinicians, we primarily target or reinforce the child's fluent responses while using a gradual increase in length and complexity of utterance strategy to establish fluency in the clinical situation. We also model a slower speech pattern and encourage the child to use it in the early steps of therapy to facilitate fluency. This slower pattern is soon faded and once fluency is established in therapy, it is transferred systematically to the child's home environment. Occasionally, the child may continue having hard or tense moments of stuttering on some words during later stages of therapy, so we teach him to stutter easily on these words.

FLUENCY GOALS

Most beginning stutterers will gain or regain spontaneous or normal fluency. This is fortunate because it is usually unrealistic to expect a young child to consistently monitor and modify his speech using controlled fluency or acceptable ways of stuttering.

FEELINGS AND ATTITUDES

As noted earlier, a beginning stutterer experiences only occasional frustration and has little or only intermittent concern about talking. He has not yet developed speech fears or avoidances. Thus, we do not believe it is necessary to focus on feelings and attitudes in therapy with the beginning stutterer.

We do believe it is beneficial, however, to desensitize the child to any fluency disrupting conditions or stimuli that remain near the end of treatment, although this is often not necessary. We countercondition the child's remaining tension responses to fluency disrupting stimuli by repeatedly pairing his new, fluent speech pattern with these stimuli. As the child talks fluently in the presence of stimuli that previously disrupted his fluency, these positive experiences countercondition (i.e., decrease) tension responses. More is said on this topic when we describe our procedures for desensitizing the child to fluency disrupters.

MAINTENANCE PROCEDURES

Our experience has indicated that the beginning stutterer usually maintains his newfound fluency without having to monitor or modify the way he talks. However, it is important to reevaluate the child's fluency periodically for a couple of years after the end of therapy. During these reevaluations, we obtain a sample of the child's speech and discuss his fluency in the "real" world with him and his parents. If possible, we also have the parents record a sample of the child's speech at home. If we find any evidence that the child has regressed, we reenroll him in therapy until his fluency is regained. The length of time between these reevaluations is increased systematically until our contact with the child is completely faded.

CLINICAL METHODS

In terms of clinical methods, our data collection procedures with the beginning stutterer are influenced more by fluency shaping therapy than by stuttering modification therapy. However, this is less true for the structure of therapy. For example, we find that some beginning stutterers respond better to a programmed instruction approach, but others to a less structured, more game-orientated approach. Thus, our establishing and transferring fluency hierarchy can be incorporated into either a programmed instruction format or a game-orientated format. We expand on this point when discussing our clinical procedures in the next section.

In terms of data collection, we believe it is very important to measure the child's frequency of stuttering and rate of speech before beginning treatment, during treatment, and after terminating treatment. Depending on whether we are using a programmed instruction approach or a game-orientated approach during treatment, we either assess all of the child's responses during the entire session or probe or take a sample of the child's responses at the end of each session. The particular measures that we use are discussed in our clinical procedures section.

Clinical Procedures: Direct Treatment of the Child

We base our direct treatment of the beginning stutterer primarily on fluency shaping strategies but include some components of stuttering modification therapy also.[1] Typically, we organize direct treatment of a child into the following four phases: (*a*) establishing and transferring fluency, (*b*) desensitizing the child to fluency disrupters, (*c*) modifying moments of stuttering (optional), and (*d*) maintaining improvement. The third phase, modifying moments of stuttering, is used only if the child is still having some hard or tense moments of stuttering toward the end of the establishing and transferring fluency phase.

ESTABLISHING AND TRANSFERRING FLUENCY

Our goal for this first phase of treatment is for the child to converse fluently with his parents in the home environment. We have found that when beginning stutterers are able to do this, many are already generalizing their fluency automatically to many other speaking situations.

To achieve this goal, we usually guide the child through the 13 steps presented in the establishing and transferring fluency hierarchy in Table 13.1. We refer to these steps simply as our fluency hierarchy. The antecedent events, responses, consequent events, and criteria in Table 13.1 depict a programmed instruction methodology. As noted earlier, some children respond well to a structured or programmed instruction form of therapy, and others do not. The latter children often perform better in a looser, game-orientated therapy. When we use this less structured approach, we follow the same sequence of steps outlined in Table 13.1, but we are not so concerned with implementing the four elements of programmed instruction methodology listed in the previous section. We are also less rigorous in our data collection procedures. We comment on both methods when we discuss our procedures for each step of the fluency hierarchy.

How do you decide whether to use a highly structured or a loosely structured approach? We suggest doing some trial therapy with the child on the first step of the hierarchy, then use the method that works best with the child.

Before discussing the fluency hierarchy in detail, we need to make a few introductory comments about antecedent events, responses, consequent events, and criteria. In our hierarchy, we systematically and gradually modify the antecedent events by doing the following:

1. Change the person to whom the child is talking from the clinician to the parent.
2. Change the physical setting from the clinic to the home.
3. Increase the length and complexity of linguistic units from a single word to a carrier phrase, to one sentence, to two to four sentences, and, finally, to conversational speech.
4. Modify our speech pattern from slow speech to normal speech.
5. Decrease our modeling from a direct model to an indirect model and then to no model at all.

All of these modifications specify the *antecedent events* in Table 13.1 and are defined when we discuss the procedures involved in each step of the hierarchy.

---

[1] For an earlier version of integrating stuttering modification and fluency shaping therapies with the beginning stutterer, the reader is referred to Guitar, B., & Peters, T.J. (1980). The preschool child who stutters. In B. Guitar and T.J. Peters, *Stuttering: An integration of contemporary therapies.* (pp. 65–76). Memphis: Speech Foundation of America.

what clinician does or says

Table 13.1. Outline of Establishing and Transferring Fluency Hierarchy

Antecedent Events	Response	Consequent Events	Criterion
Clinician—Single word. Slow speech. Direct model.	Single word. Fluent, slow speech.	Social. Token (optional). Continuous.	19/20 fluent responses for 5 successive strings of 20.
Clinician—Single word. Slow speech. Indirect model.	"	"	"
Clinician—Carrier phrase + word. Slow speech. Indirect model.	Carrier phrase + word. Fluent, slow speech.	"	"
Clinician and parent— Carrier phrase + word. Slow speech. Indirect model.	"	"	"
Parent—Carrier phrase + word. Slow speech. Indirect model.	"	"	"
Parent at home—Carrier phrase + word. Slow speech. Indirect model.	"	"	"
Clinician—Sentence. Slow speech. Indirect model.	Sentence. Fluent, slow speech.	"	95% fluent responses for 2 successive sessions.
Clinician—Sentence. Normal speech. Indirect model.	Sentence. Fluent, normal speech.	"	"
Clinician—2 to 4 sentences. Normal speech. Indirect model.	2 to 4 sentences. Fluent, normal speech.	"	"
Clinician—Conversation. Normal speech. No model.	Conversation. Fluent, normal speech.	Social. Token (optional). Intermittent.	1 SW/M or less for 2 successive sessions.
Clinician and parent— Conversation. Normal speech. No model	"	"	"
Parent—Conversation. Normal speech. No model.	"	"	"
Parent at home— Conversation. Normal speech. No model.	"	"	"

SW/M, stuttered words per minute.

19 fluent for 100 words
-if 19 or 20 correct, move to next step

Responses are what the child does in responding to the antecedent events we provide. First of all, we want the child's responses to be fluent. Second, we want them to approximate the length and complexity of the antecedent event's linguistic unit. Finally, we want the child's speech to resemble the pattern that is modeled. All these do not always occur, and we comment on the acceptable limits of the child's responses when we discuss the steps of the hierarchy.

Consequent events are the stimuli we present contingent on the child's responses. We generally ignore any stuttering as the child progresses through the hierarchy, but we reinforce fluent responses. We always use social reinforcement and token reinforcement when necessary. Our experience suggests that token reinforcement is not always needed. In early steps, we typically use a continuous reinforcement schedule, which changes to an intermittent schedule in later steps. We'll say more about the type and schedule of reinforcement later.

The *criterion* in Table 13.1 specifies how well the child must speak before going to the next step. We believe it is important for the child to be exhibiting a high percentage of fluent responses on a sufficient number of trials or for an adequate period of time before we move on. In other words, we want the child to establish a fairly solid foundation of fluency at one level of difficulty before advancing to the next. Ultimately, we want his speech to contain no more than an occasional easy repetition or prolongation when he has completed the fluency hierarchy. This is compatible with our fluency goal for the beginning stutterer of spontaneous or normal fluency. We will have more to say about criterion levels when we discuss the various steps of the hierarchy (Fig. 13.1).

Discussion of the procedures we use for each step of the fluency hierarchy proceeds as follows: first, we share our experiences and recommendations about the antecedent events, responses, consequent events, and criteria to use. Then, we comment on data collection procedures. Finally, we describe a typical activity that could be used for that step. Throughout, we comment on how we would vary the procedures depending on whether we are using a programmed instruction approach or a more game-orientated style of therapy.

Clinician, Single-Word, Slow-Speech, Direct Model

As suggested earlier, the clinician may want to do some trial therapy during this first step of the fluency hierarchy to determine whether the child will work better in a programmed instruction format or in a less structured, more game-orientated approach. Our experience suggests that although some children prefer one and some the other, both will work.

In terms of antecedent events, the first two are easy to define: "clinician" indicates that only the clinician is present in the therapy room with the child, and "single word" is self-explanatory. "Slow speech," is characterized by a slow rate that is achieved by slightly prolonging or stretching all the sounds in the word. A gentle onset of phonation is used to

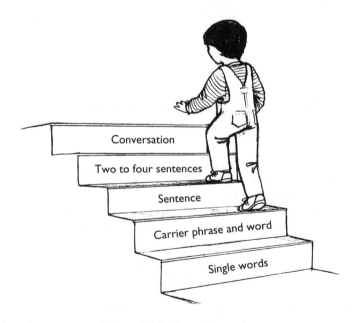

Figure 13.1. Fluency hierarchy.

initiate the word, and soft or relaxed articulatory contacts are used in producing the rest of it. This is similar to the speech pattern we taught the advanced stutterer in Chapter 9. (See Using Fluency Enhancing Behaviors and Modifying the Moments of Stuttering, in Chapter 9.) We find this slow speech pattern to be very facilitative of fluency in the beginning stutterer. In addition to modeling this slow speech pattern, we instruct the child to say the word "slow and smooth" or "slow and easy," just as we said it. We believe that "slow and smooth" is more appropriate for the child who is having a lot of effortless repetitions, while "slow and easy" is better for the child who is doing more struggling.

We should comment at this time about our overall speaking pattern during therapy sessions. We speak in a slow, relaxed manner, but not so slow that it sounds abnormal. Like Mr. Rogers on television, we use normal intonation and plenty of pauses to convey to the child that we are not in a hurry. We continue to use this rate throughout all the steps of the fluency hierarchy.

A "direct model" provides the child with both the linguistic unit, in this case a single word, and the speech pattern, in this case slow speech, that he is to imitate. For example, we might show the child a picture of a car and say "car," using a slow speech pattern. The child is then expected to say "car," using the same slow speech pattern we modeled.

"Responses" are what the child does in responding to the antecedent events just discussed. In terms of the continuity dimension of fluency, we expect the child's responses to be fluent, but there are two other aspects of a response that we need to comment on here. The first is the linguistic unit produced by the child. We expect the child to produce a linguistic unit that is similar in length and complexity to our models. At the single word level, obviously there is no problem with the length of the child's utterance. Sometimes, however, a problem arises when the child makes comments between responses and these asides contain moments of stuttering. Keep in mind that we are trying to establish a basal level of fluency and do not want stuttering mixed in with it. At such times, it is important to instruct the child not to talk between turns. We may even tell him that we will be taking a break soon and that he can then tell us whatever he wishes.

A second aspect of responses that warrants comment is the speech pattern produced by the child. We expect the child to imitate our slow speech pattern during these early steps of the fluency hierarchy. Although some children accurately imitate our slow speech pattern and are fluent. However, other children don't, but are fluent anyway. We believe that an effort should be made during these first steps to get the child to modify his speech pattern to some degree. For example, we may say "Don't forget to talk slow and smooth like I am," or "That was smooth, but make it just a little slower next time." We find that, if the child modifies his speech pattern during early steps of the hierarchy, his fluency is more stable on later steps.

Now, for some comments on consequent events. As indicated earlier, we generally ignore any stuttering the child may have, but reinforce fluent responses. Typically, we use two types of reinforcement in our approach with the beginning stutterer. We always use social reinforcement, and we sometimes use token reinforcement. When socially reinforcing or praising the child for fluent responses, we keep varying our choice of words. We say, "That's great," "You're really doing well," "Good job," and so on. We do not want to keep saying "good" over and over until it loses its impact or influence on the child's behavior. We also think it is beneficial to appropriately and frequently incorporate "slow and smooth" or "slow and easy" into our reinforcement and comments to the child because we believe this helps the child to become more aware of the appropriate speech pattern and to acquire it more readily.

We do not use token reinforcement routinely with a beginning stutterer. Our experience suggests it is often not necessary. However, when the child is not motivated to come or participate in treatment, token reinforcement procedures can be very helpful (Fig. 13.2). The clinician needs to be alert to such motivational problems, particularly during these early steps of the hierarchy. We have found that the more game- or play-orientated the therapy, the less the need for token reinforcement. In this situation, motivation is provided by innately enjoyable activities. Conversely, the more drill-like the therapy, the greater the need for token reinforcement to provide motivation. Thus, how to set up and run a token reinforcement procedure is discussed next.

First of all, we explain to the child and his parents that the child will earn a token, (i.e., a chip, bean, or tally mark) for each fluent response or utterance he produces in therapy. We then discuss the sorts of things or activities the child enjoys and go on to explain that when the child earns a predetermined number of tokens, he will win one of these prizes or the opportunity to engage in an enjoyable activity. It is important that the child truly wants these "prizes" or backup reinforcers, because if he does not, he will not be motivated to work for the tokens.

Backup reinforcers do not need to be expensive and parents provide us with many of them. We have used pieces of gum, balloons, inexpensive toys and trinkets, opportunities to draw on the blackboard or to play a computer game, and so on. Once a "menu" of backup reinforcers is established, we determine the "price" or number of tokens needed to win each item. With younger beginning stutterers, we find it effective to set prices at a level that allows them to win a prize every session. This maintains interest and motivation in therapy. With an older beginning stutterer, prices can usually be set higher because this child does not need to receive backup reinforcers as frequently to maintain interest in earning tokens. It also enhances motivation if the child receives frequent feedback regarding the number of tokens he still needs to win a prize. Such techniques as transferring tokens from one cup to another help the child maintain motivation.

We typically use a continuous reinforcement schedule in the early steps of the hierarchy by reinforcing every fluent response. If we are using a programmed instruction for-

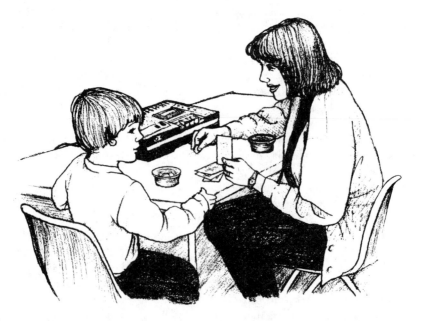

Figure 13.2. Token reinforcement procedures can be very helpful at times.

mat, we typically use a criterion level of at least 19 fluent responses in 20 consecutive responses for 5 successive strings of 20 responses before moving to the next step. In this case, we will need to record every response to determine whether or not the child meets the criterion. A somewhat less rigorous procedure we sometimes use is to score a probe of 20 responses at the end of a therapy session. In this case, if the child is fluent in 19 of 20 responses, we go on to the next step. If we are not using a programmed instruction approach, we expect the child to have no more than four or five stuttered responses during an entire therapy session and keep track of them in our head. In our experience, most beginning stutterers can meet the latter criteria within one or two therapy sessions.

A typical activity for this step is "picture identification." This requires only a stack of picture cards. Most often we use a variety of clinician-made and commercially available objects, pictures, parts of articulation and language kits, and children's games. The pictures should depict objects that can be named with a single word and should include all word-initial phonemes in the language. We name a picture, using slow speech, and ask the child to name the same picture while using slow, fluent speech. If the child does it, we reinforce him enthusiastically and let him know that his speech was either "slow and smooth" or "slow and easy," depending on which one we decided to use. If the child needs token reinforcement for motivational purposes, we also give him a token. Depending on whether we use a programmed or less structured therapy, we record the child's responses, more or less rigorously, to determine whether he is meeting criteria. This is an example of the kinds of activities we use for this step. In fact, we usually have three or four different activities like this planned for each session to help maintain the child's interest and involvement in therapy.

Clinician, Single-Word, Slow-Speech, Indirect Model

This step differs from the first step in only one aspect—the model that is provided for the child. We now provide the child with only an "indirect model." An indirect model involves our providing the child with the speech pattern he is to reproduce but not the exact linguistic unit he is to say. For example, we may name an object, using a slow speech pattern. The child then names a different object, also using our slow speech pattern. With the indirect model, the child hears the slow speech pattern between each of his responses, but all the other antecedent events remain the same.

The responses, consequent events, and criteria that were used in the first step also continue to apply here. Likewise, the same methods, therapy structure, and data collection procedures continue to be used in this step. We are beginning to gradually move up our more easy to more difficult hierarchy by modifying one antecedent event at a time. This same strategy will continue to be used, with only one exception, as we progress from step to step in the hierarchy.

A representative activity for this step is "surprise box." This requires only a box with various objects in it. We close our eyes, pick an object from the box, and name it, using slow speech. We then ask the child to close his eyes, pick another object from the box, and name it, using slow, fluent speech. If the child says the word, using slow, fluent speech, we reinforce him as before. If he is fluent but doesn't use the slow speech pattern, we tell him, "That's good and smooth, but remember to talk slowly on the next word." If the child stutters, we either ignore it or we remind him to talk slow and smooth or slow and easy on the next word. Again, depending on which structure of therapy works best for the child, we implement the surprise box activity in either a programmed instruction format or a less structured, more game-orientated style of interaction. Most beginning stutterers complete this step in one or two therapy sessions.

Clinician, Carrier Phrase + Word, Slow-Speech, Indirect Model

We begin to increase the difficulty of the task by having the child say something longer and a little more complex. We now use "carrier phrase + word." A carrier phrase is a pre-determined sequence of words that precedes the stimulus word. For example, "I see the _____," or "I think this is a _____." All the other antecedent events remain the same.

We expect the child's response to be slow and free of stutters. We also want his responses to use the same carrier phrase that we model. However, we are providing an indirect model, so the child needs to use a different stimulus word. The consequent events, criteria, and clinical methods for this step do not change.

A good activity for this step is "flashlight," which involves our placing different picture cards around the therapy room. We turn off the lights and when the child spots a picture card with the flashlight, we say, "I see the _____," using slow speech. Then, the child shines the light on a different picture card and says, "I see the _____," using slow, fluent speech. We use several similar activities in a typical therapy session, but should offer a word of caution at this point. In selecting carrier phrases for these activities, it is important to vary them. We have seen a few children's fluency become associated with specific carrier phrases, but varying the carrier phrases avoids this problem. Most beginning stutterers can meet our criteria for this step in one or two therapy sessions.

Clinician and Parent, Carrier Phrase + Word, Slow-Speech, Indirect Model

We now begin transferring the child's fluency to the parent. We have one of the parents join us in the therapy room. Everything else about this step, the other antecedent events, responses, consequent events, and criteria, are similar to those of the previous step.

We believe it is beneficial to begin transferring or generalizing the child's use of slow, fluent speech to the home early in the hierarchy, rather than waiting until he is fluent at the conversational level with us. Our experience suggests that this may facilitate the transfer process in the long run, as well as providing some additional benefits for the parent counseling process. First, it gets parents directly involved early in their child's treatment. Second, when parents have to use the slow speech pattern while interacting with their child in therapy, they begin to appreciate how difficult it can be to change the way we talk, providing them with some insight into what their child is going through.

When the parent joins the child in therapy, there are a couple of tasks we need to accomplish initially. First, we need to teach the parent to use the slow speech pattern. If he or she has been observing our therapy sessions, the task will be much easier. If not, we will need to spend some time explaining and modeling the slow speech pattern. We have found it beneficial to have the child help us teach parents and evaluate their use of slow speech. Children love to teach parents how to do something! Second, we need to teach the parent to evaluate, reinforce, and record the child's responses correctly. This involves some explaining and modeling on our part. During the first session or two with the parent in the therapy room, we take the lead. Then, over the next session or so, we gradually turn the responsibility for the session over to the parent. Thus, the parent provides the slow speech model and reinforces and records the child's responses. We remain a participant in therapy activities, but the parent is now functioning as the clinician.

An activity that we use at this point in therapy is "concentration." This is a game that involves placing matched pairs of picture cards face down on a table. The parent turns over two cards, one at a time. Before turning each card the parent says, using slow speech, "I think this is a _____." If the two cards match, the parent keeps the pair. If they don't, the cards are placed face down again on the table; we or the child take our respective turns, using slow, fluent speech. As on other steps, three or four such activities are used for each therapy session. Once the parent has helped the child meet the predetermined criterion level, we move on to the next step.

Parent, Carrier Phrase + Word, Slow-Speech, Indirect Model

The only change we make in this step of the hierarchy is to remove ourselves physically from the therapy room. Everything else remains the same. In our work environment, we have the ability to observe the parent conduct therapy with the child through a one-way mirror. If these facilities were not available to us, we would observe the parent and child while sitting quietly in a corner of the room.

There are a couple of reasons for including this step in the hierarchy. First, we want to make sure that the child continues to be fluent when we are not present. Second, we want to make sure that the parent is reinforcing fluent responses and counting stuttered responses just as we have been up to this point in therapy. In short, we want to be certain that the parent can carry out the same clinical methods we have been using with the child without our being present. This is very important for the successful implementation of the next step of the hierarchy.

Good activities for this step include games like "Go Fish" and "Old Maid," because they require players to use a carrier phrase when taking their turn. These games are also readily available, and most parents and children are familiar with them.

Once the child has met the criterion for this step and the parent is performing well in the role of a clinician, we move on to the next two steps.

Parent-Home, Carrier Phrase + Word, Slow-Speech, Indirect Model

With two exceptions, this step is the same as the previous one. The first exception is that the parent now conducts therapy sessions at home, not in the clinic. All other antecedent events stay the same, as do consequent events. For example, the parent engages in the same activities and games, or similar ones, that were used in the three previous steps. If the child has been receiving token reinforcement, this continues. The tokens he earns at home are added to those earned with the clinician to buy backup reinforcers.

The second exception is that the child does not move up the hierarchy as soon as he reaches the criterion. Instead, he continues on this step, practicing carrier phrases and words with an indirect model at home with his parent until therapy with the clinician has prepared him for the leap to conversational speech. We ask parents to engage in this transfer activity with their child for 10 or 15 minutes a day, 4 or 5 days a week. The clinician and child continue up the hierarchy until the child is ready to engage in fluent conversation with his parents at home.

We believe this frequent home practice is beneficial to the outcome of the treatment program and is reasonable in terms of the time required. In our experience, it does not become burdensome for either the parents or the child. We regularly check with parents to see if there are any problems and if the child continues to be fluent during practice sessions. After sessions have been going well for a while, some parents have asked us if the other parent can become involved in these activities. This is fine if the child continues to be fluent.

Clinician, Sentence, Slow-Speech, Indirect Model

In this step, we move up the hierarchy by increasing the length, complexity, and spontaneity of the linguistic unit as we move to the "sentence" level. This requires the child to make up his own sentences in response to objects, pictures, or questions. In keeping with our strategy of changing only one antecedent event at a time, all other antecedent events remain the same.

In terms of the child's responses, we count a sentence as fluent only if it contains no moments of stuttering. Sentences must be completely fluent to be fluent. We also want the child to generate grammatically complete sentences. However, if the child doesn't give us a grammatically complete sentence, we do not make an issue of it. Our prime goal is a fluent sentence.

Sometimes, the child gets stuck in a linguistic rut and repeatedly produces sentences that are similar in grammatical form. It is as if the child is stuck back at the carrier phrase level. For example, the child may say, "I see the ball," "I see the car," "I see the house," and so on. We do not want the child's fluency associated with only one form. So, if this occurs, we suggest other types of responses and use a variety of sentences as examples in our indirect modeling. We have found that it will not be long before the child gets out of this rut.

At this step, we use a continuous reinforcement schedule for the child's fluent responses, but we change some of the criteria. In our experience, it is more difficult for children to be fluent while generating their own sentences than when saying carrier phrases + words. For this reason, we think it is important that our criteria be more rigorous on this step and for the child practice more at this level. Thus, the child has to maintain a high level of fluency for at least two sessions before we move on to the next step. If we are using a programmed instruction approach, we ordinarily require the child to have 95% fluent responses for two successive therapy sessions. This requires us to score and record each sentence so that we can compute the percentage of correct responses for the session. If we are just taking a probe of response performance toward the end of each session, we may score only 10 to 20 sentences and calculate the percentage of correct responses from these. In this case, we still want the child to be successful for at least 2 consecutive days. If we are using a less structured form of therapy, the child is allowed only four or five sentences that contain moments of stuttering during a therapy session. We can keep track of these in our head. Again, we still want at least two successive days of successful fluency.

"Barrier games" are good activities for this step. These games require a barrier, such as a piece of cardboard, between the clinician and the child. The barrier only needs to be large enough so that the clinician and child cannot see the other's sheet of paper on the table in front of her or him. When we use a barrier game, we instruct the child to draw something on his paper. For example, we may say, "Draw a horse in the bottom right corner of your page." We then draw the same thing in the same location on our sheet. Next, the child tells us to draw something somewhere on our sheet of paper. At the same time, he draws the same item in the same place on his sheet. After each of us has taken a number of turns, we remove the barrier and compare our pictures. In this activity, the child still hears us model (indirect model) slow speech during our turns, but generates his own sentences.

Clinician, Sentence, Normal-Speech, Indirect Model

It is now time to fade out the slow speech pattern and to begin modeling a "normal speech" pattern for the child's responses. Our normal speech models are relaxed and are spoken at a slow, normal rate. We tell the child that he can talk just a little bit faster now and listen carefully to our speech. We also remind the child to continue to talk "smooth" or "easy," whichever we have been using with him. Usually, we have no problem getting the child to change his slow speech pattern to normal speech. In fact, many are likely to have increased their rate somewhat over the last few steps of the hierarchy. All the other antecedent events, consequent events, and criteria for this step remain the same as for the preceding one.

An activity we sometimes use on this step is "scrapbook." Here, the child and the clinician paste pictures of things we both like. We may make just one scrapbook for the two of us, or each of us may have our own. We begin by cutting a picture from a magazine, think of something to say about it, and model normal speech. Then, we glue the picture in the scrapbook. The child then cuts out a different picture; makes up a sentence, using fluent, normal speech; and glues his picture in the scrapbook. If necessary, we instruct the child to slightly increase his speaking rate and reinforce responses that are fluent, normal speech. This activity may continue for 10 to 20 minutes and is usually only one of several activities that we use during a given therapy session.

Clinician, Two to Four Sentences, Normal-Speech, Indirect Model

Once again we increase the length and complexity of the linguistic unit, this time to two to four sentences. First, the clinician generates two to four sentences about one or more pictures or objects. Then the child produces two to four sentences in response to different pictures or stimuli. Thus, the clinician is still providing an indirect model of a normal speech pattern between each of the child's responses. On this step, we want the child's response to be longer than just one sentence, but we do not want him to go on talking forever. This is a transitional step, which immediately precedes the move to conversation. All the other aspects of the step remain the same.

A good activity for this step is "sequencing cards," using the cards found in many commercially available language kits. We begin by arranging a set of cards, usually three to five, in a sequence, then telling a two- to four-sentence story based on the cards while providing the child with an indirect model of fluent, normal speech. The child takes the next set of cards, arranges them in a sequence, and tells a story using fluent, normal speech. As usual, we reinforce his fluent responses that are two to four sentences long. The child has come a long way from the first step of the hierarchy, when he was reinforced for saying a fluent word. When the child meets the criterion for this step, we move on to conversation.

Clinician, Conversation, Normal Speech, No Model

Unlike all of the preceding steps, we change two antecedent events on this step. First, the linguistic task is "conversation" while we interact with the child in games or play activities. Second, we provide the child with "no model." We continue to speak in a relaxed manner at a slow, normal rate, but we no longer take turns while interacting with the child. Thus, the child does not hear us model a normal speech pattern between each of his responses.

During the conversation step, we also begin to use intermittent reinforcement. We now reinforce the child after he has completed a half-dozen or so fluent utterances or sentences. It is important to present reinforcement during pauses in the conversation so as not to interrupt the child while he is speaking. As he experiences more and more success on this conversation step, we gradually increase the amount of fluency required before he is reinforced, beginning the process of fading our reinforcement of the child's fluency.

We also change the measure we use for the criterion on this step. Instead of percentage of fluent responses, we begin to use stuttered syllables per minute (SS/M) or stuttered words per minute (SW/M), both of which are much easier to calculate at the conversational level. For example, all one needs to do to compute SS/M is to count the number of stuttered syllables the child has during a therapy session, measure his talking time with a stopwatch during the session, and divide the stuttered syllables by the time. If we are using a programmed instruction approach, we typically use 1 SS/M or less for two successive sessions as our criterion. If we decide not to measure fluency over the entire session, we usually take probes of the child's fluency during the last 5 or 10 minutes of each therapy session and determine his SS/M for these periods. Of course, we still want him to exhibit 1 SS/M or less during the probes for two successive therapy sessions. If we choose not measure the child's talking time during therapy sessions, we expect him to have no more than 5 or 10 stuttered syllables per session for 2 successive therapy sessions.

As the reader may remember, we said that the beginning stutterer gains or regains spontaneous or normal fluency. We further stated that it is unrealistic to expect a child this young to consistently monitor and modify his speech to use controlled fluency. At about this point in the fluency hierarchy, the child occasionally seems to be monitoring his speech to use a fluent, smooth or easy speech pattern, but often he is not monitoring. He is just being spontaneously fluent.

We sometimes use "art projects" as an activity during this step of the hierarchy. We engage the child in conversation while we work together on one of these projects. The projects are often related to a central theme, such as holidays, or the seasons of the year. We find it very easy to reinforce and measure the child's fluency during these activities.

Clinician and Parent, Conversation, Normal Speech, No Model

For some time, one of the parents and the child have been practicing fluent, slow speech in carrier phrases + words at home. Now, it is time to transfer fluent, normal conversational speech to the parent. At this point, we bring the parent back to the therapy room. This is the only aspect of this step that differs from the preceding step.

When we bring the parent back to therapy, we need to familiarize him or her with the new, normal speech pattern. Again, if the parent has been observing the therapy, this is usually a relatively easy task. If the parent has not been observing the therapy, this may require some explaining and modeling. Usually, getting the parent to use a slow, normal rate and a relaxed manner of speaking is not a problem. The only trouble comes when the parent seems to be an innately rapid speaker. In such cases, we most likely have already been discussing this problem with the parent during our counseling sessions. We also find it helpful to have the child critique his parent's speech rate during therapy. Children love this role, and parents usually respond well to it. We must also spend time explaining the new, intermittent reinforcement schedule and the new criterion level to parents. They will need practice in using these, too.

Activities that seem to work well in therapy at this time include open-ended conversations with the child about what he did at school that day or what he plans to do that evening; spontaneous conversations that arise while playing such games as Candyland or checkers; and conversations that develop while playing with toy farm sets, doll houses, computer games, and so on.

Parent, Conversation, Normal Speech, No Model

As we did on the steps that transferred fluent, slow speech in carrier phrases + words to the parent, we again remove ourselves from the therapy situation. We do this by observing the parent and child through a one-way mirror or from the corner of the therapy room. All the other components are identical with the previous step.

This step is important for two reasons. One, we want to make sure that the child maintains his fluency in conversation when we are no longer present. Two, we want to make sure that the parent is reinforcing and evaluating the child's fluency accurately. To evaluate these two sets of behaviors, we observe the interaction between the parent and the child in conversational activities. We reinforce the parent for the things that are going well and suggest ways to improve those things that may not be going well.

When the child has met the criterion for this step and the parent is working well as the clinician, we move to the last step of the hierarchy, "parent-home, conversation, normal speech, no model," as well as to the next phase of our direct treatment of the child, "desensitizing the child to fluency disrupters."

Parent-Home, Conversation, Normal Speech, No Model

This step is similar to the previous step, except that the parent now engages the child in conversation at home, not in the therapy room. We ask the parent to engage in a transfer step with the child for 10 or 15 minutes a day, 4 or 5 days a week. This replaces the earlier "parent-home, carrier phrase + word, slow speech, indirect model" step in daily practice sessions at home. Besides using some of the conversational activities that were used in the preceding steps, many parents simply set aside a specific period each day for their child to practice using his smooth or easy speech. Typical practice periods include the times after school, after dinner, or before bed. We want the child to maintain the same level of fluency during these periods that he was having in therapy, and we regularly check with the parent to make sure he is doing so. Some parents gradually get the other parent involved in these activities, and they continue these practice sessions at home until the child is into the "maintaining improvement" phase of therapy.

We find that many beginning stutterers are already transferring their fluency, usually spontaneous fluency, to many other speaking situations when they reach this point in treatment. Thus, just completing this hierarchy is all that is necessary. However, in some cases a child's fluency does not transfer automatically to all situations, and additional steps are needed. These may include bringing siblings or playmates to therapy sessions, having the child's teacher attend several sessions, bringing grandparents to therapy, or conducting therapy in other physical settings, such as the child's favorite fast-food restaurant. These additional steps vary for each child, but there is a common theme: the clinician and the child meet with other persons or in other physical settings, and the child practices his smooth or easy speech. The other persons involved should be aware of the purpose of such sessions, and the child's fluency should be treated openly and matter-of-factly.

The activities used during these sessions should be appropriate for the situation. For example, if one of the child's playmates comes to a therapy session, it is appropriate for everyone to play a game that the children enjoy. During the game, the beginning stutterer practices his smooth or easy speech, and the clinician reinforces it. By going through these additional steps, the child's fluency continues to generalize to speaking situations throughout his speaking day. The establishing and transferring fluency phase of therapy comes to an end when the child is exhibiting spontaneous or controlled fluency, but usually spontaneous fluency, in all speaking situations.

DESENSITIZING THE CHILD TO FLUENCY DISRUPTERS

As we indicated before, when the child has completed the "parent, conversation, normal speech, no model" step of the fluency hierarchy, we usually begin the desensitization phase of our direct treatment. With some children it is not necessary. Our goal is to desensitize the child to any remaining fluency disrupting stimuli that still precipitate stuttering for him. Many such fluency disrupters have already been eliminated or significantly reduced as part of our parent counseling, and we talk about this process soon. However, some fluency disrupters, because of their nature, cannot be eliminated from the child's life. The child needs to live with them. For example, some parents report at this time that when their child gets excited, he still has some stuttering. They also report that other conditions, such as visits from relatives or the child's recounting of a long story, still tend to disrupt his fluency. It varies with the child. We believe that these children can be "inoculated" against relapse by being desensitized to these remaining fluency disrupters.

Our procedures are similar to those developed by Van Riper (see Chapter 12), but with some variations. As you may recall, Van Riper created a basal level of fluency or a few minutes of fluent speech by providing simple fluency models for the child, by engaging the child in rhythm or timing activities, and by reinforcing the child for fluency without him being aware of it. We, on the other hand, by taking the child through our fluency hierarchy, already have him conversing fluently with us for an entire therapy session. This is our basal level of fluency.

Suppose the child's fluency does break down when he becomes excited. How do we desensitize him to this excitement? We are very open with the child regarding our goal. We tell him that we are going to try to get him excited and his job is to use his smooth or easy speech in spite of it. We then engage the child in an activity that excites him. For example, we saw a child with beginning-level stuttering in a therapy room that we emptied of furniture except for a trash can, which served as a basket for a foam rubber basketball. At first, we kept the tempo of our basketball game slow, and the child was reminded to use his slow and easy speech. When he was fluent, we praised his smooth speech. When he stuttered, we reminded him to use smooth and easy speech. When the excitement seemed too great for him to monitor his speech, the game was slowed down. We did not want to push the child beyond his fluency's breaking point. When the child was fluent for several minutes, we sped up the tempo of the game. Finally, after a number of therapy sessions like this, arms and legs and the ball were flying all over the therapy room, but the child remained fluent. Excitement no longer disrupted his fluency. We were on the way to desensitizing the child to excitement.

We are confident that the clinician will be able to think of other, individually tailored activities for desensitizing a beginning stutterer to fluency disrupters. Whatever the activity, it is important to do the following: let the child know you are going to be introducing the fluency disrupter, tell him he is to use his smooth or easy speech, reinforce him for using it, and gradually and systematically expose him to stronger and stronger doses of the fluency disrupter. Be careful not to overexpose him to a fluency disrupter. We do not want his fluency to substantially break down. This desensitization process should continue until the child is in the "maintaining improvement" phase of treatment or until there are no more fluency disrupters.

MODIFYING THE MOMENTS OF STUTTERING (OPTIONAL)

Modifying the child's moments of stuttering is an optional phase of our treatment program for the beginning stutterer. Most beginning stutterers respond well to the fluency hierarchy just described and do not need this phase. A few, however, may still have some tense moments of stuttering during later steps of the hierarchy. These residual stutters are not as hard or as tense as they were originally, but some tension is still present. They are milder versions of the child's earlier stuttering. We believe it is important to give these children a tool for coping with these remaining stutters. Thus, we teach them how to stutter easily. During therapy sessions, we alternate teaching the child to stutter easily with work on the remaining steps of the hierarchy. Once the child has learned to stutter easily, we can work on a step of the hierarchy and easy stuttering at the same time. The child can be practicing his fluent, easy speech pattern; if he happens to have a tense moment of stuttering, he can practice stuttering easily on it.

In teaching the child with beginning stuttering to stutter easily, we adopt some of Van Riper's (1973) and Dell's (1979) ideas for treating the intermediate stutterer, whom Van Riper calls the young, confirmed stutterer and Dell calls the confirmed stutterer. We explain to the child that there are two ways of stuttering on a word, a "hard way," and an "easy way." Then we model both ways for him. The hard way should resemble the child's typical, tense, residual moments of stuttering; this may vary from child to child. The easy way consists of saying a word slowly and loosely, slightly stretching out each sound in the word. A gentle onset of phonation is used to initiate the word, and soft articulatory contacts are used throughout the remainder of the word. We remind the child of the "slow and easy"[2] speech we used in the early steps of the fluency hierarchy. We point out that the slow and easy speech is similar to this easy way of stuttering.

When the child understands what we mean by hard and easy stuttering, we engage him in some enjoyable activities during which we repeatedly put easy stuttering into our speech. We also encourage the child to practice using voluntary, easy stuttering in his own speech. At first, we do this with single words or short utterances; later, it is beneficial to practice while we are conversing. We want the child to develop the ability to use slow movements, gentle onsets, and soft articulatory contacts on individual words in connected speech. We also want him to feel comfortable producing words this way, so we strongly reinforce him for using voluntary easy stuttering. Some children who develop the ability to use these forms of voluntary easy stuttering automatically begin to replace tense moments of stuttering with easy ones. When this doesn't occur, we teach the child to modify his moments of stuttering as he is experiencing them. To do this, we suggest the following progression of procedures.

First, we model how a modification will look and sound. We begin by simulating the child's typical, residual moment of stuttering. Then we ease out of it with slow, relaxed movements. We will need to provide this model for the child many times. In essence, this is a Van Riper pull-out, but we call it easy stuttering when talking with a child.

Second, we have the child join us in simulating his stuttering and ease out of it with slow, relaxed movements. In other words, both of us stuttering easily in unison. We want the child to feel what it is like to turn a hard stutter into an easy stutter. We give the child lots of support and reinforcement, because it often is not easy for a child to deal directly with his moments of stuttering in this way.

Third, we help the child catch himself in a moment of stuttering and then ease out of it into the rest of the word, using slow, relaxed movements. We have found it helpful to squeeze the child's arm when he is caught in a moment of stuttering. When we squeeze his arm, he is to hang on to his stutter. Then, as we slowly release our grip on his arm, he is to ease out of the moment of stuttering and complete the rest of the word, using slow, relaxed articulatory movements. We may even join the child at this time and help him ease out of his stutter. We give the child a lot of support and reinforcement during this procedure. It takes time and practice to develop this skill, but once the child learns to develop it, he is well on his way to learning easy stuttering.

---

[2] Because this child still has some mild, tense, residual stutters, it is likely that he had some tense struggle behaviors when he began therapy; thus, we probably used "slow and easy" with him, instead of "slow and smooth."

MAINTAINING IMPROVEMENT

After the child is exhibiting spontaneous fluency or controlled fluency in all speaking situations, we move into the maintaining improvement phase of therapy. We do not dismiss the child at this point; rather, we gradually reduce our active treatment, beginning with scheduling a therapy session weekly for a month, then biweekly for 1 or 2 months. If things continue to go well, we begin to see him for a series of reevaluations.

During these reevaluations, we obtain a sample of the child's speech and talk with the child and his parents about how his speech has been since the last appointment. We begin monthly reevaluations for several months, then every other month for several more months, then, once a semester for 1 year, after which we dismiss the child. Many times, we have the parents bring us a recorded sample of the child talking at home. If the child seems to be regressing at any point in this process, we return him to active, more intensive treatment. The nature of this treatment depends on what the child's problem seems to be, but it usually involves the child spending more time in one or more of the three phases of treatment he has previously completed. Most beginning stutterers spend approximately 2 years in this last phase of treatment.

Clinical Procedures: Family Counseling

We have a number of objectives in mind when we counsel families of a beginning stutterer as his direct treatment is proceeding. These include (*a*) explaining the treatment program and the parents' role in it, (*b*) discussing the possible causes of stuttering, (*c*) identifying and reducing fluency disrupters, and (*d*) identifying and increasing fluency enhancing situations.

We may begin to work on some of these objectives, especially the first two, during the initial evaluation. Then we focus on the others in later counseling sessions. We let families' most immediate concerns dictate the topics of our conversations. By showing respect for families' concerns first, we increase the likelihood that they will be amenable to changing some of their habits and household routines later on. Some topics may be covered only briefly at first, then discussed repeatedly over several sessions. As we learn more about the child and his family and as parents learn more about stuttering and its treatment, old issues are revisited from new points of view. For example, we may feel the need to explore some aspect of the child's life further, or the family may have more questions about a specific topic. Thus, counseling the family of a beginning stutterer is not a step-by-step set of procedures; it is an ongoing, dynamic process (Fig. 13.3).

EXPLAINING THE TREATMENT PROGRAM AND THE PARENTS' ROLE IN IT

Most parents want to know the nature of a treatment program and how long it is going to take. They want to have a good idea of what is involved. After all, it is likely to have a considerable impact on their time and activities for the next year or two. At this point, we describe the fluency hierarchy and their role in transfer steps in particular. We may also comment briefly on their role in identifying and reducing fluency disrupters, to be discussed shortly. Ordinarily, we do not explain desensitizing the child to fluency disrupters or modifying his moments of stuttering at this time. We can explain these phases later at a more appropriate time. We usually tell parents that it is best if we see their child two or three times per week for 30 to 45 minutes each time. We tell them that therapy may take anywhere from 6 months to 2 years.

Parents often ask what they should tell their child about coming to speech therapy. Many times, parents have been told or have read that they should not mention stuttering to him.

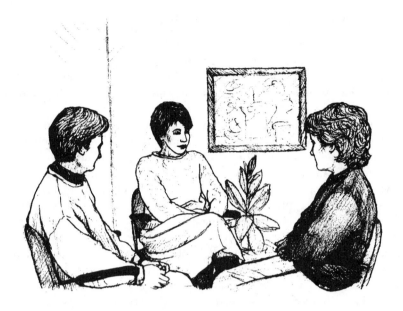

Figure 13.3. Parent counseling is an ongoing process.

We believe this is unwise. In our experience, most children with beginning stuttering know that they have problems talking and are not deeply embarrassed by it or ashamed of it. They are aware that they have trouble getting words out on occasion, and they often know that they "stutter." When significant adults in their lives don't talk about it, children often begin to think that their speech must be so terrible that even their mother and father are too ashamed to talk about it. This is an awful message to give a child. It is wiser to talk openly about stuttering. We suggest that parents tell their child that he will be going to speech school to get help with his stuttering or talking. Usually, we use the word stuttering; it is a commonly used and descriptive word. Occasionally, we may not use the word if the child is very young and seems unaware of the term. Moreover, we suggest that the family tell the child that a lot of young children need help in learning to talk smoothly, and this is what he is going to do at speech school. We also suggest that they tell the child that, with this help, he will grow up talking like everybody else, and this is most likely true.

Another question that parents often ask is, "What should I do when my child is having many episodes of hard stuttering and seems upset by it?" Again, we recommend that they talk openly about stuttering. We point out that if their child came into the house with a bloody nose, they would not ignore it; rather, they would acknowledge it and help the child. Thus, we suggest that they should acknowledge it when their child seems to be having a difficult time with his stuttering and be reassuring. A statement such as "Oh, that was a hard one, wasn't it; at speech school you will learn to say those easily" is an example. Family members will need to express these thoughts and feelings in ways that are comfortable for them.

One additional bit of information about stuttering that we share with parents is the research data on spontaneous recovery, presented in Chapter 1. As you may recall, of the children who begin to stutter, between 50% and 80% will recover without any formal treatment. We tell the parents that, with treatment, these percentages go up substantially. Although we cannot guarantee success with every beginning stutterer, this information is very reassuring for most parents. We tell them that they have good reason to be hopeful!

EXPLAINING THE POSSIBLE CAUSES OF STUTTERING

Everything said in Chapter 11 about explaining stuttering to the parents of the intermediate stutterer applies here as well. We believe it is very important for the parents of a child whose stuttering is at a beginning level to be given an explanation of its possible causes, and we share with them our understanding of the current theoretical and research literature.

What do we tell the family of the child with beginning stuttering about the possible causes of the disorder? We discuss, in language appropriate to their background, the type of information covered in Section I of this book. We explain that although no one knows for sure what causes stuttering, we have some educated guesses based on recent research. We believe that children who stutter may have a slightly different organization of their brain. This leads to some problems in coordinating the fine motor skills needed for speech, resulting in the repetitions and prolongations that we often see when stuttering just begins. The child's temperament may predispose him to respond to stress with increased tension and hurry in his speech. These two factors—discoordination and vulnerability to stress may—both of which may have genetic roots, interact with the stresses and pressures of growing up in a normal home and immature speech and language skills to produce the kinds of stuttering we see in their child. Some stuttering, we point out, is the result of motor discoordinations, and some from the child's reactions to the frustration and embarrassment of having his speech get stuck.

We also explore with the parents the developmental and environmental influences reviewed in Chapter 3. These influences may interact with predisposing physiological factors to cause the child to stutter. In some cases, we do not find any developmental or environmental factors that seem to be contributing to the problem. However, when we do find some possible factor, we try to reduce its influence. For example, if we learn that the child's stuttering got worse soon after the birth of a baby sister or brother, we suggest to parents that this may be contributing to the problem. We point out how none of us function as well when we are under stress and how their child's speech may be especially vulnerable to it. We note that, when he is under stress, his fine timing or coordination of his speech mechanism tends to break down. We then explore with the parents ways to reduce the disrupting influence of the child's new rival for their love and attention. For example, it would be especially important for the parents to give much love to the child who is beginning to stutter during this time. After exploring other options with us, parents usually come up with a number of other things they can do to reassure the child of their love and affection during this transition period.

Our experience suggests that solutions for reducing the impact of these developmental and environmental influences are fairly straightforward. In a few cases, it is more difficult. In such cases, referral for counseling to a private psychotherapist or mental health agency is necessary.

IDENTIFYING AND REDUCING FLUENCY DISRUPTERS

We believe it is important to explore with parents one special group of environmental influences that often interact with the child's physiological predisposition to worsen stuttering. These influences arise from the child's speech and language environment. They include the parents' speech and language patterns and circumstances in which the child often speaks. These two broad headings encompass many specific variables: high rate of speech, advanced speech and language models, unrealistic speech and language expectations, calling negative attention to the stuttering, competition for the floor, interruptions, listener loss, demanding speech, time pressures, display speech, excitement, and other emotionally laden situations. These variables are discussed in Chapter 3, and the reader may wish to refresh his or her understanding of them.

We begin by explaining to the family what we mean by fluency disrupters: that certain situations in the child's speech and language environment may cause him to be more disfluent. We then discuss some of the more common fluency disrupters with them. If family members' speech rate appears to be too rapid to provide a good fluency model for their child, we recount how other families have found that a slower rate facilitates their child's fluency. We offer to help them speak more slowly around their child. We also ask family members to observe their child carefully for the next week or so and to note those situations that seem to cause him to stutter more. When we get together at our next counseling session, we help them search for patterns in these situations. Sometimes the family comes to the next session having already figured out what types of situations seem to give their child the most trouble. Other times, it may take several weeks of observation and brainstorming with us to identify any patterns. In some cases, there does not appear to be a pattern to the situations that appear to disrupt the child's fluency.

Once one or more patterns have been identified, we explain to the family that our goal is to reduce the fluency disrupters in their child's life as much as is realistically possible. We do not have any specific recommendations of how to do this; rather, we explore with the family possible ways they might do this. After all, family members are the ones who have to make the modifications in their child's speech and language environment. We can only give suggestions and help them consider possible alternatives. Once parents decide how they are going to modify a given situation, we support and encourage their efforts. We also monitor on a regular basis their progress in changing the child's environment and their observation of the effect this change has on the child's fluency. Two examples may be helpful here.

The first example involves a father who had unrealistic speech and language expectations for his 4-year-old son. This father was an engineer who was well educated in the physical sciences and believed that it was important for his son to know the physical laws of nature. Unfortunately, even though this father was well intentioned, he was not well informed about child development. This became apparent when we were discussing situations in which his son was most disfluent. For example, the father reported that his son had been very disfluent on the previous night when they had been discussing the law of gravity. The father related that the son had said, "I-I-I-Is gra-gra-gravity the rea-rea-reason I ca-ca-ca-can ju-ju-jump higher on the-the-the moo-moo-moo-moon tha-than I ca-ca-can on earth?" This, and many other examples, soon illustrated that this father was attempting to teach his son scientific concepts that were well beyond his son's understanding. When this was pointed out to him, he replied, "I just wanted my son to be ready for kindergarten." To relieve his concern, we evaluated his son with several tests of cognitive and language development. As we expected, he performed a year or two above his chronological age on each of them. When the father learned this, he no longer felt it necessary to teach his son such difficult concepts at this time. The father modified his interactions with his son, and the son's fluency soon began to improve.

The next example involves a mother who constantly, but unknowingly, interrupted her 6-year-old son. She often interrupted everybody else, including us. When we asked her to look for situations at home when her son was most disfluent, she was unable to identify any. We then asked her to tape-record a conversation with her son at home for our next counseling session. We listened to the tape together and noted that her son was quite disfluent and that she was interrupting him every third sentence or so. She began talking before he had finished many sentences, asked him questions in the middle of his utterances, and interrupted and corrected the content of his statements at times. After listening to about half the tape she said, "Do I always do that? I'm constantly interrupting him!" She was obviously unaware of her behavior, but once she became aware of it, she tried very hard to change. It was difficult, but she improved and so did her son. We believe the changes she made contributed to his improvement.

These two examples also illustrate another point we need to make. Most parents want to help their children improve their fluency. Neither the father nor the mother in these examples was engaging in these behaviors to be cruel. Each was simply unaware of the influence these behaviors seemed to have on their child. When it was suggested that they change, they did their best to do so. Accordingly, we do not want to make such parents feel guilty for their past mistakes. We tell them that we know they love their child, that it was an understandable mistake, and that we know they want to help their child. We accept past errors and encourage them to change in the future.

IDENTIFYING AND INCREASING FLUENCY ENHANCING SITUATIONS

We not only want to identify and reduce fluency disrupting situations, but we also want to identify and increase fluency enhancing situations. Most children with beginning stuttering are usually fluent in some situations. These are often relaxed, one-on-one situations with the parent, perhaps while sharing a story with mother before going to bed or while working on a quiet project with father. Just as we ask family members to identify fluency disrupting situations, we also have them look for those situations in which the child is often fluent. Once these situations are identified, we encourage the family to engage the child in these activities as often as possible, at least on a daily basis. The more practice the child has in being fluent, the more solid his fluency will become.

We also talk with the family about the fact that beginning stuttering is often cyclic in nature. Children with beginning stuttering have "good days" and "bad days." On the child's good days, we encourage the family to engage him in a lot of talking so that he will experience more fluency. On the child's bad days, we suggest to the parents that they attempt to find quiet activities for him to do. We do not want him to experience the struggle and possible frustration involved in such stuttering. We realize families will not be able to apply these suggestions perfectly, but to the extent that they are able to have their child experience a lot of fluency on his good days and less stuttering on bad days, we believe their efforts will be helpful.

This concludes our integration of stuttering modification and fluency shaping therapies for the beginning stutterer. Let us now look at how other clinicians integrate these two approaches.

OTHER CLINICIANS

Hugo Gregory and Diane Hill

Hugo Gregory and Diane Hill (1980) believe that stuttering develops from an interaction between the child and environmental variables. They include five treatment objectives for the beginning stutterer or the child who is "atypically disfluent with or without complicating speech, language, or behavioral factors." These objectives are (a) to avoid increasing the child's awareness of his stuttering, (b) to increase the amount of the child's fluency, (c) to increase the child's tolerance for fluency disrupters, (d) to increase the child's self-acceptance, and (e) to help the child gain competence in areas, such as articulation or syntactic development, that may interfere with his fluency development. The fifth objective is discussed in the next section of this chapter when we consider the treatment of concomitant speech and language problems. Gregory and Hill also recommend that the child's parents be involved in a parent counseling program.

With regard to the first objective, Gregory and Hill do not call attention to the child's stuttering; however, if the child brings it up, they acknowledge it and reassure him. To increase the child's fluency, Gregory and Hill model "easy, relaxed speech," which is characterized by "smooth movements into and between words." The child's dependence on their modeling is systematically reduced through the following hierarchy: direct model, delayed model, intervening model, no model, and question model. At the same time, the length and complexity of the child's utterances are increased from single-word responses to phrases to sentences, and finally, to conversation. Concurrently with these procedures, the child's use of easy, relaxed speech is systematically generalized to other physical settings and other people.

Gregory and Hill typically generalize the use of easy, relaxed speech at a linguistic level to other physical and social conditions before moving on to longer and more complex linguistic utterances. They reinforce easy, relaxed speech responses and use criterion levels for moving on to more difficult steps. To increase the child's tolerance for fluency disrupters, Gregory and Hill use desensitization procedures similar to those of Van Riper, which are applied at various length-of-response levels. In meeting the next objective, increasing the child's self-acceptance, Gregory and Hill may engage the child in such activities as art projects, and they deliberately make mistakes. They are then very accepting of these mistakes.

Among Gregory and Hill's goals for parents during parent counseling are the following: to provide the parents with information on how stuttering may develop, to help the parents identify moments of stuttering, to help the parents identify factors that increase their child's stuttering, and to help the parents develop a problem-solving approach for reducing those factors that increase their child's stuttering.

Meryl Wall and Florence Myers

Meryl Wall and Florence Myers (1995) believe that stuttering results from a lack of synergism among psycholinguistic, physiological, and psychosocial factors in children. They characterize their therapy as "eclectic" and argue that all three factors—psycholinguistic, physiological, and psychosocial—need to be taken into account in both the direct treatment of the child and in parent counseling.

With regard to psycholinguistic factors, Wall and Myers' therapy has a "language-based orientation," regardless of whether the child has a concomitant speech and language disorder or not. In their basic approach to therapy for all children who stutter, Wall and Myers interact with the child in a loosely structured activity while, at the same time, controlling the length and semantic-syntactic complexity of the child's utterances. They usually begin by eliciting one- or two-word utterances from the child. They do this in a variety of ways, such as eliciting responses during parallel or interactive play, asking either/or or yes/no questions, and naming objects or pictures during play. When the child is fluent at this level, he gradually begins to work on longer and more complex linguistic tasks in the following sequence: two- and three-word phrases, simple sentences, complex sentences, picture descriptions, storytelling, and conversation. Throughout all these tasks, the clinician gradually puts greater linguistic demands on the child. The child needs to be fluent or almost fluent at one level before the clinician moves on to the next level. Wall and Myers also include pragmatic aspects of discourse as the child proceeds through therapy in order to foster increased fluency during different communication tasks and in different settings. We discuss their views on dealing with concomitant speech and language problems in the next section of this chapter.

In terms of physiological factors, Wall and Myers provide the child with an "easy speech" model to facilitate fluency during the language-based tasks just described. Easy speech is characterized by a slow-normal rate, relaxed articulation, gentle voice onset, and slightly reduced volume. If the child still has blocks on some words, Wall and Myers teach the child techniques, such as Van Riper pull-outs, to modify these stutters.

Among the tactics that Wall and Myers use to deal with psychosocial factors are the following: share information about stuttering with the parents, help the parents talk with their child about his stuttering, help the parents reduce fluency disrupters in the child's environment, and help the child deal with any teasing he may be experiencing.

SUMMARY OF INTEGRATION OF APPROACHES

Earlier in this chapter, we stated that stuttering modification and fluency shaping therapies are similar in their treatment of the beginning stutterer. Some stuttering modification clinicians teach the child to modify his moments of stuttering, but others reinforce fluency in ways similar to those of fluency shaping clinicians. Stuttering modification clinicians also tend to give some attention to the child's feelings and attitudes about his speech, whereas fluency shaping clinicians do not. From the discussion of our clinical procedures and our descriptions of Gregory and Hill's and Wall and Myers' clinical procedures, the reader should recognize that it is easy to incorporate some work on modifying the moment of stuttering and some work on attending to feelings and attitudes with a basic fluency shaping program in the treatment of the beginning stutterer.

TREATMENT OF CONCOMITANT
SPEECH AND LANGUAGE PROBLEMS

One of the clinical issues discussed in Chapter 6 is the management of concomitant speech and language problems in the beginning stutterer. Research has indicated that some of these children are delayed in their speech and language development, especially in their articulation development. A number of clinicians have recommended treating these concomitant speech and language problems in the beginning stutterer. We strongly support these developments and discuss the recent contributions of Conture, Louko and Edwards, Gregory and Hill, Bernstein Ratner, Wall and Myers, and Riley and Riley.

In discussing the contributions of these clinicians, we limit our remarks primarily to their views on the clinical management of concomitant speech and language problems as they interface with the treatment of the stuttering, not on their overall treatment approach to stuttering. We conclude the section with a discussion of our own experiences in integrating the treatment of stuttering with the treatment of concomitant speech and language problems.

Edward Conture, Linda Louko, and Mary Louise Edwards

Conture, Louko, and Edwards (1993) developed a treatment approach for children with fluency and phonological problems that tempers the demands of articulation therapy while providing support for increased fluency. These researchers work on both problems at the same time, but use an indirect approach for the articulation problems. This avoids the demands of traditional "corrective" articulation therapy. Their approach provides the child with plenty of models of target phonemes through extensive auditory stimulation and opportunities for improved production. This is done in an accepting environment rather than correcting the child when he is wrong and asking him to try again with more attention and effort. Thus, this approach does not stress the child's production capacities as much as a traditional approach. Conture, Louko, and Edwards also incorporate a variety of fluency facilitating techniques, such as slow speaking rate, relaxed manner of speaking, reduced interruptions, and increased interspeaker pause time. This is done while they work on articulation to enhance the child's fluency overall when under the stress of attempting to produce new phonological structures. This approach is contrasted with others in the section in Bernstein Ratner's overview of these therapies.

Hugo Gregory and Diane Hill

Hugo Gregory and Diane Hill (1980) believe that concomitant speech and language problems may contribute to maintaining or increasing stuttering in the young stutterer. Thus, in treating the "child atypically disfluent with complicating speech, language, or behavioral factors," they believe it is important to target these problems in therapy as well.

As you may recall, one of Gregory and Hill's objectives was "to increase the amount of the child's fluency." They systematically increased the length and complexity of the child's utterances from single-word responses, to phrases, to sentences, and, finally, to conversation. Gregory and Hill suggest that this strategy readily lends itself to working on syntactic or articulation errors. For example, depending on the developmental level of the child's language, various syntactic structures can be practiced at the same time that the child is practicing fluent speech. In other words, by using the appropriate instructions and materials, the clinician has the child practice a specific syntactic structure and easy, relaxed speech at the same time. Gregory and Hill also indicate that this applies equally well to articulation therapy. Depending on where the child is in articulation therapy, he could be practicing his new phoneme in a response of a given length and complexity at the same time he is practicing his fluency.

Gregory and Hill report that a significant percentage of the young stutterers they see have word retrieval problems. Their first goal is to help these children feel comfortable with pauses in their speech. So, they model delays in responding to naming tasks, then say something like, "I can't think of what that is called; everybody has problems like this sometimes." Of course, they also give the child ample time to recall words. Their second goal is to provide the child with a strategy for retrieving words. They do this by helping the child learn to build associations between objects and their semantic attributes, such as function, size, shape, color, and other characteristics. Then they create situations for the child to practice using this strategy to retrieve words.

Gregory and Hill also work with parents to improve the speech and language models to which the child is exposed at home. For example, if the parents speak too rapidly, ask too many questions too fast, or do not listen to the child, Gregory and Hill instruct and model more appropriate speech and language behaviors for the parents to use around the child.

Nan Bernstein Ratner

Bernstein Ratner identifies several models for working with children who stutter and have concomitant speech or language disorders (Bernstein Ratner, 1995). The sequential model typically treats the language or articulation problem first, with the hope that once this problem is resolved, stuttering will no longer be a problem for the child. If it is not improved, the child's stuttering may become more severe, more chronic, and more resistant to treatment, either because of the demands of the language or articulation therapy used or simply because it remains untreated for an extended period of time.

The concurrent model avoids this problem by beginning treatment of fluency simultaneously with treatment of the other disorders. When this approach is used effectively, two principles are followed. First, the child practices fluency only with language and phonological structures that he has already mastered. Second, phonological or language therapy procedures avoid demands that may make the child excessively self-conscious of his errors. This can prevent him from excessive physical or mental efforts in the production of the forms targeted for therapy (see Conture, Louko, & Edwards, 1993).

A third model, the blended model, also works on both fluency and the other disorder or disorders at the same time. This provides extra support of fluency. The clinician and child speak with slow rate, gentle onsets, relaxed movements, ample pausing within and between utterances, and careful turn-taking. Training and modeling of this style of speaking are crucial for success. As new phonological and linguistic structures are mastered, they are practiced with more normal speech characteristics (normal rate, and so on). A particular advantage of the blended approach is that it gives the child an opportunity to tackle difficult utterances (complex language; challenging phonology) with the support of fluency facilitators. Thus, the child learns to maintain fluency in the face of high demands (see Conture, Louko, & Edwards).

The fourth and final model is the cyclic model, in which fluency treatment is alternated with language or phonology therapy over the course of the year. Bernstein Ratner points out that this allows initial periods of concentrated learning of new skills, followed by opportunities for spontaneous generalization of these skills in other settings.

Glyndon and Jeanna Riley

Glyndon and Jeanna Riley (1984) advocate a "component model" of treatment for the child at their "intervention level II: chronic stuttering." By treating underlying components of the stuttering, they report that the child regains normal fluency in most cases. At this intervention level, they do not attempt to modify the child's moments of stuttering nor reinforce his fluent responses. They only treat what they see as the underlying and maintaining components of the stuttering.

There are nine components in the Riley model. Four are "neurogenic" components, and five are "traditional" components. The neurogenic components are attending disorders, auditory processing disorders, sentence formulation disorders, and oral motor disorders. The five traditional components are disruptive communicative environment, unrealistic parental expectations, abnormal parental need for the child to stutter, high self-expectations by the child, and manipulative stuttering. It seems to us that three of these components may be viewed as concomitant speech and language problems. They are auditory processing disorders, sentence formulation disorders, and disruptive communicative environment.

Riley and Riley report that approximately 27% of their young stutterers have auditory processing disorders. By auditory disorders, they mean that the child has problems receiving and manipulating auditory information. Such children may have any of the following problems: retaining auditory images, making figure-ground distinctions, or selecting meaningful from nonmeaningful auditory signals. Treatment goals depend on the child's particular auditory processing problem, but often include increasing the child's auditory memory or increasing his ability to follow directions. Riley and Riley recommend a number of commercially available programs for improving children's receptive language abilities.

Sentence formulation disorders may include the following types of problems: word retrieval problems, word order problems involving reversals and transpositions, and formulation problems involving incomplete and fragmented sentences. They report that approximately 30% of their young stutterers have such problems. Treatment goals depend on the child's particular problems. A number of commercially available materials based on generative grammar, not those based simply on length of utterances, are recommended for treating these expressive language difficulties. Riley and Riley also stress the importance of a careful analysis of the child's syntax so that treatment is targeted at the child's level of language abilities.

Riley and Riley report that 53% of their young stutterers come from disruptive communicative environments. By this, they are referring to fluency disrupters in the child's environment, such as the child has difficulty getting the parents' attention, being interrupted while talking, or being rushed while speaking. Riley and Riley counsel parents regarding the importance of reducing such fluency disrupters.

Meryl Wall and Florence Myers

Meryl Wall and Florence Myers (1984) note that some clinicians are reluctant to work on a young stutterer's concomitant speech or language problem because they fear that calling attention to the child's speech and language will exacerbate stuttering. They believe, however, that this fear is largely unjustified.

As you may recall, Wall and Myers' (1995) basic approach to therapy for all children who stutter has a "language-based orientation," in which they control the length and semantic-syntactic complexity of the child's utterances. They typically go through the following sequence: two- and three-word phrases, simple sentences, complex sentences, picture descriptions, storytelling, and conversation. Wall and Myers indicate that this method of sequencing linguistic tasks ensures that the length and semantic-syntactic complexity of therapy activities are kept within the child's capacity. In the early stages of therapy, vocabulary should consist of words already in the child's repertoire. In the later stages of therapy, new words can be added to the child's lexicon. In a similar manner, syntactic structures already in the child's repertoire should be used in the early stages of treatment. Later on, new grammatical structures can be gradually introduced in their normal developmental sequence. Wall and Myers recommend that the clinician move the child through this sequence of linguistic tasks, with easy speech or pull-outs being incorporated with the work on new vocabulary or new syntactic structures.

What about the child with a phonological or articulation disorder? Wall and Myers recommend that such problems be treated after fluency has been stabilized if the child's disability is mild and not interfering with intelligibility. However, if disability is severe and interfering with intelligibility, the problem should be dealt with immediately, because it may be adding considerable stress to the child's communicative attempts. If treatment of a phonological or articulation disorder is begun, Wall and Myers recommend that the phoneme or phoneme group selected for treatment be one that is the easiest for the child to produce. Words and syntactic structures selected for practice material should be ones with which the child can easily cope. Work on sound production can be integrated with work on fluency. For example, practice of a new sound in a word can be integrated with practice of easy speech.

Wall and Myers also have suggestions for parents of the child with both a beginning stuttering problem and a delayed speech and language problem. If the parents talk fast, they are asked to talk more slowly around the child. If they use language that clearly exceeds the child's semantic-syntactic level, they are asked to simplify their language when talking to the child. To help parents make these changes and become better fluency models for their child, they are encouraged to watch the clinician working with their child and observe how she modifies her rate and language to enhance the child's fluency.

Besides improving the fluency models that parents present to the child, Wall and Myers also discuss with them other ways to use language at home to enhance their child's fluency. They point out that questions that requiring short responses usually elicit more fluency than do open-ended questions, which require longer and more complex answers. For example, "Did you have fun at Ted's birthday party?" usually elicits a shorter and more fluent response than does "What did you do at Ted's birthday party?" By using these and other strategies, Wall and Myers help parents provide their child with a linguistic environment that is more conducive to fluency.

Our Experience

We believe it is important to treat a beginning stutterer's concomitant speech or language problems or both. As the child gains more competence and confidence in speaking, treatment has a positive effect on his fluency. Moreover, we haven't found that treating the other speech or language problem has exacerbated the child's stuttering.

The most common concomitant speech and language problems we find in beginning stutterers are phonological and syntactic disorders. We integrate our treatment of the child's fluency with treatment of these other problems much as do Conture, Louko, and Edwards, Gregory and Hill, and Wall and Myers. As we move up our fluency hierarchy, we target both the child's fluent responses and his phonological or syntactic responses and often have the child practice both smooth, fluent speech and correct phonemes and syntactic structures at the same time. However, there are two issues that we typically encounter in integrating work on the child's fluency with work on other speech and language problems. One issue deals with sequencing, the other deals with terminology. Let's first discuss the issue of sequencing.

In most cases, the children we see are referred to us because someone, usually the family, is concerned about the child's stuttering. Thus, we begin our treatment by responding to this concern. That is, we begin by increasing the child's fluency use of our fluency hierarchy. After successfully completing several steps of this hierarchy, we begin working on a concomitant speech or language problem. Sometimes, the child cannot work on a concomitant problem at the same level of linguistic difficulty he is practicing in the fluency hierarchy. For example, if the child is at the "carrier phrase + word" level in the fluency hierarchy when we begin working on a misarticulated phoneme, he may not be able to use this phoneme correctly at the carrier phrase + word level. We may need to begin teaching this phoneme at the nonsense syllable or word level, so the child is not practicing fluency and correct articulation at the same time in the same response. Rather, part of each therapy session is spent practicing fluency in the fluency hierarchy, and part of each session is spent practicing correct articulation. Only when the child can be successful with both fluency and articulation at the same linguistic level are they worked on together. These same principles apply when we integrate therapy for fluency with therapy for syntactic problems. Thus, work on fluency sometimes coincides with work on the other concomitant speech and language problems, and sometimes one precedes the other.

Let us now consider the issue of terminology. As mentioned before, we use verbal reinforcers, such as "that's great" or "good job," when a child produces a fluent response. We also refer to these fluent responses as being "smooth" or "easy." So, what do we do when working on both fluency and another speech or language problem at the same time? Suppose we are working with a child on both fluency and a specific syntactic structure, and he produces a response that is fluent but not syntactically correct. If we say "good," we are reinforcing fluency, but we are also reinforcing a response that is syntactically incorrect. We do not want to do this. If we label the target responses differently, however, we seldom have significant problems. For example, we worked with one 4-year-old beginning stutterer who also had phonological and syntactic problems. When we worked on both fluent and correct syntactic responses at the same time, we referred to a fluent response as being "smooth" and a syntactically correct response as being "a good sentence." In addition to this verbal feedback, we also used token reinforcement with the boy. On any given response, he might earn two, one, or zero tokens, depending on whether his response was both fluent and syntactically fluent or either fluent or syntactically correct, or neither fluent nor syntactically correct. When we targeted both fluent and correct phonological responses at the same time, the procedures were the same but we referred to phonologically correct responses as "having the good sound." We found that by using these procedures with this boy, he did not have any problem keeping things straight.

Like the other clinicians we discussed in this section, we believe it is important to work with the parents of a young stutterer to improve, when necessary, the speech and language models to which the child is exposed at home and to temper their expectations for immediate changes in his language or phonology.

SUMMARY OF TREATMENT OF CONCOMITANT SPEECH AND LANGUAGE PROBLEMS

There appears to be substantial support for integrating work on a beginning stutterer's fluency with his other speech or language problems. None of the latter clinicians reported observing adverse effects on the child's stuttering. Furthermore, it appears that this integration can be successfully accomplished by gradually and systematically increasing the length and complexity of the child's responses.

STUDY QUESTIONS

1. List the four phases of our therapy for the beginning stutterer. What is the goal of each phase?
2. Briefly describe our establishment and transfer fluency hierarchy.
3. Describe our procedures for the following phases of treatment: (a) desensitizing the child to fluency disrupters, (b) modifying the moments of stuttering, and (c) maintaining improvement.
4. Describe our counseling with the family of children with beginning stuttering.
5. Based on Conture, Louko, and Edwards', Gregory and Hill's, Wall and Myers', and our own experiences, describe how the treatment of beginning stuttering and other speech and language disorders can be integrated.
6. What are the four approaches to treating concomitant problems described by Bernstein Ratner?

SUGGESTED READINGS

Bernstein Ratner, N. (1995). Treating the child who stutters with concomitant language and phonological impairment. *Language, Speech, and Hearing Services in Schools,* **26(2), 180–186.**
In this insightful overview of the treatment of children with concomitant disorders, Bernstein Ratner identifies several models that have evolved.

Conture, E., Louko, L., & Edwards, M.L. (1993). Simultaneously treating stuttering and disordered phonology in children: Experimental therapy, preliminary findings. *American Journal of Speech-Language Pathology, 2,* **72–81.**
This article details how to use indirect articulation therapy with children at both beginning and intermediate levels of stuttering.

Gregory, H.H. (1986). *Stuttering: Differential evaluation and therapy.* **Austin, TX: Pro-Ed.**
This is a good overview of Gregory, Hill, and Campbell's therapy for stuttering.

Gregory, H.H., & Hill, D. (1980). Stuttering therapy for children. *Seminars in Speech, Language and Hearing, 1,* **351–363.**
This is a good reference for dealing with children who have both language delay and stuttering.

Riley, G.D., & Riley, J. (1984). A component model for treating stuttering in children. In M. Peins (Ed.), *Contemporary approaches in stuttering therapy.* **Boston: Little, Brown, & Company.**
This chapter describes treatment for oral motor, language, and other problems that may be components of stuttering in children.

Wall, M.J., & Myers, F.L. (1995). *Clinical management of childhood stuttering,* **2nd ed. Austin, TX: Pro-Ed.**
This new edition includes a complete treatment approach for beginning and intermediate stutterers.

Borderline Stutterer: A Consensus

Fluency shaping and stuttering modification therapies become more and more similar as we move from advanced to intermediate to beginning stuttering. At the level of borderline stuttering, the two approaches are essentially alike. Both approaches make extensive use of the family in the therapy process, according to the belief that stuttering emerges from interactions between the environment and the child's predispositions. Both work, at least initially, to increase the child's fluency without focusing on stuttering. The goal of both fluency shaping and stuttering modification therapies is spontaneous fluency. Neither works directly on the child's feelings or attitudes about stuttering, and both gradually fade contact over a period of time while continuing to assess the child's speech to make sure it remains normally fluent.

Because of their similarity, we have combined the discussion of the two therapy approaches into a single chapter. This chapter begins with our own integrated approach, then describes a variety of other approaches. The other approaches, rather than being designated as fluency shaping or stuttering modification therapies, are characterized as "more indirect" or "more direct."

Indirect approaches loosely correspond to the family-oriented counseling that stuttering modification clinicians use with beginning level stuttering. Such approaches try to increase the child's fluency by working with the family to create an environment that is conducive to fluent speech. Direct approaches follow the fluency shaping tradition of reinforcing fluency and ignoring or punishing stuttering. The two approaches are blended when clinicians using an indirect approach do not see progress after several weeks of treatment and supplement their indirect therapy with more direct methods.

OUR INTEGRATED APPROACH

Our integration of approaches for a borderline stutterer combines two principles: working with the environment to decrease stress and working with the child to increase fluency. We begin with the environment, using family counseling. If the child's family can discover ways to facilitate the child's fluency, they become confident in their power to observe and effect change and are able to assume long-term responsibility for the child's fluency. If this is not effective or is slow to take effect, we work directly with the child as well, taking our cue from fluency shaping.

Clinician's Beliefs

NATURE OF STUTTERING

As described in Chapter 4, we believe that borderline stuttering occurs as a result of the interplay between the child's constitutional predispositions and the stresses resulting from developmental demands and the environment. Our treatment for a borderline stutterer is based on the assumption that if we can decrease the child's stresses, his stuttering will taper off and he will become normally fluent. We believe that the plasticity of normal neural maturation allows most of these children to compensate for constitutional predispositions toward stuttering. For such flexibility in development to blossom into normal fluency, however, we must provide an environment that fosters fluency and diminishes negative experiences with speaking. And we must do it promptly. If we wait too long, the child may become aware of his stuttering and become frustrated by it. If this happens, awareness and frustration, combined with the child's concern about negative listener reactions, may push his stuttering beyond the borderline level into beginning and even intermediate stuttering. Both levels of stuttering are usually more resistant to treatment.

With borderline stuttering, we seldom treat the child directly, at least not at first. Instead, we work with the child's family to help them reduce environmental stresses. We assume that stress is normal in the life of every child, but that the child with borderline stuttering is simply more vulnerable to fluency breakdown under normal stresses. As you will see in the description of our clinical procedures, we usually begin by informing and educating family members about ways they can reduce stresses and foster fluency. We demonstrate a facilitating style of communicative interaction as a model for the family to try, and we meet with them once a week to support and guide their efforts in finding ways to help their child.

If indirect therapy is not effective in reducing stuttering after 6 weeks or if the child's stuttering proves to be more advanced than initially thought, we add more direct procedures. Our more direct approach, which assumes that the child is aware of stuttering, consists of a hierarchy of activities that focus on playing with stuttering and changing the stuttering to a milder form.

SPEECH BEHAVIORS TARGETED FOR THERAPY

Because we don't treat the child's speech directly, no speech behaviors are specifically targeted for therapy in our treatment of the borderline stutterer. Instead, we target the family's interaction styles, including both speech and nonspeech behaviors. We encourage family members to speak fluently, but in a slow and relaxed manner. We support their efforts to make other aspects of their interactions with the child who stutters as unstressful as possible. If we need to use a more direct approach to treatment, we target the child's repetitions and prolongations.

FLUENCY GOALS

We believe that all children at the borderline level can achieve spontaneous fluency. With effective early intervention, this goal is readily achievable because the borderline stutterer's developing nervous system increases his capacity for fluent speech.

FEELINGS AND ATTITUDES

Our main focus of treatment is on the behaviors of family members and others who interact frequently with the child. Consequently, we do not deal directly with the child's feelings and attitudes. However, as we monitor his fluency, we try to ensure that he is not developing negative attitudes about speaking or about his disfluencies. If the child's borderline stuttering persists and shows periodic worsening, he may become more aware of it and frustrated when it is at its worst. In these cases, the addition of more direct intervention is used to deal with such feelings.

MAINTENANCE PROCEDURES

Many borderline stutterers achieve fluent speech soon after their families have made some environmental modifications. Most maintain fluency without further treatment. However, we keep in contact with the family even after formal treatment has stopped to prevent backsliding into old, more stressful interaction patterns. This contact, through telephone calls or letters, is gradually faded.

CLINICAL METHODS

Our clinical approach to borderline stuttering—working with the child's family—includes elements of both fluency shaping and stuttering modification. We begin with a counseling approach for the family, exploring factors that may be related to the appearance and maintenance of the child's stuttering and supporting their efforts to foster his fluency. Such counseling and support are more aligned with stuttering modification therapies. If we need to use modeling and instruction to help families change their interaction styles, we are likely to use a more programmed format, borrowing procedures from fluency shaping. In addition, we typically collect data on the child's progress and the changes a family makes, which is typical of a fluency shaping approach.

With some children, reinforcement of fluency (a procedure borrowed from fluency shaping) is suggested. For direct therapy procedures, we use the modeling and differential reinforcement strategies of stuttering modification.

Clinical Procedures: Indirect Treatment

Our indirect treatment begins during evaluation and diagnostic sessions. At that time, we study family interactions, listen to descriptions of the home environment, and ask about factors that may be associated with fluctuations in the child's fluency.

STUDYING FAMILY INTERACTION PATTERNS

The family's interaction patterns, which are gleaned from tapes sent to us before the evaluation or observed at the time of the evaluation, often give us clues about possible stresses in the child's environment. Thus, one of the first things we do in treating the borderline stutterer is to decide which family-child interaction variables should be discussed with the family and considered for change. Here are some aspects of conversational interactions that are "normal" in busy homes but may put pressure on a borderline stutterer:

1. High rates of speech
2. Rapid-fire conversational pace (lack of pauses between speakers)
3. Interruptions
4. Frequent open-ended questions
5. Many critical or corrective comments
6. Inadequate or inconsistent listening to what the child says
7. Vocabulary far above the child's level
8. Advanced levels of syntax

After observing 10 or 15 minutes of family-child interaction, an experienced clinician usually has some hypotheses about which variables might be important to help the family change. For example, family members' speech rates may be unusually fast, or they may interrupt each other frequently when conversing, or they may convey high expectations of the child through critical or corrective comments.

Less experienced clinicians may want to follow the suggestions in Table 14.1 in developing their skills for assessing family interaction variables. As described in Chapter 7, it is helpful to have a recording of a family interaction before the evaluation. Ask the family to record 10 minutes of a typical conversational interaction with the child when he is likely to stutter. This might be a time, for example, when one or more family members are playing together with the child.

In some cases, it will not be possible for the family to make a recording before the evaluation; or, it may be that a noisy recording prevents assessment of key variables. In these instances, the family interaction recorded in the clinic can be used. Family members are asked to interact with the child in a room outfitted with an array of quiet materials (paper, crayons, dolls, games) to ensure an audible recording. Once a good recording is in hand, the clinician can make a transcript of a 10- or 15-minute interaction and quantify the 8 variables listed previously (see Table 14.1).

INVOLVING THE FAMILY IN CHANGE

During the diagnostic evaluation (see Chapter 7 for details) we also gather information about other important aspects of the child's environment. These include such things as the busyness of the family's daily schedule, the amount of individual attention the child receives, and how the family reacts to the child's stuttering. Using this information, we develop some tentative hypotheses about what factors may be important in influencing this child's stuttering. We keep these hypotheses to ourselves for the moment, first because they may be wrong and second because it is more effective for the family to lead

Table 14.1. Suggestions for Quantifying Family-Child Interaction Patterns

1. High rates of speech. Count the number of syllables spoken by each family member interacting with the child. Next, using a stopwatch, measure the amount of time each individual speaks. Be sure to stop timing whenever they stop speaking or pause for more than 2 seconds. Resume timing as soon as the speaking continues. Then, calculate the time in minutes to hundredths of a minute (e.g., 1 minute and 13 seconds would be 1.22 minutes). Divide the total number of syllables spoken by the time in minutes to obtain number of syllables per minute (SPM). For example, if a family member speaks 366 syllables in 1.22 minutes, their rate of speech is 300 SPM. Normal adult speaking rates are 180 to 220 SPM. Thus, this is a fast rate of speech.

2. Rapid-fire conversational pace (lack of pauses between speakers). Using a stopwatch, measure intervals from when the child stops speaking and when another family member begins. If these intervals average less than 1 second, the pace of conversation is rapid.

3. Interruptions. Count the number of sentences or sentence-like utterances the child speaks during the sample and the number of times a family member interrupts the child. Divide the number of interruptions by the total number of sentences. If there are more than 10% of interruptions, the child may feel pressure to speak quickly.

4. Frequent questions. Count the number of sentences spoken by family members to the child and the number of sentences that are questions. Divide the number of questions by the total number of sentences. If there are more than 25% of questions, the child may feel pressure from having to answer questions.[a]

5. Many critical or corrective comments. Each sentence of family members should be characterized as being either "critical" or "accepting." Sentences characterized as critical would be (a) those that convey that the speaker does not unconditionally accept the child, his actions, or his words; (b) those that pressure the child to speak or direct the child's activity; (c) those spoken with a tone of voice that is stern or incredulous. The number of sentences that are critical should be divided by the total number of sentences. If the percentage of critical comments is higher than 50%, the child may feel stress from high standards in the family.

6. Inadequate or inconsistent listening to what the child says. Assess the content of family members' sentences during each speaking turn. Note whether family members are responding to the content of the child's utterances. If more than 50% of family members' utterances ignore the topic the child has been speaking about, the child may feel he is not being heard.

7. Vocabulary far above child's level. Compare the vocabulary level of family members' speech with that of the child. If more than only a small amount of the family members' vocabulary exceeds the child's receptive level, the child may feel pressure when trying to understand family members' vocabulary.

8. Advanced levels of syntax. Assess the syntax used by family members when speaking to the child. If more than only a small amount is considerably above the child's current receptive level, the child may feel pressure not only to understand family members, but also to use syntax that he has yet to master.

---

[a]Recent research (Wilkenfeld & Curlee, 1997) suggests that the length of a child's utterance, rather than the number of questions he is asked, is related to the child's frequency of stuttering. Thus, open-ended questions, requiring longer answers from the child, might be a source of stress for a child with borderline stuttering.

the way in choosing what and how to change. Toward the end of a diagnostic session, we summarize our findings about the child's speech, concluding with a description of his borderline level of stuttering. We then help the family decide how to facilitate the child's fluency.

We begin by telling the family, in an appropriate vocabulary, that research suggests that stuttering first arises from an innate predisposition toward disfluency. Therefore, the child's stuttering wasn't caused by their doing something wrong or not doing something they should have. We point out that the child who has a predisposition to stutter may be especially sensitive to certain speech pressures that are typical of a normal home environment. Such pressures may trigger the appearance of stuttering in the first place or may make it harder for the child to outgrow it. We note that other children have improved when their families have been able to create an environment that is especially helpful to

Table 14.2. Things Families Can Do to Help the Borderline Stutterer

1. Listening time. All children benefit from feeling that what they have to say is important. This is especially true for the child who is beginning to stutter. Set aside some time each day as "listening time" with your child. Make it 15 to 20 minutes at about the same time each day, so your child can depend on it. During that time, refrain from making suggestions or giving instructions. Merely "be there" for the child, listening attentively to what he or she says or quietly playing alongside the child, if he or she chooses not to talk.

2. Slow rate. Family members may reduce their conversational rate of speech to a slow, soothing style. Speech should sound relaxed and calm, with comfortable pauses throughout. Fred Rogers on the television show "Mr. Rogers' Neighborhood" is a good model.[a]

3. Pauses. The pace of conversation can be kept appropriately slow if the speaker pauses at least 1 to 2 seconds before starting to talk. This also helps to keep the speaker from interrupting another speaker.

4. Positive comments. Make many positive and accepting comments about what your child is saying and doing. Limit corrections or criticisms to important issues. Changes for the better usually happen more quickly when someone feels they are okay as they are. The child who feels good about himself will be better able to use "listening time," "slow rate," and "pauses" to gain more fluency.

5. Fewer questions. It is natural to ask the child many questions, to encourage him to learn new things, and to display that knowledge. However, this makes some children feel "under the gun." So, it may be a good idea to decrease demanding questions and instructions. If you are worried that your child won't learn enough if you are too laid-back, keep in mind that learning comes naturally to children. They learn best from your interest in things, especially from your interest and positive comments about the things they do and say.

[a]Fred Rogers' speech rate, based on a small sample of "Mr. Rogers' Neighborhood," is about 165 syllables per minute, a comfortably slow rate for most adults. Mr. Rogers also pauses frequently in his speech, sometimes for several seconds.

fluent speech. We make it clear that, although they did not cause the child's stuttering, there is much they can do to help him overcome it.

We ask the child's family to observe and make notes about his stuttering and fluency for 1 week. Then we schedule a second session. We also suggest specific areas for the family to observe, such as their speech rate and conversational pace, based on our experience with other families. We also suggest areas that we hypothesize may be important to their child. We try to be nondirective, but give them guidance with suggestions such as those in Table 14.2 and in published materials for parents of children who stutter.[1]

THE FIRST TREATMENT SESSION

In the first session after a diagnostic evaluation, we help the family begin to change the child's environment. We discuss their observations and readings with them, maintaining a supportive, nonjudgmental relationship and remaining alert to comments that suggest they feel they caused their child's stuttering. Such feelings are not unusual and need to be acknowledged as natural. However, we always suggest reasons why it is unlikely that they caused their child's stuttering. For example, we may point out that their other children, who grew up in the same environment, don't stutter. We have found that reducing family members' guilt and anxiety makes it easier for them to focus on the changes in family interactions and household routines that we will be discussing. In the sharing of ideas to facilitate the child's fluency, we usually talk about changes in both family-child

---

[1] Examples of helpful booklets for parents are: *If Your Child Stutters: A Guide for Parents* and *Stuttering and Your Child: Questions and Answers* (publications 11 and 22 by the Stuttering Foundation of America), as well as *Understanding Stuttering: Information for Parents* (The National Easter Seal Society). Two useful videotapes for parents are *Stuttering and Your Child: A Video for Parents* (Stuttering Foundation of America) and *Preventing Stuttering in the Preschool Child: A Video Program for Parents* (Communication Skill Builders).

interactions and the household routine. Changes in interaction patterns are often more subtle and may be difficult to make. Therefore, we offer to model the interactions that we and the family mutually consider important to try to change.

MODELING INTERACTION

We ask the family to observe us playing with the child as we model one or two changes, such as a slower rate of speech and increased pausing.

If we have a room with a one-way mirror, the family can observe from another room. If another clinician or a student is available, we have this person observe with the family and point out good examples of the interaction style we are modeling. We also ask the other clinician or student to point out bad examples. The family trying to change is rarely helped by a perfect model. Sometimes we model interactions without a one-way mirror or another clinician by playing with the child while the family sits nearby and observes (Fig. 14.1). After the interaction, we discuss the things we have been trying to model for them.

After 5 or 10 minutes of letting the family observe, we invite them to participate. Sometimes we have only one family member participate at a time. At other times, both parents or other family members participate. This participation depends on what we are working on as well as which family members have attended the session. When a family member participates in the play session, we pull back and let him or her be the primary player. As we observe family members, we note whether they are demonstrating the desired behaviors. If they are, we continue to observe and let them practice. If not, we usually rejoin the interaction and provide further models of the desired behavior.

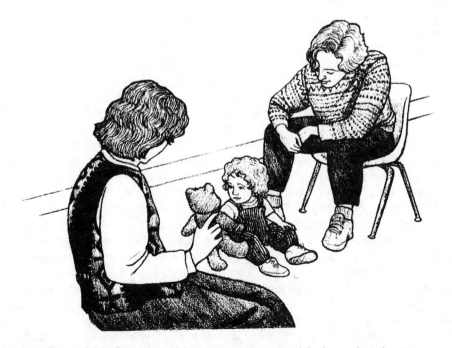

Figure 14.1. Clinician models interaction patterns while the mother observes.

After another 5 or 10 minutes of observing a parent or other family member play with the child, we arrange to talk with the family briefly in private toward the end of the session. Knowing how difficult such changes can be, we give as much positive feedback as we can about the interaction, even if we can praise only their efforts to change. Gordon Blood (personal communication, 1994), an accomplished stuttering clinician, says that he tries to use a 5:1 ratio of positive comments to corrective comments. Even if a family member has shown little change, we try to find ways of making the experience of trying to change as positive as possible.

DISCUSSING CHANGES IN FAMILY ROUTINE

In addition to changing conversational interaction patterns, a family may identify other stresses on the child that need to be changed. These include such things as the amount of individual attention the child receives and the "busyness" of the family schedule. Our main function in helping families work on these stresses is to give them information about areas of changes that others have found helpful and to be a sounding board for their plans for changing. We encourage them to assess the effects of these changes, informally, on the child's fluency and his overall adjustment. Although our praise and appreciation may help, a significant change in the child's stuttering is the real motivator.

We need to expand here on one change that we believe is of particular importance. The attention the child receives from his parents contributes immensely to his self-esteem, which, in turn, affects fluency. When the child senses that his mother or father genuinely cares about him—what he likes to do, what he thinks about things, and how he feels—the child feels comfortable with himself, is less anxious, and is better able to speak easily. For many children with borderline stuttering, a little one-on-one time spent with a parent each day can boost fluency tremendously. The time need not be long—15 to 30 minutes—but the parent needs to be with the child in a place where they won't be interrupted.

The child should choose what to play or what to talk about, and the parent should follow the child's lead, participating as the child directs. As a parent becomes more and more comfortable with this nondirective play, he or she may want to explore ways of helping the child to feel really understood. One of the parents we worked with, for example, would "mirror" her child's momentary emotions as they built a tower of blocks together. When the child placed a block on the tower and it fell off, she would quietly murmur a word of disappointment, echoing the facial expression shown by the child. This child made impressive gains in fluency in only a few weeks, and we believe that this deep attention by the parent may have contributed significantly to this change.

Attentive play can become child-directed conversations as the child grows older. These conversations can continue the process of helping the child develop a sense of being loved, understood, and appreciated. An excellent description of one-on-one time between parents and school-age children can be found in the article "Making Time for Your Child" by Stanley Greenspan, M.D., in *Parents* (August, 1993). With the borderline stutterer, we often work with families on changing the family-child interaction style as well as setting aside a one-on-one time each day. This combination gives family members a specific time to practice fluency facilitating verbal interactions, which may carry over to other times of the day.

At the end of the first therapy session, we help the family to formulate plans for implementing changes and for continuing to note conditions associated with the child's fluency and stuttering. We encourage the family not to take on too much, but to concentrate on just one or two changes. Then we arrange to meet with them again within 1 or 2 weeks to continue assessing, guiding, and supporting their attempts to help the child.

FOLLOW-UP SESSIONS

In sessions that follow the initial therapy session, we are eager to find out whether family members have tried to change aspects of the environment. However, we avoid asking them directly when we first greet them. Even "how's it going," asked routinely at the beginning of every session, may make our expectations weigh heavily on them. Instead, we endeavor to maintain a positive, low-pressure interaction style, as a model of what we want them to use with their child and allowing them to decide how they'd like to begin. As family members discuss what they have been observing and doing since the last session, we look for things to praise. As we've said before, families often feel that they are to blame for their child's stuttering; therefore, it is vital to give them sincere, positive feedback about what they are *doing well.* It is also the best way to help anyone learn new skills.

Sometimes families report that their attempts to make changes have been fairly successful. For example, they have been able to slow their speech rates and simplify their language, and they see improvement in their child. We let them know that their changes have been key factors and stress the importance of continuing them. It is easy to resume old patterns after some improvement occurs, whether it's the challenge of losing weight or that of helping the child become more fluent.

Each child and family are unique in how they respond to treatment, but it is possible to note some common trends. For example, some children become much more fluent soon after the family makes one or two changes in his environment. Occasionally, the child may become immediately fluent after an initial session, possibly because the family is much less anxious about his disfluencies after sharing their concerns with a professional. Whatever the cause, early and immediate fluency gains should be viewed with cautious optimism. We share the family's pleasure at this dramatic change, but suggest that such fluency may be fragile and will need to be nurtured by our continued efforts to create a facilitative environment.

Sometimes the path toward fluency is rough and irregular. The child may make a little or no progress. He may improve for awhile, then return to his old pattern of disfluency. When this happens and the family or the clinician feels frustrated by slow progress, further exploration of the family's feelings about the child's stuttering is called for. Many times family members worry about the child's future, afraid that stuttering will be a serious handicap for him. Sometimes there is lingering guilt about having caused the stuttering. Often it is hard for parents to accept the blemish they feel that stuttering is on the family image.

Whatever the source of a family's anxieties, their concern about stuttering may easily radiate to the child in their reactions to his stutters. Unwittingly, family members may show their anxiety or disappointment through facial expressions or body language that may make the child "hesitate to hesitate," and thus stutter more severely. Open and frank discussions with the family about their feelings and concerns may be more helpful at this point than simply trying to change their reactions. In such discussions, the clinician's role is to make it easier for the family to talk about their concerns; so we listen carefully, try our best to understand them, and convey our understanding with acceptance and respect.[2] When family members feel understood and accepted, it is easier for them to share

---

[2] For those who would like to improve their skills in family counseling, much can be learned from reading such books as Carl Roger's *Counseling and Psychotherapy* (1942), David Luterman's *Counseling Persons with Communication Disorders and Their Families* (1996), and a special issue of *Seminars in Speech and Language* (vol. 9, 1988) edited by Richard Curlee, which is devoted to counseling. Workshops, conferences, and institutes can also provide training. In addition, many of us have found that seeking psychotherapy for ourselves has improved our ability to help families.

their feelings and accept them. When this occurs, some feelings may change and, in turn, the child's stuttering may decrease, possibly because his stuttering no longer seems so terrible.

Another barrier to changing a family's interaction patterns is the fact that some styles of interaction reflect important cultural values. For example, in the urban eastern United States, family members frequently finish each others' sentences, conveying a closeness and solidarity within the family that is highly valued. If they are asked to speak more slowly, with pauses between speakers, such changes would be in conflict with one of the family's cultural values. Another example might be parents who frequently teach, correct, and criticize their children's behavior. This "instructional" mode of interaction may reflect the value that the family's culture places on education.

We believe it is important to explore how the family feels about changes we are considering. In some cases, we can find ways to change other variables that will be as effective, thereby leaving unchanged those that are of value to the family. Recently, we worked with a parent who spoke very rapidly to her child who was showing some borderline stuttering. She resisted changing her rate because "it isn't the way we talk." In addition, she was frequently critical of her child's behavior. Consequently, we trained her to use positive reinforcement for fluency, as described in Onslow, Andrews, and Lincoln (1994) and asked her to let her child know, with an upbeat statement of praise, that she liked his smooth fluency. The child's stuttering diminished almost immediately, and the parent was delighted with her ability to help her child.

Sometimes we encounter a family who resists change. There may be psychological issues that need to be resolved through referral to another professional, or the family may have other, more serious problems to cope with. In these cases, we let the family know that we remain available to them, by occasional phone calls or postcards, so that they can return if they wish to.

MAINTENANCE

Indirect treatment of a borderline stutterer is often effective within five or six sessions. The child's speech becomes markedly less disfluent. Part-word repetitions become whole-word repetitions or phrase repetitions, and the family's concerns about the child's speech diminish. When this happens, we review the changes the family has made with them and the changes in their child's stuttering that reflect his improvement. Using this information, we help the family develop a plan to deal with periods of stress that may prompt stuttering to reappear. Most families feel that they have a handle on how to reduce stress on their child at this stage of therapy, and their experiences in observing and changing their behaviors has given them confidence. If their child's stuttering suddenly increases, they know how to examine their speech rates or attentiveness when talking to the child or to examine other aspects of their interactions and negotiate a change.

Effective maintenance, in our view, is the result of two things: (a) helping the family to view the child's stuttering more objectively, without guilt or panic, and (b) building the family's faith in their own ability to respond constructively to increases in the child's disfluency. Sometimes, however, despite a family's best efforts to respond constructively, stuttering returns. This may occur after an increase in stress from some trauma or from normal life events, such as moving to a new house. On the other hand, it may accompany a growth spurt in the child's language, or it may be unexplainable. Whatever the cause, the family should feel comfortable getting back in contact with the clinician. We let each family know at the end of therapy, that relapse is possible, is not abnormal, and that we would look forward to seeing the child again if our help is needed.

Clinical Procedures: Direct Treatment

We do not use direct treatment with every child who is a borderline stutterer, but it is a powerful alternative when indirect treatment is not immediately effective. The causes of our failure with an indirect approach are often unknown. Sometimes the family seems unable to change or may modify the child's environment as planned, but the child's stuttering persists. In these few cases, if we continue our indirect treatment for several months without seeing change, borderline stuttering may escalate in severity and become beginning stuttering.

DIRECT TREATMENT FOR MILD BORDERLINE STUTTERING

Most children with borderline stuttering are only slightly aware of their disfluencies. Their repetitions appear relaxed, and they show no signs of extra effort or attempts to "fight" their stutters. These children also are normally fluent a great deal of the time and have, we think, the capacity to "choose" between normal fluency and stuttering. Consequently, when we decide to work directly on their speech, we focus on reinforcing their fluency. We follow much of Onslow's behavioral management of stuttering therapy (Onslow, Andrews, & Lincoln, 1994), described in Chapter 12. However, we just reinforce fluency and ignore disfluencies.

We usually begin by commenting positively on the child's fluent utterances, choosing words that are in his vocabulary. For instance, we might say "Gee, you said that really smoothly." We might also echo what the child said, emphasizing its smoothness. If the child appears puzzled, or if this strategy doesn't seem to work, we may use some of the ideas suggested by Fosnot and Woodford (their program is discussed in the following text) and others to make sure the child understands the concepts of smoothness and bumpiness. Even though we use bumpiness to help the child understand its opposite—smoothness—and give examples of fluent and disfluent speech, we comment only on the child's fluent speech. We believe that positive reinforcement is powerful enough to be used alone and that the potential for punishment to create negative emotion, which would interfere with learning, is too great.

We are careful also not to make too many comments on the child's speech. We use our clinical judgment to help us know when we have used enough positive reinforcement to make the child feel good about his fluency and not too much reinforcement to make him think "enough already!"

During this part of direct therapy, we ask parents to observe us, either through a one-way mirror or in the room with us. Afterward, we talk to them about what they have seen and help them get a feel for how, when, and how often to reinforce fluency. When the child is talking in the clinic with normal levels of fluency (about 90%), we have the parents join our play activity in therapy and ask them to positively reinforce their child's fluency. Once we are satisfied that they have a good sense of how to reinforce fluency, we have them try it at home. We stay in close contact with them at first, in case questions arise. However, we find that with our continued support parents usually can carry on most of this treatment on their own.

DIRECT TREATMENT FOR MORE SEVERE BORDERLINE STUTTERING

Some children with borderline stuttering are beginning to have negative feelings about their disfluencies but are not showing the full-blown signs of physical tension or escape behaviors that characterize beginning stutterers. Still they may occasionally express real frustration with their stuttering. Others may evidence signs of both borderline and beginning stuttering: predominantly easy repetitions that become physically tense and abrupt under stress. As a result, the child shows signs of alarm. These are children whom we feel are very vulnerable to stress and who need to be inoculated against the negative emotions that they attach to stuttering unless these emotions are addressed without delay.

Typically, we work with children with more severe borderline for about 45 minutes each week. We continue to provide encouragement and support to the family in helping them make the child's environment as facilitating to fluency as possible. Our direct treatment activities are presented in a hierarchy that the clinician and child can ascend as far as is necessary to bring the child's disfluencies into the range of normal. Progressive steps are taken when the clinician senses that the child is feeling competent at the previous step. Thus, progress may be rapid or slow, sudden or gradual, depending on the child's feeling of comfort and mastery, session by session, with the tasks at hand. There is no need to hurry this process. It should take place within the context of games and activities that make the focus on stuttering casual. The clinician has to remain alert to the child's immediate sense of confidence and self-esteem in selecting the moment to take the child to the next step.

Modeling Easy Stutters

Our direct treatment begins rather indirectly, with the clinician providing models of easy stuttering in her speech.[3] If the child's repetitions are fast and abrupt, the clinician's models are slow with gradual endings. If the child has many repetitions or long prolongations, the clinician repeats only a few times or prolongs sounds briefly. These models are done casually, as we play with the child. We don't produce them immediately after the child stutters, but insert them randomly about once every two or three sentences, as if we were stuttering as we talked.

Once the child has become acclimated to the models of easy stuttering after 10 or 15 minutes of play, the clinician can begin to make accepting comments about them. She might say, for example, "Hmmmm, I bounced a bit on that word, didn't I?" or "That word stuck a little, but that's okay." Most children will appear shyly interested in what the clinician is talking about, and direct therapy can continue to develop. A few, however, will react negatively, saying, "Don't do that!" or "I don't like it when you stutter." For them, direct therapy needs to proceed slowly, letting the clinician's acceptance and support during play activities gradually counteract their anxiety.

If the child has begun to experience the first pangs of frustration from stuttering (which can be inferred from his questions or complaints about getting stuck on words), the clinician can help the child vent. Even though she is making comments that show acceptance of her own stuttering, she occasionally may produce a longer than usual stutter and say, "Sometimes they go on for a long time. That feels weird." The clinician should continue to try to sense what the child is feeling and to empathize as naturally as possible. This should be done not only when the clinician is modeling easy stutters, but throughout direct treatment.

For children who evidence periods of acute frustration with their stuttering, parents should be coached on how to make empathic statements in a calm, soothing, slow style when the child is going through a difficult time.

---

[3] Many of the ideas in this section were inspired by the writings of Van Riper (1973) and Dell (1979) and conversations with my colleague, Julie Reville.

The Child Begins Active Participation—Catch Me

When the clinician senses that the child is comfortable with her easy stuttering models, she might see if the child will take part. She may say, "Can you help me? Sometimes when I get stuck on a word, it goes on and on. I try to make my stuck words real slow and loose, but sometimes I forget. If you hear me go on and on like thi-thi-thi-thi-thi-this, just say, 'There's one,' and I'll try to make it slow and loose."

Praise should flow liberally when the child catches one of the clinician's modeled stutters. This provides a first sense of competence for the child, associated with something previously felt to be out of control. For many children, tangible rewards are important motivators and should be used along with praise to establish the child's ability to catch the clinician's stutters.

The Child Begins Active Participation—Play

This stage can either follow or precede "Catch Me." It depends on the clinician's judgment about which activity would be more comfortable for the child. Sometimes we start one of these two stages, find the child is not ready, and switch to the other. The "Play" stage engages the child in following the clinician's lead in playfully imitating disfluencies similar to his own—repeated or prolonged sounds. The purpose is to desensitize the child to the frustration that can arise sometimes in borderline stuttering, a process that may take place because play can give the child a sense of mastery without the risk of failure.[4]

Take, for example, the child who stutters primarily in a repetitive fashion. The clinician might say, "Let's play a game of saying some sounds over and over. Let's see how many times we can say them. I bet I can say a sound five times! Watch this. Ba-ba-ba-ba-ba! Can you do it five times?" Or, it can begin with making sounds for animals, puppets, or other objects: "Hey, this is a zebragella! It goes 'llllllllllllllllllla!' Then it jumps around like this (jump-jump-jump) and eats carpet (eat-eat-eat)."

The clinician and child can keep incorporating such play into their routine as long as the child finds it fun. From playing with repeated or prolonged sounds, the clinician can build a bridge to playing with repeated or prolonged sounds in conversation and, in time, to the child's actual stutters.

The Child Produces Intentional Stutters

After the child is able to catch the clinician's stutters and appears comfortable doing it, the clinician should look for an opportunity to ask the child to produce a stutter intentionally. This is done most easily by pretending to have trouble producing a slow and loose stutter. The clinician might say, "I can't seem to make this one slow and loose. Can you show me how to do it?" Again, this should be done intermittently and casually, mixed in with other activities.

Praise and, if needed, tangible rewards are used to help the child feel confidence. When the child is able to produce slow and loose stutters, the clinician can let the parent know, in the child's presence, about this accomplishment, focusing on the child's ability to teach the clinician. If the child seems proud of this accomplishment, the clinician might take advantage of this opportunity and have the child show intentional stutters to

---

[4] Many scientists speculate that childrens' play is an opportunity for them to practice and master skills that are needed in adulthood. Playing with stuttering may take advantage of a child's natural tendency to play and provide him with the pleasure of mastery and control over something that has been frustrating and, sometimes, even frightening.

the parent. This not only desensitizes the child to stuttering with the parent, but also desensitizes the parent to the child's stuttering, and models "acceptance" for the parent toward the child's stuttering.

The Child Changes His Own Real Stutters

For many children whose stuttering fluctuates between borderline and beginning levels, the previous stages of direct therapy, combined with a facilitating environment provided by parents, may be enough to advance fluency into the normal range within a few months. For those whose stuttering persists, still another stage of direct therapy may be necessary. In these cases, the clinician needs to look for opportunities when the child seems ready to modify his own stutters.

The clinician can begin by responding to a few of the child's real stutters with accepting comments to help the child feel comfortable with his stutters. She might say, "Oh, that was a good one on 'my-my-my car . . . ,'" then return to the business of playing. After further play, when the child stutters again, the clinician can model an easier and slower style of stuttering and comment positively about it. This is intended to suggest to the child that an easier, slower style of stuttering will be rewarded.

Then the clinician looks for slightly slower and easier stutters in the child's speech and rewards them. Even intentional stutters produced to get a reward should always be rewarded. From this point on, the clinician uses a combination of modeling and reinforcement to shape the child's stuttering. It is the slowness and "easyness" with which repetitions or prolongations are produced, along with the sense of playing with stuttering, that make it possible for the child to begin to feel a sense of control. This, in turn, should reduce frustration and fear, further diminish tension, and enable the child to move through stutters with minimal effort.

After the child is able to make his stutters slower and easier in the clinic, generalization may occur without the need for formal transfer activities. Such "spontaneous" generalization may be the result of the child's increased self-esteem from gaining mastery over what he previously felt was uncomfortable and out of his control. Consequently, emphasis should be placed on the stutters that the child handles successfully, rather than on the times when he loses control.

If generalization is not occurring automatically, the clinician can work with family members to make the child's ability to play with and modify stutters a point of pride at home. Initially, the child can teach parents and siblings to stutter in the clinic, under the clinician's guidance. Then the clinician can work with the child at home and involve family members when appropriate. Finally, parents can be taught to use positive reinforcement selectively to increase slow and easy stutters and to let the child know he is appreciated.

OTHER CLINICIANS

More Indirect Approaches

RICHARD CURLEE

Curlee (1993, 1998) believes that most children who begin to stutter will recover within 2 years of onset without needing treatment. Consequently, his approach to borderline stuttering focuses on identifying which children should be treated and which should not be treated, but systematically monitored. His diagnostic and evaluation procedures, described in the suggested readings, consist of parent interviews, analysis of parent-child interactions, evaluation of the child's stuttering, and screening of the child's articulation and language. If the child has been stuttering for less than 1 year and has no other speech or language problems and neither the family nor the child is distressed by the child's stuttering, Curlee institutes a program of monitoring the child's speech until the stuttering has stopped or appears to be persistent, therefore requiring treatment.

Monitoring consists of asking the family to record on audiotape or videotape the child's speech during various interactions and to analyze these recordings monthly. Clinic visits are scheduled every 2 or 3 months. However, if analysis of the recordings and reports from parents indicate that stuttering is decreasing, the clinic visit is delayed until 6 months have passed.

When evaluating the child's stuttering on the initial visit and subsequent recordings, Curlee makes careful observations of the child's stuttering pattern. Taking into account research by Yairi (1997a) and others, Curlee suggests that a child's stuttering is more likely to be chronic if these disfluency types are increasing: multiple-unit repetitions (li-li-li-li-like this), prolongations, and tense pauses with fixed articulatory postures (blocks). In addition, he notes that muscle tension associated with stuttering, escape, and avoidance behaviors, as well as negative emotional reactions to stuttering, are signs that stuttering may be worsening. If recordings show that these signs are consistent or increasing as the child is monitored over a period of 6 months, he recommends treatment.

For some children, Curlee does not use systematic monitoring, but initiates treatment immediately after the initial evaluation. These are children for whom a critical number of factors suggest persistent stuttering; such factors include the presence of other speech or language disorders, family history of persistent stuttering, and consistent stuttering-like disfluencies that are not diminishing over a period of a year. Curlee also initiates treatment if the family asks for therapy instead of systematic monitoring. With some families, Curlee may begin therapy by working with family-child interaction patterns if his analysis of their speech rate, length and complexity of utterances, and turn-switching pauses appear to place stress on the child. In other cases, he may use a home-based direct treatment such as Onslow's approach, described in Chapter 12, or he may opt for a two- or three-session-per-week treatment in his clinic.

BARBARA HEINZE AND KARIN JOHNSON

Johnson and Heinze (1994) begin with an assessment of the disfluent child (*The Fluency Companion*, Chapter 3). If the child is found to have borderline stuttering, therapy is indirect, primarily family counseling. Handouts[5] are given to guide the family in practices that reduce stuttering (e.g., "Speak slowly to the child"; "Let the child decide when to speak.") and that increase fluency (e.g., "Recite nursery rhymes with the child"; "Set up a schedule of daily activities."). The family is given written materials and videos and asked to fill out a weekly calendar for monitoring the child's speech. The parents are urged to set aside a daily quiet time to practice fluency enhancing activities.

After an initial postassessment meeting with the family, the clinician sets up a series of four counseling sessions. In the first session, the family is given information about normal speech characteristics, including normal disfluency. The parents are taught how various stresses in the home may exacerbate stuttering and how certain interaction styles may reduce stuttering. The child's speech, which has been recorded in the weekly cal-

---

[5] In the publications cited in "Suggested Readings," the authors provide a wealth of material that can be copied as handouts for families. A "Materials Book" accompanies the *Easy Does It* therapy manual and provides stimulus items for treatment.

endar, is reviewed. Next, the family and the clinician explore possible communication stresses that may account for times when the child was disfluent during the week. The family is then helped to formulate plans that will counteract these stresses.

The second and third sessions follow similar patterns, each session starting with a supportive discussion of changes in the home environment and in the child's disfluencies. This discussion is followed by the introduction of new information, such as how language and cognitive development and social-emotional pressures may affect the child's speech. After the new material is introduced, handouts are provided, and the family is guided in planning of further changes in the home environment to relieve pressures in these areas.

After the third session, the family is asked to record on videotape or audiotape a conversation with the child at home and to bring him in for a reevaluation. The fourth session is used to review the child's and the family's progress, and a decision is made regarding whether to dismiss the child from therapy because of adequate progress, to continue counseling alone, or to combine counseling with therapy for the child. If it is decided to dismiss the child, the clinician and the family talk over how to deal with possible relapses and difficult situations, including the beginning of school.

If the child has not made satisfactory progress, counseling continues and the child receives therapy. Treatment for a borderline stutterer is "indirect modeling" in which the clinician models slow, easy speech, and the child's fluency increases as he imitates the clinician's model. Heinze and Johnson caution, in *Easy Does It,* that clinicians should not call attention to the child's speech by directly reinforcing fluency, but should reinforce progress *indirectly* by expressing pleasure during the activities they are doing together. Therapy progresses from nursery rhymes and songs performed in unison, to words, phrases, and sentences in a conversational format—all in fluent, easy speech.

After the child is fluent in conversational speech, the clinician introduces fluency disrupters to toughen the child's fluency and to prepare for transfer. Because the family has been involved throughout therapy, some transfer has already been achieved. Nonetheless, structured transfer activities ensure that the child can maintain fluency not only in typical daily situations, but in difficult, emotional circumstances as well. The therapy program ends with a careful fading of contact with the child and family.

LOIS NELSON

Lois Nelson's intervention approach to the child with borderline stuttering is focused on the verbal interaction patterns that adults use when talking with the child (Nelson, 1985). She relies on a style of simpler language, slow rate, and reduction of fluency disrupters. After getting a baseline of the child's disfluency, she uses this style as she interacts with him during the evaluation. If it is successful in reducing disfluencies, she asks parents to use this interaction pattern at home. Parents vary greatly in their need for support in changing their verbal interaction patterns. Some elect to try it immediately on their own, with Nelson providing guidance over the telephone. Others prefer to work jointly with Nelson for several sessions, then try it on their own with her intermittent guidance.

Nelson recommends the following seven strategies:

1. Adults should slow their speech rate around the child. They should also convey to him, both verbally and nonverbally, that there is no reason to hurry when he talks—adults have time to listen.
2. Adults should reduce the number of questions they ask the child by commenting instead of questioning. Comments should be brief statements about what the child may be thinking, doing, or feeling. For example, "You seem to like that red truck. It goes really fast on the carpet."

3. Let the child decide when he wants to talk in a social situation. Avoid putting him on the spot by asking him to recite or tell an adult about an event that happened.
4. Stay in the "here and now" when talking with the child. Talk about what is right in front of the child, rather than talking about things or events that are far removed in time or space.
5. Help the child feel that he is being heard and understood by echoing part of what he has just said. This will also make talking fun for the child because he will feel that he can determine the topic.
6. As much as possible, adults should try to convey nonverbally that they are listening to the child by keeping good eye contact when the child is talking.
7. Reduce language pressure on the child. Refrain from teaching him; just enjoy being in his presence. Use short, simple sentences. Pause frequently so he can talk. Allow time for silences.

Nelson also notes that some children with borderline stuttering have a great deal of awareness, frustration, and embarrassment. Often, even after children with borderline stuttering have apparently recovered, they still have some doubts about their speech. Nelson is careful to let parents know about these doubts. She asks them to continue showing enthusiasm for and attention to their child's talking so that his negative feelings continue to decline. In addition, Nelson works directly with the child, verbalizing what she perceives their feelings to be, if they are older borderline stutterers and showing interest and enthusiasm for the content of their speech if they are younger.

JULIE REVILLE

Julie Reville's approach with young borderline stutterers, age 2 to 4 years, is family-centered and takes place in the child's home (Reville, 1988). Reville begins with a careful assessment of the child's speech, the history of the problem, and a study of the family's interaction with the child. During one or two initial visits with the family without the child present, Reville obtains information about the child's history, his current stuttering, and the family's response to it. She provides information about stuttering, answers questions, and shares reading material about stuttering to prepare family members for the work ahead. Before her first visit with the family, Reville requests that the parents record on videotape or audiotape samples of the child's speech during interactions with the family. That way, she can take the tape with her and make a careful analysis of the child's speech and the family's interaction before her next meeting with the family.

After studying the tape and making preliminary hypotheses about how the child's fluency may be facilitated, Reville arranges another home visit. For this session, she brings some attractive toys for the child and observes while key family members play and interact with the child. After observing for awhile, Reville begins to play with the child, modeling the kinds of fluency facilitating interactions that she hypothesizes will help him. These interactions often include a slow speech rate, simple language, and adequate pausing, among other things. She is careful also to let the child lead the conversation and to reflect whatever he is saying in her responses. If the child is reluctant to talk, she talks aloud about what she is doing and may comment on what the child is doing. Usually, the child grows comfortable with her and begins to talk spontaneously. Reville records both the family's interactions and her own with the child to assess the effect of her facilitating style.

After Reville analyzes the tape, she telephones the parents to discuss her observations, explore possibilities for change, and provide support for their efforts. In her next visit, Reville meets alone with the parents to review the changes that have occurred in both family interactions and in the child's stuttering. Together, they examine other aspects of the child's life that might influence stuttering. For example, Reville and the family may decide that the family's hectic lifestyle may be a factor in the child's stuttering, and they may develop a plan for changing it, which Reville helps them to do.

In subsequent telephone contacts, Reville provides support and suggestions for continued change. In later home visits, she continues to record on audiotape or videotape family members and herself playing and talking with the child. In some cases, she plays selected portions of these tapes for the family so they can observe and comment on their own interaction style. Self-observation on audiotape or videotape is often a powerful motivator for families who seem unaware of their rapid speech or their critical responses to the child.

If the child has language or articulation problems in addition to stuttering, Reville blends language stimulation or articulatory modeling with the fluency enhancing interactions that the family is learning. With Reville's continued support, most families develop a facilitating environment and become aware of key variables that may be responsible for reductions in the child's stuttering. By providing treatment in the home environment and working primarily through parents, Reville reports that improvement is usually permanent and that families know what steps to take if stuttering reappears.

C. WOODRUFF STARKWEATHER, SHERYL GOTTWALD, AND MURRAY HALFOND

Starkweather, Gottwald, and Halfond rely on three treatment strategies for helping the borderline stutterer: individual parent counseling, group parent counseling, and modification of the child's speech (Starkweather, Gottwald, & Halfond, 1990).

The initial component, individual parent counseling, provides parents with information about the nature of stuttering. For example, the clinician discusses the fact that stuttering is highly variable and that many factors may influence its increases and decreases, including factors that they may be able to change. The family is introduced to a model of stuttering that explains it as emerging from the interactions between the child's capacities and the demands placed on him. The clinician also helps the family to find ways of talking about stuttering to their child. They learn to support the child by commenting sensitively when he has a hard time getting a word out. Open acknowledgment of stuttering reduces the child's and the family's negative feelings about stuttering.

During individual counseling, families are also taught to change other aspects of their behavior that may be affecting their child's fluency. For example, family members may learn to respond to their child's stuttering without interrupting, looking away, or otherwise conveying impatience. To decrease pressure from the family's speech and language environment, family members may be taught to slow their speech rates, pause more frequently, and simplify their language when talking with the child. To increase the child's self-esteem, families may be urged to create times each day when the child has a parent's full attention. Sometimes, family members may be bombarding the child with questions or otherwise pressing him for speech. As a remedy, they are shown how to talk about what they are thinking and doing as they play with the child, thereby modeling the behavior they want to encourage.

In addition to changing behavior directly related to speech, families are also counseled about other stresses in the home. For example, Starkweather and his colleagues note that a hectic pace of life can exacerbate the child's stuttering. Once parents understand that a too-busy family schedule may be a factor in their child's stuttering, they are often able to reduce the hustle and bustle in their home and are gratified when their child's stuttering diminishes. In addition, a slower pace and a slower lifestyle are often relief for all family members.

Starkweather, Gottwald, and Halfond's approach uses group parent counseling to supplement individual counseling. As members of a group, parents get support from one another and can share ideas for helping their children. The clinician's role is to help the group develop a sense of mutual trust by modeling concern, acceptance, and respect for all group members and their ideas and feelings. Generally, the group discusses topics that they select, although the clinician also may suggest certain topics that are often a concern to all members, such as regression during treatment and termination of treatment.

The third component of this therapy, modification of the child's speech, incorporates both parent and clinician modeling as well as the clinician's direct instruction, when needed, and reinforcement. The procedures, which we think they would use with the child who has borderline stuttering, would proceed as follows. First, when an evaluation indicates that the child is talking faster than usual for his age or is using more complex language, the clinician and parent model speech rates and language that are appropriate for the child. The aim is to influence the child to talk in ways that do not stress his ability. Second, the clinician uses modeling, instruction, and reinforcement to help the child change multiple repetitions into slow, smooth, and slightly stretched productions of words.

Individual and group counseling and modification of the child's speech continue until the family environment and the child's speech have met two criteria. First, the environment has changed enough so that major stresses have diminished and the family seems to understand the dynamics that may exist between environmental stresses and the child's stuttering. Second, the child's stuttering has decreased to the point at which he is normally disfluent, with an occasional mild instance of stuttering.

Starkweather and his colleagues report that most of the children they have treated have regained normal fluency. Using this approach, the average child requires about 12 sessions of therapy, although some children require much more before therapy can be terminated.

STUTTERING FOUNDATION OF AMERICA (SFA)

Ainsworth and Fraser's booklet, *If Your Child Stutters: A Guide for Parents* (1989), helps families to differentiate between normal disfluency and stuttering and provides guidelines to help families create a fluency facilitating environment. Parents are urged to seek help from a speech-language pathologist if the child's disfluencies are of concern to them or the child. The SFA material can be used also to supplement clinical treatment.

Guidelines for changing home environments focus first on talking and listening. Ainsworth and Fraser encourage families to provide appropriate speech models, to make the child feel that he has ample opportunity to talk and be understood, and to give the child pleasurable speaking experiences. Families are urged to decrease stress in daily living, such as from rigid or inconsistent discipline, competitive pressure, and high expectations. Ainsworth and Fraser also suggest ways that family members can respond to the child's disfluencies so that both they and the child do not make things worse. If the child expresses concern, parents are encouraged to talk with him about his disfluencies and help him vent his emotions.

Conture and Fraser's *Stuttering and Your Child: Questions and Answers* (1989) provides families, teachers, and others with information about stuttering and how children who stutter can be helped. It covers a wide range of issues, including stuttering versus normal disfluency, the possible causes of stuttering, changing the home environment, dealing with others' responses to the child's stuttering, and treatment. Although formal aspects of treatment are left to professionals, specific advice on how parents, babysitters, day care centers, and teachers can help children is given in highlighted pages. Parents are instructed how to be good listeners for their children, how to increase times when the child feels he is being heard, and how to reduce both conversational and lifestyle pressures.

Babysitters and day care centers are advised to react as normally as possible to the child, treating him like other children while ensuring that he has plenty of time to say what he wants to say without feeling rushed. Teachers are encouraged to give the child support for oral recitations, allow him the same speaking opportunities as other children, and help the entire class to develop good speaking and listening practices.

Stuttering and Your Child: A Videotape for Parents (Conture, 1994) is a 30-minute presentation of information and advice in which viewers are shown examples of normal disfluency and various types of stuttering to get an idea of whether their child is stuttering or not. Then, factual information about stuttering is given in the context of parent interviews. In the final section of the video, the narrator discusses ways in which family members can change their conversational patterns to facilitate the child's fluency. These include pausing before speaking; speaking more slowly; using short, simple sentences; and talking about what the child is talking about. All are illustrated through clips of parent-child interactions and comments by parents. Several other suggestions are also made to help parents keep the child from feeling stress on his speech.

Both the latter booklets and the video are designed for families with a child who may be at the borderline level of stuttering. Many of these suggestions are also applicable to children with beginning or even intermediate levels of stuttering. In all cases, they are best used as a supplement to consultation or treatment with a speech-language pathologist who has extensive, successful experience working with children who stutter.

More Direct Approaches

SUSAN MEYERS FOSNOT AND LEE WOODFORD

Fosnot and Woodford's (1992) approach has three major components: differential assessment, treatment of the child, and parent counseling.

In the differential assessment component, the clinician first obtains background information through a telephone interview with parents and a case history form. Then, she arranges to observe the child interacting with each parent and screens the child's language, articulation, voice, and hearing. The parent-child interaction is recorded on videotape or audiotape and subjected to a "microanalysis." Fosnot and Woodford detail how to transcribe and score the bidirectional interaction between parent and child. Assessment results in one of the following decisions about treatment: Normally disfluent children without other speech, language, or hearing disorders are followed up for several years to ensure that fluency is stabilized. Normally disfluent children with other speech-language disorders are given appropriate treatment that incorporates fluency monitoring. Children who stutter are enrolled in fluency therapy, and their parents are counseled to help them change the child's environment.

The child treatment component of Fosnot and Woodford's program uses cognitive and behavioral principles to teach children three rules for facilitating fluency. The first rule is to use slow speech, which is taught using stories, activities, and puppets to help young children grasp the concept of slow versus fast talking and to practice speaking slowly with normal intonation and stress. The second rule is to talk smoothly, so that part-word repetitions and sound prolongations are transformed into an effortless, easy style of speech. The concept of smooth versus bumpy is taught with foods, finger paints, and picture books. The third rule is to take turns when talking; this is an outgrowth of research that suggests that young children stutter more when they interrupt someone. The clinician teaches turn-taking with a story book, a "Mr. Turn-Taker" animal, and games that incorporate turn-taking with speaking slowly and beginning speech smoothly.

After the child has learned the three rules for fluency and can remain fluent in spontaneous conversation, the clinician introduces the concept of "pressure" that disrupts fluent speech. Games and activities using a "Mr. Pressure" mask are used to help the child understand and resist pressure on fluency from fast talkers and from interruptions. After the child has learned to remain fluent in the face of pressures used during these games, the clinician introduces the child's parents into the therapy setting. Using data from the child's initial assessment, the clinician selects parents' behaviors that are most in need of change and coaches the parents on how to make their interactions more facilitating to their child's fluency. Parents take what they have learned in therapy sessions and apply it in interactions at home, with feedback and reinforcement from the clinician.

Fosnot and Woodford's approach also has a data collection component, which is used to assess the success of treatment and determine when to move from one stage of therapy to the next. The authors provide instructions for assessing and charting fluency at each stage, preparing the child for "graduation" from therapy, and planning follow-up procedures. While the child is in direct therapy, the parents receive group counseling to help them understand their child and his problem better and how to make their home a fluency facilitating environment. The authors carefully structure activities and topics for parent counseling.

Beatrice Stocker and Robert Goldfarb

The Stocker Probe is an assessment tool and a treatment approach. It is based on evidence that children's stuttering varies with the level of communicative demand. For example, they stutter less when asked, "Is this hot or cold?" than they do when they're asked to make up a story. The assessment phase measures how much stuttering occurs at each of five different levels of communicative demand: (a) choosing of alternatives to describe an object, such as "Is it round or square"; (b) simple "wh-" questions, such as, "What is it"; (c) more complex "Wh-" questions, such as "What do you do with it"; (d) open-ended descriptions, such as "Tell me everything you know about this," and finally (e) a request to make up a story about an object. The clinician records how much stuttering occurs on each level of demand.

Treatment begins at a level of demand in which the child showed no disfluency. The clinician rewards the child for successively longer periods of fluent speech (timed by a stopwatch) at this level until the child is fluent for "three consecutive sixty-second periods of fluency." Then the child moves to the next higher level of demand, and the clinician continues rewarding the child for fluency at that level. If the child is disfluent, the clinician simply resets the stopwatch to zero and has the child respond to another question or probe. Gradually, by successive approximations, the child learns to be fluent for longer and longer periods of time at higher and higher levels of communicative demand.

Clinicians are given substantial leeway in using materials, other than those provided, to keep therapy interesting for the child. In addition to direct treatment of the child, the clinician councils the parents to lower demands on the child's speech at home, until the child has moved far enough up the demand hierarchy in therapy to remain fluent at highest levels of demand in all situations.

SUMMARY OF APPROACHES TO BORDERLINE STUTTERING

Fluency shaping and stuttering modification therapies are highly similar in their approaches to borderline stuttering. Both work with family members to reduce stress and to create an environment that is conducive to fluency; both may provide a "scaffold" for the child's fluency by modeling and reinforcing an easy, slow, smooth style of speech. Differences between approaches are largely in terms of whether clinicians are more indirect, meaning that they begin with family counseling and work directly with the child only if needed, or more direct, meaning that they begin working with the child and counsel the family only as an adjunct to the child's direct treatment.

Our own therapy for borderline stuttering begins with an analysis of a family's interaction patterns to identify factors that may be contributing to the child's stuttering. We then work cooperatively with the family, share information about stuttering, and suggest possible areas for change. As the family takes the lead in determining which interaction patterns to change, we provide modeling, support, and feedback to support their efforts. If this approach does not result in improvements in the child's stuttering within 6 weeks, we initiate more direct therapy with the child, which ranges from reinforcement of fluency, for mild borderline stuttering, to helping the child explore, discuss, and modify his stutters, for children with severe borderline stuttering.

STUDY QUESTIONS

1. What are some aspects of family conversational interactions that may put pressure on the child with borderline stuttering?

2. What changes can a family make in their home to relieve speech and language pressures?

3. Discuss how the clinician can facilitate changes in family routines that may help the child's fluency.

4. What are some of the barriers to change that are found in some families? How can the clinician help the family overcome these barriers?

5. Compare our direct approach to a mild borderline stutterer with an approach for a severe borderline stutterer.

6. Compare one of the other clinician's more indirect therapies with one of the more direct therapies.

SUGGESTED READINGS

Ainsworth, S., & Fraser, J. (1989). *If your child stutters: A guide for parents,* **3rd rev. ed. Memphis: Stuttering Foundation of America.**

This inexpensive booklet gives advice to parents who think their child is beginning to stutter.

Conture, E. (Producer). (1994). *Stuttering and your child: A videotape for parents.* **Memphis: Stuttering Foundation of America.**

This video, available from the Stuttering Foundation for $5.00, depicts a variety of stuttering behaviors, provides information on stuttering, and portrays ways in which parents can facilitate fluency.

Conture, E., & Fraser, J. (Eds.). (1989). *Stuttering and your child: Questions and answers.* **Memphis: Stuttering Foundation of America.**
This booklet gives answers to commonly asked questions about stuttering.

Curlee, R.F. (1993). Identification and management of beginning stuttering. In R.F. Curlee (Ed.), *Stuttering and related disorders of fluency.* **New York: Thieme Medical Publishers.**
This chapter describes procedures to evaluate children who may be stuttering, to select those who need therapy, and to follow up when appropriate.

Curlee, R.F. (in press). Identification and case selection guidelines for early childhood stuttering. In R.F. Curlee (Ed.), *Stuttering and related disorders of fluency,* **2nd ed. New York: Thieme Medical Publishers.**
This chapter updates Curlee's procedures for evaluation and case selection, but does not provide the specifics on therapy given in the 1993 version.

Fosnot, S.M., & Woodford, L.L. (1992). *The fluency development system for young children.* **Buffalo: United Educational Services, Inc.**
This kit supplies all the props and materials needed to evaluate stuttering in young children, provide therapy, and counsel their parents.

Gottwald, S., & Starkweather, C.W. (1995). Fluency intervention for preschoolers and their families in the public schools. *Language, Speech, and Hearing Services in Schools, 26,* **115–126.**
This article describes assessment and treatment procedures used by a variety of clinicians for young children who stutter.

Guitar, B. (1984). Indirect treatment of childhood stuttering. In J. Costello (Ed.), *Speech disorders in children: Recent advances.* **San Diego: College-Hill Press.**
This chapter is an overview of various approaches to therapy that do not directly change the way the child speaks.

Guitar, B., Kopff-Schaefer, H., Donahue-Kilburg, G., & Bond, L. (1992). Parent verbal interaction and speech rate. *Journal of Speech and Hearing Research, 35,* **742–754.**
This article describes therapy with parents of a young child who stutters and the analysis of parent-child interactions.

Heinze, B., & Johnson, K. (1985). *Easy does it: Fluency activities for young children.* **East Moline, IL: LinguiSystems.**
This manual provides instructions and materials for establishing fluency and transferring it to everyday situations. Desensitization to fluency disrupters is also part of the program.

Johnson, K., & Heinze, B. (1994). *The fluency companion: Strategies for stuttering intervention.* **East Moline, IL: LinguiSystems.**
This manual provides instruction and materials for both direct and indirect stuttering therapy for children, from toddlers to teenagers.

Nelson, L. (1985). Language formulation related to dysfluency and stuttering. In *Stuttering therapy: Prevention and intervention with children.* **Memphis: Stuttering Foundation of America.**
This chapter delineates Lois Nelson's treatment strategies for preschoolers who stutter. It is a distillation of many years of experience with stuttering children.

Reville, J. (1988). *The many voices of Paws*. Princeton Junction, NJ: Speech Bin.
This is a manual for speech-language pathologists and parents to help them work with preschool children who stutter. A slow, easy style of speaking is taught with the help of a poem about a cat named "Paws."

Starkweather, C.W., Gottwald, S.R., & Halfond, M.H. (1990). *Stuttering prevention: A clinical method*. Englewood Cliffs, NJ: Prentice-Hall.
This book details a program of assessment and treatment for children who stutter and for their parents.

Stocker, B., & Goldfarb, R. (1995). *The Stocker probe for fluency and language*. Vero Beach, FL: The Speech Bin.

References

Adams, M. (1977). A clinical strategy for differentiating the normally nonfluent child and the incipient stutterer. *Journal of Fluency Disorders, 2,* 141–148.

Adams, M.R. (1980). The young stutterer: Diagnosis, treatment and assessment of progress. *Seminars in Speech, Language and Hearing, 1,* 289–299.

Adams, M. (1990). The demands and capacities model I: Theoretical elaborations. *Journal of Fluency Disorders, 15,* 135–141.

Adams, M.R., & Hayden, P. (1976). The ability of stutterers and nonstutterers to initiate and terminate phonation during production of an isolated vowel. *Journal of Speech and Hearing Research, 19,* 290–296.

Adams, M.R., & Runyan, C.M. (1981). Stuttering and fluency: Exclusive events or points on a continuum? *Journal of Fluency Disorders, 6,* 197–218.

Ahlbach, J., & Benson, V. (1994). *To say what is ours: The best 13 years of "Letting Go."* San Francisco: National Stuttering Project.

Ainsworth, S., & Fraser, J. (1989). *If your child stutters: A guide for parents,* 3rd rev. ed. Memphis: Stuttering Foundation of America.

Alfonso, P.J., Story, R.S., & Watson, B.C. (1987). The organization of supralaryngeal articulation in stutterers' fluent speech production: A second report. *Annual Bulletin Research Institute of Logopedics and Phoniatrics, 21,* 117–129.

Allen, S. (1988). *Durations of segments in repetitive disfluencies in stuttering and nonstuttering children.* Unpublished manuscript, E.M. Luse Center, University of Vermont, Burlington.

Ambrose, N., & Yairi, E. (1995). The role of repetition units in the differential diagnosis of early childhood incipient stuttering. *American Journal of Speech-Language Pathology, 4,* 82–88.

Ambrose, N., Yairi, E., & Cox, N. (1993). Genetic aspects of early childhood stuttering. *Journal of Speech and Hearing Research, 36,* 701–706.

Andrews, G., & Craig, A. (1988). Prediction of outcome after treatment for stuttering. *British Journal of Psychiatry, 153,* 236–240.

Andrews, G., Craig, A., Feyer, A.-M., et al. (1983). Stuttering: A review of research findings and theories circa 1982. *Journal of Speech and Hearing Disorders, 48,* 226–246.

Andrews, G., & Cutler, J. (1974). Stuttering therapy: The relation between changes in symptom level and attitudes. *Journal of Speech and Hearing Disorders, 39,* 312–319.

Andrews, G., & Harris, M. (1964). *The syndrome of stuttering.* Clinics in Developmental Medicine, no. 17. London: Spastics Society Medical Education and Information Unit in association with W. Heinemann Medical Books.

Andrews, G., Howie, P.M., Dozsa, M., & Guitar, B.E. (1982). Stuttering: Speech pattern characteristics under fluency-inducing conditions. *Journal of Speech and Hearing Research, 25,* 208–216.

Andrews, G., & Ingham, R. (1971). Stuttering: Considerations in the evaluation of treatment. *British Journal of Communication Disorders, 6,* 129–138.

Andrews, G., Morris-Yates, A., Howie, P., & Martin, N.G. (1990). The genetic nature of stuttering. *Archives of General Psychiatry, 48*(11), 1034–1035.

Arthur, G. (1952). Arthur adaptation of the Leiter International Performance Test. Los Angeles: Western Psychological Services.

Bandura, A. (1977). Self-efficacy: Toward a unifying theory of behavioral change. *Psychological Review, 84*(2), 191–215.

Bates, E., Dale, P., & Thal, D. (1995). Individual differences and their implications for theories of language development. In P. Fletcher & B. MacWhinney (Eds.), *The handbook of child language.* Oxford: Basil Blackwell.

Beitchman, J., Nair, R., Clegg, M., & Patel, P.G. (1986). Prevalence of speech and language disorders in 5-year-old kindergarten children in the Ottawa-Carleton region. *Journal of Speech and Hearing Disorders, 51,* 98–110.

Berk, L.E. (1991). *Child development,* 2nd ed. Boston: Allyn & Bacon.

Bernstein, N.E. (1981). Are there constraints on childhood disfluency? *Journal of Fluency Disorders, 6,* 341–350.

Bernstein Ratner, N. (1995). Treating the child who stutters with concomitant language and phonological impairment. *Language, Speech, and Hearing in Schools, 26*(2), 180–186.

Bernstein Ratner, N. (1997). Stuttering: A psycholinguistic perspective. In R. Curlee & G. Siegel (Eds.), *Nature and treatment of stuttering: New directions,* 2nd ed. (pp. 97–127). Boston: Allyn & Bacon.

Bernstein Ratner, N., & Sih, C.C. (1987). Effects of gradual increases in sentence length and complexity on children's dysfluency. *Journal of Speech and Hearing Disorders, 52,* 278–287.

Bernthal, J. (1994). *Child phonology: Characteristics, assessment, and intervention in special populations.* New York: Thieme Medical Publishers.

Bernthal, J., & Bankson, N. (1998). *Articulation and phonological disorders,* 4th ed. Needham Heights, MA: Allyn & Bacon.

Berry, M.F. (1937). *The medical history of stuttering children.* Unpublished doctoral dissertation, University of Wisconsin, Madison.

Berry, M.F. (1938). Developmental history of stuttering children. *Journal of Pediatrics, 12,* 209–217.

Bloch, E.L., & Goodstein, L.D. (1971). Functional speech disorders and personality: A decade of research. *Journal of Speech and Hearing Disorders, 36,* 295–314.

Bloodstein, O. (1944). Studies in the psychology of stuttering: XIX. The relationship between oral reading rate and severity of stuttering. *Journal of Speech Disorders, 9,* 161–173.

Bloodstein, O. (1948). *Conditions under which stuttering is reduced or absent.* Unpublished doctoral dissertation, University of Iowa, Iowa City.

Bloodstein, O. (1950). Hypothetical conditions under which stuttering is reduced or absent. *Journal of Speech and Hearing Disorders, 15,* 142–153.

Bloodstein, O. (1958). Stuttering as an anticipatory struggle reaction. In J. Eisenson (Ed.), *Stuttering: A symposium.* New York: Harper & Row.

Bloodstein, O. (1975). Stuttering as tension and fragmentation. In J. Eisenson (Ed.), *Stuttering: A second symposium.* New York: Harper & Row.

Bloodstein, O. (1987). *A handbook on stuttering,* 4th ed. Chicago: National Easter Seal Society.

Bloodstein, O. (1993). *Stuttering: The search for a cause and a cure.* Boston: Allyn & Bacon.

Bloodstein, O. (1995). *A handbook on stuttering,* 5th ed. San Diego: Singular Publishing Group, Inc.

Bloodstein, O. (1997). Stuttering as an anticipatory struggle reaction. In R.F. Curlee & G.M. Siegel (Eds.), *The nature and treatment of stuttering: New directions,* 2nd ed. (pp. 169–181). Boston: Allyn & Bacon.

Boberg, E. (1984). Intensive adult/teen therapy program. In W.H. Perkins (Ed.), *Stuttering disorders.* New York: Thieme-Stratton.

Boberg, E., & Kully, D. (1994). Long-term results of an intensive treatment program for adults and adolescents who stutter. *Journal of Speech and Hearing Research, 37,* 1050–1059.

Boehmler, R.M. (1994). *The treatment of stuttering as a speech-flow disorder.* Unpublished manuscript.

Boone, D., & McFarlane, S. (1988). *The voice and voice therapy*, 4th ed. Englewood Cliffs, NJ: Prentice-Hall.

Bouton, M.E., & Bolles, R.C. (1985). Contexts, event-memories, and extinction. In P.D. Balsam & A. Tomie (Eds.), *Context and learning.* Hillsdale, NJ: Lawrence Erlbaum Associates.

Branigan, G. (1979). Some reasons why successive single word utterances are not. *Journal of Child Language, 6,* 411–421.

Braun, A.R., Varga, M., Stager S., et al. (1996). $H_2^{15}O$ positron emission tomography studies in developmental stuttering: Comparisons of brain activity during non-linguistic orolaryngeal motor activity, fluency- and dysfluency-evoking language conditions. Paper presented at the Third International Conference on Speech Motor Production and Fluency Disorders, Nijmegen, The Netherlands.

Brown, S.F. (1937). The influence of grammatical function on the incidence of stuttering. *Journal of Speech Disorders, 2,* 207–215.

Brown, S.F. (1938a). A further study of stuttering in relation to various speech sounds. *Quarterly Journal of Speech, 24,* 390–397.

Brown, S.F. (1938b). Stuttering with relation to word accent and word position. *Journal of Abnormal Social Psychology, 33,* 112–120.

Brown, S.F. (1938c). The theoretical importance of certain factors influencing the incidence of stuttering. *Journal of Speech Disorders, 3,* 223–230.

Brown, S.F. (1943). An analysis of certain data concerning loci of "stutterings" from the viewpoint of general semantics. *Papers from the Second American Congress of General Semantics, 2,* 194–199.

Brown, S.F. (1945). The loci of stutterings in the speech sequence. *Journal of Speech Disorders, 10,* 181–192.

Brown, S.F., & Moren, A. (1942). The frequency of stuttering in relation to word length during oral reading. *Journal of Speech Disorders, 7,* 153–159.

Brundage, S., & Bernstein Ratner, N. (1989). The measurement of stuttering frequency in children's speech. *Journal of Fluency Disorders, 14,* 351–358.

Brutten, G.J. (1970). Two-factor behavior theory and therapy. In *Conditioning in stuttering therapy: Applications and limitations.* Memphis: Speech Foundation of America.

Brutten, G.J. (1975). Stuttering: Topography, assessment and behavior change strategies. In J. Eisenson (Ed.), *Stuttering: A second symposium.* New York: Harper & Row.

Brutten, G.J., & Dunham, S. (1989). The Communication Attitude Test: A normative study of grade school children. *Journal of Fluency Disorders, 14,* 371–377.

Brutten, G.J., & Shoemaker, D. (1967). *The modification of stuttering.* Englewood Cliffs, NJ: Prentice-Hall.

Calkins, S. (1994). Origins and outcomes of individual differences in emotion regulation. In N.A. Fox & J. Campos (Eds.), *The development of emotional regulation: Biological and behavioral considerations.* Chicago: Society for Research in Child Development.

Calkins, S.D., & Fox, N.A. (1994). Individual differences in the biological aspects of temperament. In J.E. Bates & T.D. Wachs (Eds.), *Temperament: Individual differences at the interface of biology and behavior.* Washington, DC: American Psychological Association.

Caruso, A.J. (1988). Childhood stuttering: A review of behavioral, acoustical, and physiological research. (Abstract). *ASHA, 30,* 73.

Caruso, A.J., Abbs, J.H., & Gracco, V.L. (1988). Kinematic analysis of multiple movement coordination during speech in stutterers. *Brain, 111,* 439–455.

Caruso, A.J., Chodzko-Zajko, W., & McClowry, M. (1995). Emotional arousal and stuttering: The impact of cognitive stress. In C. W. Starkweather & H.F.M. Peters (Eds.), *Stuttering: Proceedings of the First World*

Congress on Fluency Disorders. Nijmegen, The Netherlands: International Fluency Association.

Caruso, A.J., Chodzko-Zajko, W., Bidinger, D., & Sommers, R. (1994). Adults who stutter: Responses to cognitive stress. *Journal of Speech and Hearing Research, 37,* 746–754.

Chase, C.H. (1996). Neurobiology of learning disabilities. *Seminars in Speech and Language, 17*(3), 173–181.

Clarke-Stewart, A., & Friedman, S. (1987). *Child development: Infancy through adolescence.* New York: John Wiley & Sons.

Colburn, N., & Mysak, E.D. (1982a). Developmental disfluency and emerging grammar. I. Disfluency characteristics in early syntactic utterances. *Journal of Speech and Hearing Research, 25,* 414–420.

Colburn, N., & Mysak, E.D. (1982b). Developmental disfluency and emerging grammar. II. Co-occurrence of disfluency with specified semantic-syntactic structures. *Journal of Speech and Hearing Research, 25,* 421–427.

Colcord, R.D., & Adams, M.R. (1979). Voicing duration and vocal SPL changes associated with stuttering reduction during singing. *Journal of Speech and Hearing Research, 22,* 468–479.

Colton, R., & Casper, J. (1996). *Understanding voice problems: A physiological perspective for diagnosis and therapy.* Baltimore: Williams & Wilkins.

Conrad, C. (1996). Fluency in multicultural populations. In L. Cole & V.R. Deal (Eds.). *Communication disorders in multicultural populations.* Rockville, MD: American Speech-Language-Hearing Association.

Conture, E., & Fraser, J. (1989). *Stuttering and your child: Questions and answers.* Memphis: Speech Foundation of America.

Conture, E., & Guitar, B. (1993). Evaluating efficacy of treatment of stuttering: school-age children. *Journal of Fluency Disorders, 18,* 253–287.

Conture, E., Guitar, B., & Williams, D. (1996). *Childhood stuttering: A videotape for parents.* (Videotape). Memphis: Stuttering Foundation of America.

Conture, E.G. (1982). *Stuttering.* Englewood Cliffs, NJ: Prentice-Hall.

Conture, E.G. (1990). *Stuttering,* 2nd ed. Englewood Cliffs, NJ: Prentice-Hall.

Conture, E.G. (1991). Young stutterers' speech production. In H.F.M. Peters, W. Hulstijn, & C.W. Starkweather (Eds.), *Speech motor control and stuttering.* (pp. 365–384). Amsterdam: Excerpta Medica.

Conture, E.G. (Producer), (1994). *Stuttering and your child: A videotape for parents.* (30-minute videotape). Memphis: Stuttering Foundation of America.

Conture, E.G., Louko, L., & Edwards, M.L. (1993). Simultaneously treating stuttering and disordered phonology in children: Experimental therapy, preliminary findings. *American Journal of Speech-Language Pathology, 2,* 72–81.

Conture, E.G., McCall, G.N., & Brewer, D.W. (1977). Laryngeal behavior during stuttering. *Journal of Speech and Hearing Research, 20,* 661–668.

Cooper, C.S. (1991). Using collaborative/consultative service delivery models for fluency intervention and carryover. *Language, Speech, and Hearing Services in Schools, 22,* 152–153.

Cooper, E.B. (1979). *Understanding stuttering: Information for parents.* Chicago: National Easter Seal Society.

Cooper, E.B., & Cooper, C.S. (1985). *Cooper personalized fluency control therapy—* revised. Allen, TX: DLM.

Cooper, E.B., & Cooper, C.S. (1993). Fluency disorders. In D.E. Battle (Ed.), *Communication disorders in multicultural organizations.* (pp. 189–211). Boston: Andover Medical Publishers.

Cooper, E.B., & Cooper C.S. (1995). Treating fluency disordered adolescents. *Journal of Communication Disorders, 28,* 125–142.

Costello, J.M. (1980). Operant conditioning and the treatment of stuttering. *Seminars in Speech, Language and Hearing, 1,* 311–325.

Costello, J.M. (1983). Current behavioral treatments for children. In D. Prins & R.J. Ingham (Eds.), *Treatment of stuttering in early childhood: Methods and issues.* San Diego: College-Hill Press.

Cox, N.J. (1988). Molecular genetics: The key to the puzzle of stuttering? *ASHA, 30*(4), 36–40.

Cox, N.J., Seider, R.A., & Kidd, K.K. (1984). Some environmental factors and hypotheses for stuttering in families with several stutterers. *Journal of Speech and Hearing Research, 27,* 543–548.

Craig, A., & Andrews, G. (1985). The prediction and prevention of relapse in stuttering. *Behavior Modification, 9,* 427–442.

Craig, A., Franklin, J., & Andrews, G. (1984). A scale to measure locus of control of behavior. *British Journal of Medical Psychology, 57,* 173–180.

Craig, A., Hancock, K., Chang, E., et al.(1996). A controlled clinical trial for stuttering in persons aged 9 to 14 years. *Journal of Speech and Hearing Research, 39,* 808–826.

Cross, D.E., & Cooke, P. (1979). Vocal and manual reaction times of adult stutterers and nonstutterers. (Abstract). *ASHA, 21,* 693.

Cross, D.E., & Luper, H.L. (1979). Voice reaction time of stuttering and nonstuttering children and adults. *Journal of Fluency Disorders, 4,* 59–77.

Cross, D.E., & Luper, H.L. (1983). Relation between finger reaction time and voice reaction time in stuttering and nonstuttering children and adults. *Journal of Speech and Hearing Research, 26,* 356–361.

Cross, D., Sweet, J., & Bates, D. (1985). Mental imagery and stuttering: Electroencephalographic and physiological characteristics. Paper presented at the American Speech-Language-Hearing Association Convention, Washington, DC.

Crystal, D. (1987). Towards a "bucket" theory of language disability: Taking account of interaction between linguistic levels. *Clinical Linguistics and Phonetics, 1,* 7–22.

Culatta, R., & Goldberg, S. (1995). *Stuttering therapy: An integrated approach to theory and practice.* Boston: Allyn & Bacon.

Cullinan, W.L., & Springer, M.T. (1980). Voice initiation times in stuttering and nonstuttering children. *Journal of Speech and Hearing Research, 23,* 344–360.

Curlee, R. (1984). A case selection strategy for young disfluent children. *Seminars in Speech, Language, and Hearing, 1,* 277–287.

Curlee, R. (1988). (Ed.) Counseling in speech, language, and hearing. (Entire issue). *Seminars in Speech and Language, 9*(3).

Curlee, R.F. (1993). Identification and management of beginning stuttering. In R.F. Curlee (Ed.), *Stuttering and related disorders of fluency.* New York: Thieme Medical Publishers.

Curlee, R.F. (in press). Identification and case selection guidelines for early childhood stuttering. In R.F. Curlee (Ed.), *Stuttering and related disorders of fluency,* 2nd ed. New York: Thieme Medical Publishers.

Curlee, R.F., & Perkins, W.H. (1969). Conversational rate control therapy for stuttering. *Journal of Speech and Hearing Disorders, 34,* 245–250.

Curlee, R.F., & Perkins, W.H. (1984). Preface. In R.F. Curlee & W.H. Perkins (Eds.), *Nature and treatment of stuttering: New directions.* San Diego: College-Hill Press.

Curlee, R. F., & Siegel, G. (Eds.). (1997). *Nature and treatment of stuttering: New directions,* 2nd ed. Boston: Allyn & Bacon.

Dalton, P., & Hardcastle, W.J. (1977). *Disorders of fluency.* New York: Elsevier.

Daly, D. (1986). The clutterer. In K. St. Louis (Ed.), *The atypical stutterer.* New York: Academic Press.

Daly, D.A. (1988). *The freedom of fluency.* East Moline, IL: LinguiSystems.

Daly, D.A. (1993). Cluttering: Another fluency syndrome. In R. Curlee (Ed.), *Stuttering and related disorders of fluency.* (pp. 151–175). New York: Thieme Medical Publishers.

Darley, F.L. (1955). The relationship of parental attitudes and adjustments to the development of stuttering. In W. Johnson & R.R. Leutenegger (Eds.), *Stuttering in children and adults.* Minneapolis: University of Minnesota Press.

Darley, F., & Spriestersbach, D. (1978). *Diagnostic methods in speech pathology,* 2nd ed. New York: Harper & Row.

Darwin, C. (1950). *Charles Darwin's autobiography.* New York: Henry Schuman.

Davis, D.M. (1940). The relation of repetitions in the speech of young children to certain measures of language maturity and situational factors: Parts II & III. *Journal of Speech Disorders, 5,* 235–246.

DeJoy, D.A., & Gregory, H.H. (1973). The relationship of children's disfluencies to the syntax, length, and vocabulary of their sentences. (Abstract). *ASHA, 15,* 472.

DeJoy, D.A., & Gregory, H.H. (1985). The relationship between age and frequency of disfluency in preschool children. *Journal of Fluency Disorders, 10,* 107–122.

Dell, C. (1979). *Treating the school age stutterer: A guide for clinicians.* Memphis: Speech Foundation of America.

Dell, C. (1993). Treating school-aged stutterers. In R. Curlee (Ed.), *Stuttering and related disorders of fluency.* New York: Thieme Medical Publishers.

De Nil, L. (1995). Linguistic and motor approaches to stuttering: Exploring unification. A panel presentation at the Annual Convention of the American Speech-Language-Hearing Association, Orlando, Florida, December.

De Nil, L., & Brutten, G.J. (1991). Speech-associated attitudes of stuttering and normally fluent children. *Journal of Speech and Hearing Research, 34,* 60–66.

De Nil, L., Kroll, R., Kapur, S., & Houle, S. (1995). Silent and oral reading in stuttering and nonstuttering adults: A positron emission tomography study. Paper presented at the Annual Convention of the American Speech-Language-Hearing Association, Orlando, Florida, December.

Denny, M., & Smith, A. (1992). Gradations in

a pattern of neuromuscular activity associated with stuttering. *Journal of Speech and Hearing Research, 35,* 1216–1229.

DiSimoni, F.G. (1974). Preliminary study of certain timing relationships in the speech of stutterers. *Journal of the Acoustical Society of America, 56,* 695–696.

Edelman, G. (1992). *Bright air, brilliant fire: On the matter of mind.* New York: Basic Books.

Emerick, L., & Haynes, W. (1986). *Diagnosis and evaluation in speech pathology,* 3rd ed. Englewood Cliffs, NJ: Prentice-Hall.

Felsenfeld, S. (1997). Epidemiology and genetics of stuttering. In R.F. Curlee & G.M. Siegel (Eds.), *The nature and treatment of stuttering: New directions,* 2nd ed. (pp. 3–23). Boston: Allyn & Bacon.

Fibiger, S. (1971). Stuttering explained as a physiological tremor. *Quarterly Progress and Status Report, 2–3,* Speech Transmission Laboratory, Royal Institute of Technology, Stockholm, Sweden.

Flugel, F. (1979). Erhebungen von Personlichkeitsmerk-malen an Muttern stotternder Kinder und Jugendicher. *dsh Abstracts, 19,* 226.

Fosnot, S.M. (1995). Clinical forum. *Language, Speech, and Hearing Services in Schools, 26*(2), 115–200.

Fosnot, S.M., & Woodford, L.L. (1992). *The fluency development system for young children.* Buffalo: United Educational Services.

Fowlie, G.M., & Cooper, E.B. (1978). Traits attributed to stuttering and nonstuttering children by their mothers. *Journal of Fluency Disorders, 3,* 233–246.

Fox N., & Davidson, R. (1984). Hemispheric substrates of affect: developmental model. In N. Fox & R. Davidson (Eds.), *The psychobiology of affective development.* Hillsdale, NJ: Lawrence Erlbaum Associates.

Fox, P.T., Ingham, R., Ingham, J., et al. (1996). A PET study of the neural systems of stuttering. *Nature, 382,* 158–162.

Frankenburg, W.K., & Dodds, J.B. (1967).

The Denver Developmental Screening Test. *Journal of Pediatrics, 71,* 181–191.

Fraser, J., & Perkins, W.H. (Eds.). (1987). *Do you stutter: A guide for teens.* Memphis: Speech Foundation of America.

Freeman, F.J. (1988). Gestural analysis of stuttering. (Abstract). *ASHA, 30,* 121.

Freeman, F.J., & Ushijima, T. (1975). Laryngeal activity accompanying the moment of stuttering: A preliminary report of EMG investigations. *Journal of Fluency Disorders, 1,* 36–45.

Freeman, F.J., & Ushijima, T. (1978). Laryngeal muscle activity during stuttering. *Journal of Speech and Hearing Research, 21,* 538–562.

Froeschels, E. (1943). Pathology and therapy of stuttering. *Nervous Child, 2,* 148–161.

Gaines, N.D., Runyan, C.M., & Meyers, S.C. (1991). A comparison of young stutterers' fluent versus stuttered utterances on measures of length and complexity. *Journal of Speech and Hearing Research, 34,* 37–42.

Gardner, H. (1983). *Frames of mind: The theory of multiple intelligences.* New York: Basic Books.

Geschwind, N., & Galaburda, A.M. (1985). Cerebral lateralization: Biological mechanisms, associations, and pathology: I. A hypothesis and a program for research. *Archives of Neurology, 42,* 429–459.

Gibson, E. (1972). Reading for some purpose. In J.F. Kavanaugh & I. Mattingly (Eds.), *Language by ear and by eye.* Cambridge, MA: MIT Press.

Glasner, P., & Rosenthal, D. (1957). Parental diagnosis of stuttering in young children. *Journal of Speech and Hearing Disorders, 22,* 288–295.

Goldberg, G. (1985). Supplementary motor area structure and function: Review and hypotheses. *Behavioral and Brain Sciences, 8,* 567–616.

Goldman-Eisler, F. (1968). *Psycholinguistics: Experiments in spontaneous speech.* New York: Academic Press.

Goodstein, L.D. (1956). MMPI profiles of stutterers' parents: A follow-up study. *Journal of Speech and Hearing Disorders, 21,* 430–435.

Goodstein, L.D., & Dahlstrom, W.G. (1956). MMPI differences between parents of stuttering and nonstuttering children. *Journal of Consulting Psychology, 20,* 365–370.

Gordon, P.A., Luper, H.L., & Peterson, H.A. (1986). The effects of syntactic complexity on the occurrence of disfluencies in 5 year old stutterers. *Journal of Fluency Disorders, 11,* 151–164.

Gottwald, S., & Starkweather, C.W. (1984). *Stuttering prevention: Rationale and method.* Short course presented at the meeting of the American Speech and Hearing Association, San Francisco, California, November.

Gottwald, S., & Starkweather, C.W. (1985). *The prognosis of stuttering.* Miniseminar presented at the meeting of the American Speech and Hearing Association, Washington, DC, November.

Gottwald, S., & Starkweather, C.W. (1995). Fluency intervention for preschoolers and their families in the public schools. *Language, Speech, and Hearing Services in Schools, 26,* 115–126.

Gould, S.J. (1996). Charles Darwin: Voyaging, by Janet Browne. (Book review). *The New York Review of Books, XLIII*(6), 10–14.

Gray, J.A. (1987). *The psychology of fear and stress,* 2nd ed. Cambridge: Cambridge University Press.

Greenspan, S.I. (1993). Making time for your child. *Parents,* (August), 111–114.

Gregory, H.H. (1968). Application of learning theory concepts in the management of stuttering. In H.H. Gregory (Ed.), *Learning theory and stuttering therapy.* Evanston, IL: Northwestern University Press.

Gregory, H.H. (1979). Controversial issues: Statement and review of the literature. In H.H. Gregory (Ed.), *Controversies about stuttering therapy.* Baltimore: University Park Press.

Gregory, H.H. (1984a). Prevention of stuttering: Management of early stages. In R.F. Curlee & W.H. Perkins (Eds.), *Nature and treatment of stuttering: New directions.* San Diego: College-Hill Press.

Gregory, H.H. (1984b). Stuttering therapy for children. In W.H. Perkins (Ed.), *Stuttering disorders.* New York: Thieme-Stratton.

Gregory, H.H. (1986a). *Stuttering: Differential evaluation and therapy.* Austin, TX: Pro-Ed.

Gregory, H.H. (1986b). Environmental manipulation and family counseling. In G.H. Shames & H. Rubin (Eds.), *Stuttering: Then and now.* Columbus, OH: Charles E. Merrill.

Gregory, H.H., & Campbell, J.H. (1988). Stuttering in the school-age child. In D.E. Yoder & R.D. Kent (Eds.), *Decision making in speech-language pathology.* Toronto: B.C. Decker.

Gregory, H.H., & Hill, D. (1980). Stuttering therapy for children. *Seminars in Speech, Language and Hearing, 1,* 351–363.

Guitar, B. (1976). Pretreatment factors associated with the outcome of stuttering therapy. *Journal of Speech and Hearing Research, 19,* 590–600.

Guitar, B. (1979). A response to Ingham's critique. *Journal of Speech and Hearing Disorders, 44,* 400–403.

Guitar, B. (1981). Stuttering. In J. Darby (Ed.), *Speech evaluation in medicine.* New York: Grune & Stratton.

Guitar, B. (1982). Fluency shaping with young stutterers. *Journal of Childhood Communication Disorders, 6,* 50–59.

Guitar, B. (1984). Indirect treatment of childhood stuttering. In J.M. Costello (Eds.), *Speech disorders in children: Recent advances.* (pp. 291–311). San Diego: College-Hill Press.

Guitar, B. (1997). Therapy for children's stuttering and emotions. In R.F. Curlee & G.M. Siegel (Eds.), *Nature and treatment of stuttering: New directions,* 2nd ed. Boston: Allyn & Bacon.

Guitar, B., & Bass, C. (1978). Stuttering therapy: The relation between attitude change and long-term outcome. *Journal of Speech and Hearing Disorders, 43,* 392–400.

Guitar, B., & Belin-Frost, G. (1995). Stuttering. In S. Parker and B. Zuckerman (Eds.). *Behavioral and developmental pediatrics: A handbook for primary care.* Boston: Little, Brown.

Guitar, B., & Conture, E. (undated). *If you think your child is stuttering.* Publication No. 41. Memphis: Speech Foundation of America.

Guitar, B., & Conture, E. (1996). *Do you stutter: Straight talk for teens.* (Videotape). Memphis: Stuttering Foundation of America.

Guitar, B., & Grims, S. (1977). Developing a scale to assess communication attitudes in children who stutter. Poster session presented at the American Speech-Language-Hearing Association Convention, Atlanta, Georgia, November.

Guitar, B., Guitar, C., Neilson, P.D., et al. (1988). Onset sequencing of selected lip muscles in stutterers and nonstutterers. *Journal of Speech and Hearing Research, 31,* 28–35.

Guitar, B., Kopff-Schaefer, H., Donahue-Kilburg, G., & Bond, L. (1992). Parent verbal interaction and speech rate. *Journal of Speech and Hearing Research, 35,* 742–754.

Guitar, B., & Peters, T.J. (1980). *Stuttering: An integration of contemporary therapies.* Publication No. 16. Memphis: Speech Foundation of America.

Hall, J.W., & Jerger, J. (1978). Central auditory function in stutterers. *Journal of Speech and Hearing Research, 21,* 324–337.

Hammond, G.R. (1982). Hemispheric differences in temporal resolution. *Brain and Cognition, 1,* 95–118.

Hand, C.R., & Haynes, W.O. (1983). Linguistic processing and reaction time differences in stutterers and nonstutterers. *Journal of Speech and Hearing Research, 26,* 181–185.

Haynes, W.O., & Hood, S.B. (1978). Disfluency changes in children as a function of the systematic modification of linguistic complexity. *Journal of Communication Disorders, 11,* 79–93.

Heinze, B., & Johnson, K. (1985). *Easy does it: Fluency activities for young children.* East Moline, IL: LinguiSystems.

Helm-Estabrooks, N. (1986). Diagnosis and management of neurogenic stuttering in adults. In K. St. Louis (Ed.), *The atypical stutterer.* New York: Academic Press.

Herrnstein, R., & Murray, C. (1994). *The bell curve: Intelligence and class structure in American life.* New York: Free Press.

Hill, H.E. (1954). An experimental study of disorganization of speech and manual responses in normal subjects. *Journal of Speech and Hearing Disorders, 19,* 295–305.

Hillman, R.E., & Gilbert, H.R. (1977). Voice onset time for voiceless stop consonants in the fluent reading of stutterers and nonstutterers. *Journal of the Acoustical Society of America, 61,* 610–611.

Hiscock, M., & Kinsbourne, M. (1977). Selective listening asymmetry in preschool children. *Developmental Psychology, 13,* 217–224.

Hiscock, M., & Kinsbourne, M. (1980). Asymmetry of verbal-manual time sharing in children: A follow-up study. *Neuropsychologia, 18,* 151–162.

Hoffman, P., Schuckers, G., & Daniloff, R. (1989). *Children's phonetic disorders: Theory and treatment.* Boston: College-Hill Press.

Howie, P.M. (1981). Concordance for stuttering in monozygotic and dizygotic twin pairs. *Journal of Speech and Hearing Research, 24,* 317–321.

Hubbard, C.P., & Yairi, E. (1988). Clustering of disfluencies in the speech of stuttering and nonstuttering preschool children. *Journal of Speech and Hearing Research, 31*(2), 228–233.

Ingham, R.J. (1979). Comment on "Stuttering therapy: The relation between attitude change and long-term outcome." *Journal of Speech and Hearing Disorders, 44,* 397–400.

Ingham, R., Cordes, A., & Finn, P. (1993). Time-interval measurement of stuttering: Systematic replication of Ingham, Cordes, & Gow (1993). *Journal of Speech and Hearing Research, 36,* 1168–1176.

Ingham, R., Cordes, A., & Gow, M. (1993). Time-interval measurement of stuttering: Modifying interjudge agreement. *Journal of Speech and Hearing Research, 36,* 503–515.

Ingham, R.J., Fox, P.T., Ingham, J.C., et al. (1996). Functional-lesion investigation of developmental stuttering with positron emission tomography. *Journal of Speech and Hearing Research, 39,* 1208–1227.

Ingham, R.J., Gow, M., & Costello, J.M. (1985). Stuttering and speech naturalness: Some additional data. *Journal of Speech and Hearing Disorders, 50*(2), 217–219.

Jacobson, E. (1938). *Progressive relaxation.* Chicago: University of Chicago Press.

Jaffe, J., & Anderson, S.W. (1979). Prescript to Chapter 1: Communication rhythms and the evolution of language. In A.W. Siegman & S. Feldman (Eds.), *Of speech and time: Temporal speech patterns in interpersonal contexts.* Hillsdale, NJ: Lawrence Erlbaum Associates.

Janssen, P., Kloth, S., Kraaimaat, F., & Brutten, G.J. (1996). Genetic factors in stuttering: A replication of Ambrose, Yairi, and Cox's (1993) study with adult probands. *Journal of Fluency Disorders, 21,* 105–108.

Jerger, J., Speaks, C., & Trammell, J. (1968). A new approach to speech audiometry. *Journal of Speech and Hearing Disorders, 33,* 318–328.

Jezer, M. (1997). *Stuttering: A life bound up in words.* New York: Basic Books.

Johnson, K., & Heinze, B. (1994). *The fluency companion: Strategies for stuttering intervention.* East Moline, IL: LinguiSystems.

Johnson, W. (1955). A study of the onset and development of stuttering. In W. Johnson & R.R. Leutenegger (Eds.), *Stuttering in children and adults.* Minneapolis: University of Minnesota Press.

Johnson, W., and associates (1959). *The onset of stuttering.* Minneapolis: University of Minnesota Press.

Johnson, W., & Brown, S.F. (1935). Stuttering in relation to various speech sounds. *Quarterly Journal of Speech, 21,* 481–496.

Johnson, W., Darley, F., & Spriestersbach, D.C. (1952). *Diagnostic manual in speech correction.* New York: Harper & Row.

Johnson, W., et al. (1942). A study of the onset and development of stuttering. *Journal of Speech Disorders, 7,* 251–257.

Johnson, W., & Inness, M. (1939). Studies in the psychology of stuttering: XIII. A statistical analysis of the adaptation and consistency effects in relation to stuttering. *Journal of Speech Disorders, 4,* 79–86.

Johnson, W., & Knott, J.R. (1937). Studies in the psychology of stuttering: I. The distribution of moments of stuttering in successive readings of the same materials. *Journal of Speech Disorders, 2,* 17–19.

Johnson, W., & Leutenegger, R.R. (Eds.). (1955). *Stuttering in children and adults.* Minneapolis: University of Minnesota Press.

Johnson, W., & Rosen, L. (1937). Studies in the psychology of stuttering: VII. Effects of certain changes in speech pattern upon frequency of stuttering. *Journal of Speech Disorders, 2,* 105–109.

Johnson, W., & Solomon, A. (1937). Studies in the psychology of stuttering: IV. A quantitative study of expectation of stuttering as a process involving a low degree of consciousness. *Journal of Speech Disorders, 2,* 95–97.

Kagan, J. (1981). *The second year: The emergence of self-awareness.* Cambridge, MA: Harvard University Press.

Kagan, J. (1994a). The realistic view of biology and behavior. *The Chronicle of Higher Education,* October 5, A64.

Kagan, J. (1994b). *Galen's prophecy: Temperament in human nature.* New York: Basic Books.

Kagan, J., Reznick, J.S., & Snidman, N. (1987). The physiology and psychology of behavioral inhibition in children. *Child Development, 58,* 1459–1473.

Kagan, J., & Snidman, N. (1991). Temperamental factors in human development. *American Psychologist, 46*(8), 856–862.

Kasprisin-Burrelli, A., Egolf, D.B., & Shames, G.H. (1972). A comparison of parental verbal behavior with stuttering and nonstuttering children. *Journal of Communication Disorders, 5,* 335–346.

Kelly, E. (1994). Speech rates and turn-taking behaviors of children who stutter and their fathers. *Journal of Speech and Hearing Research, 37,* 1284–1294.

Kelly E., & Conture, E. (1992). Speaking rates, response time latencies, and interrupting behaviors of young stutterers, nonstutterers, and their mothers. *Journal of Speech and Hearing Research, 35,* 1256–1267.

Kent, L.R., & Williams, D.E. (1963). Alleged former stutterers in grade two. (Abstract). *ASHA, 5,* 772.

Kent, R.D. (1981). Sensorimotor aspects of speech development. In R.D. Alberts & M.R. Peterson (Eds.), *The development of perception: Psycho-biological perspectives.* New York: Academic Press.

Kent, R.D. (1983). Facts about stuttering: Neuropsychologic perspectives. *Journal of Speech and Hearing Disorders, 48,* 249–255.

Kent, R.D. (1984). Stuttering as a temporal programming disorder. In R.F. Curlee & W.H. Perkins (Eds.), *Nature and treatment of stuttering: New directions.* San Diego: College-Hill Press.

Kent, R.D. (1985). Developing and disordered speech: Strategies for organization. *ASHA Reports, 15,* 29–37.

Kent, R.D., & Perkins, W. (1984). Oral-verbal fluency: Aspects of verbal formulation, speech motor control and underlying neural systems. Unpublished manuscript.

Kenyon, E.L. (1942). The etiology of stammering: Fundamentally a wrong psycho-physiologic habit in control of the vocal cords for the production of an individual speech sound. *Journal of Speech Disorders, 7,* 97–104.

Kidd, K.K. (1977). A genetic perspective on stuttering. *Journal of Fluency Disorders, 2,* 259–269.

Kidd, K.K. (1984). Stuttering as a genetic disorder. In R.F. Curlee & W.H. Perkins (Eds.), *Nature and treatment of stuttering:*

New directions. San Diego: College-Hill Press.

Kidd, K.K., Kidd, J.R., & Records, M.A. (1978). The possible causes of the sex ratio in stuttering and its implications. *Journal of Fluency Disorders, 3,* 13–23.

Kidd, K.K., Reich, T., & Kessler, S. (1973). A genetic analysis of stuttering suggesting a single major locus. *Genetics, 74*(2, Part 2): s137.

Kinsbourne, M. (1989). A model of adaptive behavior related to cerebral participation in emotional control. In G. Gianotti & C. Caltagirone (Eds.), *Emotions and the dual brain.* New York: Springer-Verlag.

Kinsbourne, M., & Bemporad, E. (1984). Lateralization of emotion: A model and the evidence. In N. Fox & R. Davidson (Eds.), *The psychology of affective development.* Hillsdale, NJ: Lawrence Erlbaum Associates.

Kinsbourne, M., & Hicks, R. (1978). Functional cerebral space: A model for overflow, transfer and interference effects in human performance: A tutorial review. In M. Kinsbourne (Ed.), *Asymmetrical function of the brain.* Cambridge, UK: Cambridge University Press.

Kline, M.L., & Starkweather, C.W. (1979). Receptive and expressive language performance in young stutterers. (Abstract). *ASHA, 21,* 797.

Kloth, S., Janssen, P., Kraaimaat, F., & Brutten, G. (1995). Speech-motor and linguistic skills of young stutterers prior to onset. *Journal of Fluency Disorders, 20,* 157–170.

Knott, J.R., Johnson, W., & Webster, M.J. (1937). Studies in the psychology of stuttering: II. A quantitative evaluation of expectation of stuttering in relation to the occurrence of stuttering. *Journal of Speech Disorders, 2,* 20–22.

Kolk, H., & Postma, A. (1997). Stuttering as a covert repair phenomenon. In R.F. Curlee & G.M. Siegel (Eds.), *Nature and treatment of stuttering: New directions,* 2nd ed. (pp. 182–203). Boston: Allyn & Bacon.

Kramer, M.B., Green, D., & Guitar, B. (1987). A comparison of stutterers and nonstutterers on masking level differences and synthetic sentence identification tasks. *Journal of Communication Disorders, 20,* 379–390.

Lazarus, A.A. (1971). *Behavior therapy and beyond.* New York: McGraw-Hill.

LeDoux, J.E. (1997). Emotion, memory and the brain. *Scientific American: Mysteries of the Mind (Special Issue), 7*(1), 68–75.

LeDoux, J.E., Cicchetti, P., Xagoraris, A., & Romanski, L.M. (1990). The lateral amygdaloid nucleus: Sensory interface of the amygdala in fear conditioning. *Journal of Neuroscience, 10*(4), 1062–1069.

Liberman, A.M., Cooper, F.S., Shankweiler, D.S., & Studdert-Kennedy, M. (1967). Perception of the speech code. *Psychological Review, 74,* 431–461.

Lidz, T. (1968). *The person: His development throughout the life cycle.* New York: Basic Books.

Lindsay, J.S. (1989). Relationship of developmental disfluency and episodes of stuttering to the emergence of cognitive stages in children. *Journal of Fluency Disorders, 14*(4), 271–284.

Logan, K., & Conture, E. (1995). Length, grammatical complexity, and rate differences in stuttered and fluent conversational utterances of children who stutter. *Journal of Fluency Disorders, 20,* 35–61.

Luchsinger, R. (1944). Biological studies on monozygotic and dizygotic twins relative to size and form of the larynx. *Archive Julius Klaus-Stiftung fur Verergungsforschung, 19,* 3–4.

Lund, N., & Duchan, J. (1988). *Assessing children's language in naturalistic contexts,* 2nd ed. Englewood Cliffs, NJ: Prentice-Hall.

Luper, H.L., & Mulder, R.L. (1964). *Stuttering: Therapy for children.* Englewood Cliffs, NJ: Prentice-Hall.

Luterman, D. (1996). *Counseling persons with communication disorders and their families,* 3rd ed. Austin, TX: Pro-Ed.

Mahr, G., & Leith, W. (1992). Psychogenic stuttering of adult onset. *Journal of Speech and Hearing Research, 35,* 283–286.

Malecot, A., Johnston, R., & Kizziar, P.A. (1972). Syllabic rate and utterance length in French. *Phonetica, 26,* 235–251.

Manning, W.H. (1996). *Clinical decision making in the diagnosis and treatment of fluency disorders.* Albany, NY: Delmar Publishers.

Martin, R., & Haroldson, S.K. (1979). Effects of five experimental treatments on stuttering. *Journal of Speech and Hearing Research, 22,* 132–146.

Martin, R., Haroldson, S.K., & Triden, K.A. (1984). Stuttering and speech naturalness. *Journal of Speech and Hearing Disorders, 49*(1), 53–58.

Maske-Cash, W., & Curlee, R. (1995). Effect of utterance length and meaningfulness on the speech initiation times of children who stutter and children who do not stutter. *Journal of Speech and Hearing Research, 38,* 18–25.

McCauley, R.J. (1996). Familiar strangers: Criterion-referenced measures in communication disorders. *Language, Speech, and Hearing Services in Schools, 27*(2), 122–131.

McClean, M., Goldsmith, H., & Cerf, A. (1984). Lower-lip EMG and displacement during bilabial dysfluencies in adult stutterers. *Journal of Speech and Hearing Research, 27,* 342–349.

McDearmon, J.R. (1968). Primary stuttering at the onset of stuttering: A reexamination of data. *Journal of Speech and Hearing Research, 11,* 631–637.

McFarland, D.H., & Moore, W.H., Jr. (1982). Alpha hemispheric asymmetrics during an electromyographic feedback procedure for stuttering. Paper presented at the Annual Convention of the American Speech and Hearing Association, Toronto, November.

McFarlane, S.C., & Prins, D. (1978). Neural response time of stutterers and nonstutterers in selected oral motor tasks. *Journal of Speech and Hearing Research, 21,* 768–778.

McKnight, R.C., & Cullinan, W.L.(1987). Subgroups of stuttering children: Speech and

voice reaction times, segmental durations, and naming latencies. *Journal of Fluency Disorders, 12,* 217–233.

McLoughlin, J., & Lewis, R. (1990). *Assessing special students,* 3rd ed. Columbus, OH: Charles E. Merrill.

Merits-Patterson, R., & Reed, C.G. (1981). Disfluencies in the speech of language-delayed children. *Journal of Speech and Hearing Research, 24,* 55–58.

Meyers, S.C., & Freeman, F.J. (1985a). Interruptions as a variable in stuttering and disfluency. *Journal of Speech and Hearing Research, 28,* 428–435.

Meyers, S.C., & Freeman, F.J. (1985b). Mother and child speech rate as a variable in stuttering and disfluency. *Journal of Speech and Hearing Research, 28,* 436–444.

Milisen, R. (1938). Frequency of stuttering with anticipation of stuttering controlled. *Journal of Speech Disorders, 3,* 207–214.

Miller, S. (1993). *Multiple measures of anxiety and psychophysiologic arousal in stutterers and nonstutterers during nonspeech and speech tasks of increasing complexity.* Unpublished doctoral dissertation, University of Texas at Dallas.

Mineka, S. (1985). Animal models of anxiety-based disorders: Their usefulness and limitations. In A.H. Tuma & J. Mase (Eds.), *Anxiety and the anxiety disorders.* Hillsdale, NJ: Lawrence Erlbaum Associates.

Moncur, J.P. (1952). Parental domination in stuttering. *Journal of Speech and Hearing Disorders, 17,* 155–165.

Moore, W.H., Jr. (1984). Central nervous system characteristics of stutterers. In R.F. Curlee & W.H. Perkins (Eds.), *Nature and treatment of stuttering: New directions.* San Diego: College-Hill Press.

Moore, W.H., Jr., & Haynes, W.O. (1980). Alpha hemispheric asymmetry and stuttering: Some support for a segmentation dysfunction hypothesis. *Journal of Speech and Hearing Research, 23,* 229–247.

Morgenstern, J.J. (1956). Socio-economic factors in stuttering. *Journal of Speech and Hearing Disorders, 21,* 25–33.

Murray, H.L., & Reed, C.G. (1977). Language abilities of preschool stuttering children. *Journal of Fluency Disorders, 2,* 171–176.

Navon, D. (1984). Resources—a theoretical stone soup. *Psychological Review, 91*(2), 216–234.

Neilson, M.D. (1980). *Stuttering and the control of speech: A systems analysis approach.* Unpublished doctoral dissertation, University of New South Wales, Kensington, Australia.

Neilson, M.D., & Andrews, G. (1993). Intensive fluency training in chronic stutterers. In R.F. Curlee (Ed.), *Stuttering and related disorders of fluency.* (pp. 139–165). New York: Thieme Medical Publishers.

Neilson, M.D., Howie, P., & Andrews, G. (1987). Does foetal testosterone play a role in the aetiology of stuttering? Paper presented at the Fifth International Australasian Winter Conference on Brain Research, Queenstown, New Zealand, August.

Neilson, M.D., & Neilson, P.D. (1987). Speech motor control and stuttering: A computational model of adaptive sensory-motor processing. *Speech Communication, 6,* 325–333.

Neilson, M.D. & Neilson, P.D. (1991). Adaptive model theory of speech motor control and stuttering. In H.F.M. Peters, W. Hulstijn, & C.W. Starkweather (Eds.), *Speech motor control and stuttering.* (pp. 149–156). Amsterdam: Excerpta Medica.

Neilson, P.D., Neilson, M.D., & O'Dwyer, N.J. (1982). Acquisition of motor skills in tracking tasks: Learning internal models. In D.G. Russell & B. Abernethy (Eds.), *Motor memory and control: The Otago Symposium, Dunedin, New Zealand, 1982.* Dunedin, NZ: Human Performance Associates.

Neilson, P.D., Neilson, M.D., & O'Dwyer, N.J. (1992). Adaptive model theory: Application to disorders of motor control. In J.J. Summers (Ed.), *Approaches to the study of motor control and learning.* Amsterdam: Elsevier Science Publishers.

Neilson, P.D., Quinn, P.T., & Neilson, M.D. (1976). Auditory tracking measures of hemispheric asymmetry in normals and stutterers. *Australian Journal of Human Communication, 4,* 121–126.

Nelson, L. (1985). Language formulation related to dysfluency and stuttering. In *Stuttering therapy: Prevention and intervention with children,* Memphis: Stuttering Foundation of America.

Netsell, R. (1981). The acquisition of speech motor control: A perspective with direction for research. In R. Stark (Ed.), *Language behavior in infancy and early childhood.* New York: Elsevier-North Holland.

Nippold, M. (1990). Concomitant speech and language disorders in stuttering children: A critique of the literature. *Journal of Speech and Hearing Disorders, 55,* 51–60.

Nippold, M.A., Schwarz, I.E., & Jescheniak, J.-D. (1991). Narrative ability in school-age stuttering boys: A preliminary investigation. *Journal of Fluency Disorders, 16,* 289–308.

Nittrouer, S., Studdert-Kennedy, M., & McGowan, R.S. (1989). The emergence of phonetic segments: Evidence from the spectral structure of fricative-vowel syllables spoken by children and adults. *Journal of Speech and Hearing Research, 32,* 120–132.

Nudelman, H.B., Herbrich, K.E., Hoyt, B.D., & Rosenfield, D.B. (1987). Dynamic characteristics of vocal frequency tracking in stutterers and nonstutterers. In H.F.M. Peters & W. Hulstijn (Eds.), *Speech motor dynamics in stuttering.* Wien: Springer-Verlag.

Okasha, A., Bishry, Z., Kamel, M., & Hassan, A.H. (1974). Psychosocial study of stammering in Egyptian children. *British Journal of Psychiatry, 124,* 531–533.

Onslow, M. (1996). *Behavioral management of stuttering.* San Diego: Singular Publishing Group, Inc.

Onslow, M., Andrews, C., & Lincoln, M. (1994). A control/experimental trial of an operant treatment for early stuttering. *Journal of Speech and Hearing Research, 37,* 1244–1259.

Onslow, M., Costa, L., & Rue, S. (1990). Direct early intervention with stuttering:

Some preliminary data. *Journal of Speech and Hearing Disorders, 55,* 405–416.

Onslow, M., & Packman, A. (1997). Designing and implementing a strategy to control stuttered speech in adults. In R.F. Curlee & G.M. Siegel (Eds.), *Nature and treatment of stuttering: New directions,* 2nd ed. (pp. 356–376). Boston: Allyn & Bacon.

Oyler, M.E. (1992). Self perception and sensitivity in stuttering adults. Paper presented at the Annual Convention of the American Speech-Language-Hearing Association, San Antonio, Texas, November.

Oyler, M.E., & Ramig, P.R. (1995). Vulnerability in stuttering children. Paper presented at the Annual Convention of the American Speech-Language-Hearing Association, Orlando, Florida, December.

Paul, R. (1995). *Language disorders from infancy through adolescence: Assessment and intervention.* St. Louis: Mosby-Year Book.

Pearl, S.Z., & Bernthal, J.E. (1980). The effect of grammatical complexity upon disfluency behavior of nonstuttering preschool children. *Journal of Fluency Disorders, 5,* 55–68.

Perkins, W.H. (1973a). Replacement of stuttering with normal speech: I. Rationale. *Journal of Speech and Hearing Disorders, 38,* 283–294.

Perkins, W.H. (1973b). Replacement of stuttering with normal speech: II. Clinical procedures. *Journal of Speech and Hearing Disorders, 38,* 295–303.

Perkins, W.H. (1979). From psychoanalysis to discoordination. In H.H. Gregory (Ed.), *Controversies about stuttering therapy.* Baltimore: University Park Press.

Perkins, W.H. (1981). An alternative to automatic fluency. In *Stuttering therapy: Transfer and maintenance.* Memphis: Speech Foundation of America.

Perkins, W.H. (1984). Techniques for establishing fluency. In W.H. Perkins (Ed.), *Stuttering disorders.* New York: Thieme-Stratton.

Perkins, W.H. (1986). Postscript: Discoordination of phonation with articulation and respiration. In G.H. Shames & H. Rubin (Eds.), *Stuttering: Then and now.* Columbus, OH: Charles E. Merrill.

Perkins, W.H., Kent, R.D., & Curlee, R.F. (1991). A theory of neuropsycholinguistic function in stuttering. *Journal of Speech and Hearing Research, 34,* 734–752.

Perkins, W., Rudas, J., Johnson, L., & Bell, J. (1976). Stuttering: Discoordination of phonation with articulation and respiration. *Journal of Speech and Hearing Research, 19,* 509–522.

Peters, H.F.M., & Hulstijn, W. (1984). Stuttering and Anxiety: The difference between stutterers and nonstutterers in verbal apprehension and physiologic arousal during the anticipation of speech and non-speech tasks. *Journal of Fluency Disorders, 9,* 67–84.

Peters, H.F.M., & Hulstijn, W. (Eds.). (1987). *Speech motor dynamics in stuttering.* New York: Springer-Verlag.

Peters, H.F.M., Hulstijn, W., & Starkweather, C.W. (1991). *Speech motor control and stuttering.* Amsterdam: Excerpta Medica.

Peters, H.F.M., & Starkweather, C.W. (1990). The interaction between speech motor coordination and language processes in the development of stuttering. *Journal of Fluency Disorders, 15,* 115–125.

Peters, T.J. (1968). Oral language skills of children who stutter. (Abstract). *Speech Monographs, 35,* 325.

Peters, T.J. (1987). *Handouts for the advanced stutterer.* Unpublished material, University of Wisconsin-Eau Claire, Center for Communication Disorders, Eau Claire, WI.

Peterson, H., & Marquardt, T. (1990). *Appraisal and diagnosis of speech and language disorders,* 2nd ed. Englewood Cliffs, NJ: Prentice-Hall.

Pindzola, R., Jenkins, M., & Lokken, K. (1989). Speaking rates of young children. *Language, Speech, and Hearing Services in Schools, 20,* 133–138.

Platt, J., & Basili, A. (1973). Jaw tremor during stuttering block: An electromyographic study. *Journal of Communication Disorders, 6,* 102–109.

Pool, K.D., Devous, M.D., Freeman, F.J., Watson, B.C., & Finitzo, T. (1991). Regional cerebral blood flow in developmental stutterers. *Archives of Neurology, 48,* 509–512.

Pool, K.D., Freeman, F.J., & Finitzo, T. (1987). Brain electrical activity mapping: Applications to vocal motor control disorders. In H.F.M. Peters & W. Hulstijn (Eds.), *Speech Motor Dynamics in Stuttering.* New York: Springer-Verlag.

Postma, A., & Kolk, H.H.J. (1993). The covert repair hypothesis: Prearticulatory repair process in normal and stuttered disfluencies. *Journal of Speech and Hearing Research, 36,* 472–487.

Prins, D. (1984). Treatment of adults: Managing stuttering. In R. F. Curlee & W.H. Perkins (Eds.), *Nature and treatment of stuttering: New directions.* San Diego: College-Hill Press.

Prins, D. (1997). Modifying stuttering—The stutterer's reactive behavior: Perspectives on past, present, and future. In R. Curlee & G. Siegel (Eds.), *Nature and treatment of stuttering: New directions.* Boston: Allyn & Bacon.

Ramig, P.R., & Bennett, E.M. (1995). Working with 7–12 year old children who stutter: Ideas for intervention in the public schools. *Language, Speech, and Hearing Services in Schools, 26,* 138–150.

Ramig, P.R., & Bennett, E.M. (1997). Clinical management of children: Direct management strategies. In R.F. Curlee & G.M. Siegel (Eds.), *Nature and Treatment of Stuttering: New Directions,* 2nd ed. Boston: Allyn & Bacon.

Rastatter, M., & Dell, C. (1987). Vocal reaction times of stuttering subjects to tachistoscopically presented concrete and abstract words: A closer look at cerebral dominance and language processing. *Journal of Speech and Hearing Research, 30,* 306–310.

Reville, J. (1988). *The many voices of Paws.* Princeton Junction, NJ: Speech Bin.

Riley, G. (1972). A stuttering severity instrument for children and adults. *Journal of Speech and Hearing Disorders, 37,* 314–322.

Riley, G. (1994). *Stuttering severity instrument for children and adults,* 3rd ed. Austin, TX: Pro-Ed.

Riley, G., & Riley, J. (1979). A component model for diagnosing and treating children who stutter. *Journal of Fluency Disorders, 4,* 279–293.

Riley, G.D., & Riley, J. (1983). Evaluation as a basis for intervention. In D. Prins & R.J. Ingham (Eds.), *Treatment of stuttering in early childhood: Methods and issues.* San Diego: College-Hill Press.

Riley, G.D., & Riley, J. (1984). A component model for treating stuttering in children. In M. Peins (Ed.), *Contemporary approaches in stuttering therapy.* Boston: Little, Brown.

Roessler, R., & Bolton, B. (1978). *Psychosocial adjustment to disability.* Baltimore: University Park Press.

Rogers, C. (1942). *Counseling and psychotherapy.* Boston: Houghton Mifflin.

Rosenbek, J. (1984). Stuttering secondary to nervous system damage. In R.F. Curlee & W.H. Perkins (Eds.), *Nature and treatment of stuttering: New directions.* (pp. 31–48). San Diego: College-Hill Press.

Rosenfield, D.B., & Jerger, J. (1984). Stuttering and auditory function. In R.F. Curlee & W.H. Perkins (Eds.), *Nature and treatment of stuttering: New directions.* San Diego: College-Hill Press.

Roth, C., Aronson, A., & Davis, L. (1989). Clinical studies in psychogenic stuttering of adult onset. *Journal of Speech and Hearing Disorders, 54,* 634–646.

Rumelhart, D., McClelland, J., & the PDP Research Group. (1986). Parallel distributed processing: Explorations in the microstructure of cognition. Cambridge, MA: MIT Press.

Runyan, C., & Runyan, S. (1986). The "fluency rules" program. *Language, Speech, and Hearing Services in Schools, 17,* 276–284.

Runyan, C., & Runyan, S. (1993). Therapy for school-age stutterers: An update on the "fluency rules" program. In R. Curlee (Ed.), *Stuttering and related disorders of fluency.* New York: Thieme Medical Publishers.

Rustin, L., & Cook, F. (1995). Parental involvement in the treatment of stuttering. *Language, Speech, and Hearing Services in Schools, 26,* 127–137.

Rustin, L., Cook, F., & Spence, R. (1995). *The management of stuttering in adolescence: A communication skills approach.* London: Whurr.

Ryan, B.P. (1971). Operant procedures applied to stuttering therapy for children. *Journal of Speech and Hearing Disorders, 36,* 264–280.

Ryan, B.P. (1974). *Programmed therapy of stuttering in children and adults.* Springfield, IL: Charles C Thomas.

Ryan, B.P. (1979). Stuttering therapy in a framework of operant conditioning and programmed learning. In H.H. Gregory (Ed.), *Controversies about stuttering therapy.* Baltimore: University Park Press.

Ryan, B.P. (1984). Treatment of stuttering in school children. In W.H. Perkins (Ed.), *Stuttering disorders.* New York: Thieme-Stratton.

Ryan, B.P. (1986). Postscript: Operant therapy for children. In G.H. Shames & H. Rubin (Eds.), *Stuttering: Then and now.* Columbus, OH: Charles E. Merrill.

Ryan, B.P. (1992). Articulation, language, rate, and fluency characteristics of stuttering and nonstuttering preschool children. *Journal of Speech and Hearing Research, 35,* 333–342.

Ryan, B.P., & van Kirk, B. (1974). The establishment, transfer, and maintenance of fluent speech in 50 stutterers using delayed auditory feedback and operant procedures. *Journal of Speech and Hearing Research, 39,* 3–10.

Sackeim, H.A., & Gur, R.C. (1978). Lateral asymmetry in intensity of emotional expression. *Neuropsychologia, 16,* 437–481.

St. Louis, K. (Ed.). (1986). *The atypical stutterer.* New York: Academic Press.

St. Louis, K. (1991). The stuttering/articulation disorders connection. In H. Peters, W. Hulstijn, & C.W. Starkweather, (Eds.), *Speech motor control and stuttering.* Amsterdam: Excerpta Medica.

St. Louis, K., & Myers, F. (1997). Management of cluttering and related fluency disorders. In R.F. Curlee & G.M. Siegel (Eds.), *The nature and treatment of stuttering: New directions,* 2nd ed. (pp. 313–332). Boston: Allyn & Bacon.

St. Onge, K. (1963). The stuttering syndrome. *Journal of Speech and Hearing Research, 6,* 195–197.

Schiavetti, N., & Metz, D. (1997). Stuttering and the measurement of speech naturalness. In R.F. Curlee & G.M. Siegel (Eds.), *Nature and treatment of stuttering: New directions,* 2nd ed. Boston: Allyn & Bacon.

Schindler, M.D. (1955). A study of the educational adjustments of stuttering and nonstuttering children. In W. Johnson & R.R. Leutenegger (Eds.), *Stuttering in children and adults.* Minneapolis: University of Minnesota Press.

Schwartz, M.F. (1974). The core of the stuttering block. *Journal of Speech and Hearing Disorders, 39,* 169–177.

Seeman, M. (1937). The significance of twin pathology for the investigation of speech disorders. *Archive gesamte Phonetik 1,* Part II, 88–92.

Seider, R.A., Gladstien, K.L., & Kidd, K.K. (1982). Language onset and concomitant speech and language problems in subgroups of stutterers and their siblings. *Journal of Speech and Hearing Research, 25,* 482–486.

Shames, G.H., & Florance, C.L. (1980). *Stutter-free speech: A goal for therapy.* Columbus, OH: Charles E. Merrill.

Shapiro, A.I. (1980). An electromyographic analysis of the fluent and dysfluent utterances of several types of stutterers. *Journal of Fluency Disorders, 5,* 203–231.

Shapiro, A.I., & DeCicco, B.A. (1982). The relationship between normal dysfluency and stuttering: An old question revisited. *Journal of Fluency Disorders, 7,* 109–121.

Shaywitz, B., Shaywitz, S., Pugh, K., et al.

(1995). Sex differences in the functional organization of the brain for language. *Nature, 373,* 607–609.

Sheehan, J.G. (1953). Theory and treatment of stuttering as an approach-avoidance conflict. *Journal of Psychology, 36,* 27–49.

Sheehan, J.G. (1970). *Stuttering: Research and therapy.* New York: Harper & Row.

Sheehan, J.G. (1974). Stuttering behavior: A phonetic analysis. *Journal of Communication Disorders, 7,* 193–212.

Sheehan, J.G. (1975). Conflict theory and avoidance-reduction therapy. In J. Eisenson (Ed.), *Stuttering: A second symposium.* New York: Harper & Row.

Sheehan, J.G., & Sheehan, V.M. (1984). Avoidance-reduction therapy: A response suppression hypothesis. In W.H. Perkins (Ed.), *Stuttering disorders.* New York: Thieme-Stratton.

Shields, D. (1989). *Dead languages.* New York: Knopf.

Shine, R.E. (1980). Direct management of the beginning stutterer. *Seminars in Speech, Language and Hearing, 1,* 339–350.

Shine, R.E. (1988). *Systematic fluency training for young children,* 3rd ed. Austin, TX: Pro-Ed.

Silverman, E.-M. (1974). Word position and grammatical function in relation to preschoolers' speech disfluency. *Perceptual and Motor Skills, 39,* 267–272.

Silverman, F.H. (1988). The "monster" study. *Journal of Fluency Disorders, 13,* 225–231.

Skinner, B.F. (1938). *The behavior of organisms.* New York: Appleton-Century-Crofts.

Skinner E., & McKeehan, A. (1996). *Preventing stuttering in the preschool child: A video program for parents.* (Videotape). San Antonio, TX: Communication Skill Builders.

Smith, A. (1989). Neural drive to muscles in stuttering. *Journal of Speech and Hearing Research, 32,* 252–264.

Smith, A. (1995). Muscle activities in stuttering. In C.W. Starkweather & H.F.M. Peters (Eds.), *Stuttering: Proceedings of the First World Congress on Fluency Disorders.* Munich: International Fluency Association.

Smith, A., & Kelly, E. (1997). Stuttering: A dynamic, multifactorial model. In R.F. Curlee & G.M. Siegel (Eds.), *Nature and treatment of stuttering: New directions,* 2nd ed. Boston: Allyn & Bacon.

Solomon, R.L., & Wynne, L.C. (1953). Traumatic avoidance learning: Acquisition in normal dogs. *Psychological Monographs, 67,* 1–19.

Springer, S., & Deutsch, G. (1981). *Left brain, right brain.* San Francisco: W.H. Freeman.

Stark, R., Tallal, C., & McCauley, R. (1988). *Language, speech and reading disorders in children.* Boston: Little, Brown.

Starkweather, C.W. (1972). *Stuttering: An account of intensive demonstration therapy.* Memphis: Speech Foundation of America.

Starkweather, C.W. (1980). A multiprocess behavioral approach to stuttering therapy. *Seminars in Speech, Language and Hearing, 1,* 327–337.

Starkweather, C.W. (1981). Speech fluency and its development in normal children. In N. Lass (Ed.), *Speech and language: Advances in basic research and practice,* vol. 4. New York: Academic Press.

Starkweather, C.W. (1982). Stuttering and laryngeal behavior: A review. *ASHA Monographs, 22.*

Starkweather, C.W. (1983). *Speech and language: Principles and processes of behavior change.* Englewood Cliffs, NJ: Prentice-Hall.

Starkweather, C.W. (1985). The development of fluency in normal children. In *Stuttering therapy: Prevention and intervention with children.* Memphis: Speech Foundation of America.

Starkweather, C.W. (1986). Talking with the parents of young stutterers. In *Counseling stutterers.* Memphis: Speech Foundation of America.

Starkweather, C.W. (1987). *Fluency and stuttering.* Englewood Cliffs, NJ: Prentice-Hall.

Starkweather, C.W. (1991). Stuttering: The motor-language interface. In H. Peters, W. Hulstijn, & C. Starkweather (Eds.), *Speech motor control and fluency*. Amsterdam: Excerpta Medica.

Starkweather, C.W. (1994). Talking with parents of young stutterers. In J. Fraser Gruss (Ed.), *Counseling stutterers*. Memphis: Stuttering Foundation of America.

Starkweather, C.W. (1997). Learning and its role in stuttering development. In R.F. Curlee & G.M. Siegel (Eds.), *The nature and treatment of stuttering: New directions,* 2nd ed. (pp. 79–95). Boston: Allyn & Bacon.

Starkweather, C.W., Givens-Ackerman, J. (1997). *Stuttering*. Austin, TX: Pro-Ed.

Starkweather, C.W., & Gottwald, S. (1990). The demands and capacities model II: Clinical application. *Journal of Fluency Disorders, 15,* 143–157.

Starkweather, C.W., Gottwald, S.R., & Halfond, M.H. (1990). *Stuttering prevention: A clinical method*. Englewood Cliffs, NJ: Prentice-Hall.

Starkweather, C.W., Hirschman, P., & Tannenbaum, R.S. (1976). Latency of vocalization onset: Stutterers versus nonstutterers. *Journal of Speech and Hearing Research, 19,* 481–492.

Starkweather, C.W., & Myers, M. (1979). Duration of subsegments within the intervocalic interval in stutterers and nonstutterers. *Journal of Fluency Disorders, 4,* 205–214.

Stemberger, J.P. (1982). The nature of segments in the lexicon: Evidence from speech errors. *Lingua, 56,* 235–259.

Stocker, B., & Goldfarb, R. (1995). *The Stocker probe for fluency and language*. Vero Beach, FL: Speech Bin.

Stocker, B., & Usprich, C. (1976). Stuttering in young children and level of demand. *Journal of Childhood Communication Disorders, 1,* 116–131.

Studdert-Kennedy, M. (1987). The phoneme as a perceptuomotor structure. In A. Allport, D. McKay, W. Prinz, & E. Scheerer (Eds.), *Language perception and production*. London: Academic Press.

Taylor, O. (1986). *Treatment of communication disorders in culturally and linguistically diverse populations*. San Diego: College-Hill Press.

Throneburg, R., & Yairi, E. (1994). Temporal dynamics of repetitions during the early stage of childhood stuttering: An acoustic study. *Journal of Speech and Hearing Research, 37,* 1067–1075.

Till, J.A., Reich, A., Dickey, S., & Sieber, J. (1983). Phonatory and manual reaction times of stuttering and nonstuttering children. *Journal of Speech and Hearing Research, 26,* 171–180.

Toscher, M.M., & Rupp, R.R. (1978). A study of the central auditory processes in stutterers using the Synthetic Sentence Identification (SSI) test battery. *Journal of Speech and Hearing Research, 21,* 779–792.

Travis, J. (1996). Let the games begin. *Science News, 149*(7), 97–112.

Travis, L.E. (1931). *Speech pathology*. New York: Appleton-Century.

Tudor, M. (1939). *An experimental study of the effect of evaluative labeling on speech fluency*. Unpublished master's thesis, University of Iowa, Iowa City.

Turnbaugh, K.R., & Guitar, B.E. (1981). Short-term intensive stuttering treatment in a public school setting. *Language, Speech, and Hearing Services in Schools, 12,* 107–114.

Turnbaugh, K.R., Guitar, B.E., & Hoffman, P.R. (1979). Speech clinicians' attribution of personality traits as a function of stuttering severity. *Journal of Speech and Hearing Research, 22,* 37–45.

Umeda, N. (1975). Vowel duration in American English. *Journal of the Acoustical Society of America, 58,* 434–445.

Umeda, N. (1977). Consonant duration in American English. *Journal of the Acoustical Society of America, 61,* 846–858.

Van Lishout, P. (1995). *Motor planning and articulation in fluent speech of stutterers and nonstutterers*. Nijmegen, The Netherlands:

Nijmegen Institute for Cognition and Information.

Van Riper, C. (1936). Study of the thoracic breathing of stutterers during expectancy and occurrence of stuttering spasm. *Journal of Speech Disorders, 1,* 61–72.

Van Riper, C. (1971). *The nature of stuttering.* Englewood Cliffs, NJ: Prentice-Hall.

Van Riper, C. (1973). *The treatment of stuttering.* Englewood Cliffs, NJ: Prentice-Hall.

Van Riper, C. (1974). Modification of behavior. In *Therapy for stutterers.* Memphis: Speech Foundation of America.

Van Riper, C. (1975a). The stutterer's clinician. In J. Eisenson (Ed.), *Stuttering: A second symposium.* New York: Harper & Row.

Van Riper, C. (1975b). *Therapy in action.* (3 videotapes). Memphis: Stuttering Foundation of America.

Van Riper, C. (1982). *The nature of stuttering,* 2nd ed. Englewood Cliffs, NJ: Prentice-Hall.

Van Riper, C. (1994). The severe young stutterer. In J. Fraser Gruss (Ed.), *Counseling stutterers.* Memphis: Stuttering Foundation of America.

Van Riper, C., & Hull, C.J. (1955). The quantitative measurement of the effect of certain situations on stuttering. In W. Johnson & R.R. Leutenegger (Eds.), *Stuttering in children and adults.* Minneapolis: University of Minnesota Press.

Wall, M.J. (1980). A comparison of syntax in young stutterers and nonstutterers. *Journal of Fluency Disorders, 5,* 345–352.

Wall, M.J., & Myers, F.L. (1984). *Clinical management of childhood stuttering.* Baltimore: University Park Press.

Wall, M.J., & Myers, F.L. (1995). *Clinical management of childhood stuttering,* 2nd ed. Austin, TX: Pro-Ed.

Watson, B.C., & Alfonso, P.J. (1987). Physiological bases of acoustic LRT in nonstutterers, mild stutterers, and severe stutterers. *Journal of Speech and Hearing Research, 30,* 434–447.

Watson, J.B., & Kayser, H. (1994). Assessment of bilingual/bicultural children and adults who stutter. *Seminars in Speech and Language, 15,* 149–163.

Weber, C., & Smith, A. (1990). Autonomic correlates of stuttering and speech assessed in a range of experimental tasks. *Journal of Speech and Hearing Research, 33,* 690–706.

Webster, R.L. (1974). A behavioral analysis of stuttering: Treatment and theory. In K.S. Calhoun, H.E. Adams, & K.M. Mitchell (Eds.), *Innovative treatment methods in psychopathology.* New York: John Wiley & Sons.

Webster, R.L. (1979). Empirical considerations regarding stuttering therapy. In H.H. Gregory (Ed.), *Controversies about stuttering therapy.* Baltimore: University Park Press.

Webster, R.L. (1980). Evolution of a target-based behavioral therapy for stuttering. *Journal of Fluency Disorders, 5,* 303–320.

Webster, W. (1990). Evidence in bimanual finger tapping of an attentional component to stuttering. *Behavioural Brain Research, 37,* 93–100.

Webster, W. (1993). Hurried hands and tangled tongues. In E. Boberg (Ed.), *Neuropsychology of stuttering.* Edmonton: University of Alberta Press.

Weiss, C., Gordon, M., & Lillywhite, H. (1987). *Clinical management of articulatory and phonologic disorders,* 2nd ed. Baltimore: Williams & Wilkins.

Weiss, D.A. (1964). *Cluttering.* Englewood Cliffs, NJ: Prentice-Hall.

West, R. (1931). The phenomenology of stuttering. In R. West (Ed.), *A symposium on stuttering.* Madison, WI: College Typing Company.

Westby, C.E. (1979). Language performance of stuttering and nonstuttering children. *Journal of Communication Disorders, 12,* 133–145.

Wexler, K.B., & Mysak, E.D. (1982). Disfluency characteristics of 2-, 4- and 6-year old males. *Journal of Fluency Disorders, 7,* 37–46.

White, P.A., & Collins, S.R.C. (1984). Stereotype formation by inference: A possible explanation for the "stutterer" stereotype. *Journal of Speech and Hearing Research, 27,* 567–570.

Wiig, E., & Semel, E. (1984). *Language assessment and intervention,* 2nd ed. Columbus, OH: Charles E. Merrill.

Wijnen, F. (1990). The development of sentence planning. *Journal of Child Language, 17*(3), 651–675.

Wilkenfeld, J., & Curlee, R. (1997). The relative effects of questions and comments on children's stuttering. *American Journal of Speech-Language Pathology, 6,* 79–89.

Williams, D.E. (1957). A point of view about stuttering. *Journal of Speech and Hearing Disorders, 22,* 390–397.

Williams, D.E. (1971). Stuttering therapy for children. In L.E. Travis (Ed.), *Handbook of speech pathology.* New York: Appleton-Century-Crofts.

Williams, D.E. (1979). A perspective on approaches to stuttering therapy. In H.H. Gregory (Ed.), *Controversies about stuttering therapy.* Baltimore: University Park Press.

Williams, D.E., Melrose, B.M., & Woods, C.L. (1969). The relationship between stuttering and academic achievement in children. *Journal of Communication Disorders, 2,* 87–98.

Williams, D.E., Silverman, F.H., & Kools, J.A. (1968). Disfluency behavior of elementary-school stutterers and nonstutterers: The adaptation effect. *Journal of Speech and Hearing Research, 11,* 622–630.

Williams, D.E., Melrose, B.M., & Woods, C.L. (1969). The relationship between stuttering and academic achievement in children. *Journal of Communication Disorders, 2,* 87–98.

Wingate, M.E. (1964). Recovery from stuttering. *Journal of Speech and Hearing Disorders, 29,* 312–321.

Wingate, M.E. (1969). Sound and pattern in "artificial" fluency. *Journal of Speech and Hearing Research, 12,* 677–686.

Wingate, M.E. (1970). Effect on stuttering of changes in audition. *Journal of Speech and Hearing Research, 13,* 861–873.

Wingate, M.E. (1983). Speaking unassisted: Comments on a paper by Andrews et al. *Journal of Speech and Hearing Disorders, 48,* 255–263.

Wingate, M.E. (1988). *The structure of stuttering: A psycholinguistic approach.* New York: Springer-Verlag.

Winitz, H. (1961). Repetitions in the vocalizations and speech of children in the first two years of life. *Journal of Speech and Hearing Disorders,* Monograph Supplement, 7, 55–62.

Winnicott, D.W. (1971). *Playing and reality.* New York: Routledge.

Wood, F., Stump, D., McKeehan, A., et al. (1980). Patterns of regional cerebral blood flow during attempted reading aloud by stutterers both on and off haloperidol medication: Evidence for inadequate left frontal activation during stuttering. *Brain and Language, 9,* 141–144.

Woods, C.L., & Williams, D.E. (1976). Traits attributed to stuttering and normally fluent males. *Journal of Speech and Hearing Research, 19,* 267–278.

Woolf, G. (1967). The assessment of stuttering as struggle, avoidance, and expectancy. *British Journal of Disorders of Communication, 2,* 158–171.

Yairi, E. (1981). Disfluencies of normally speaking two-year old children. *Journal of Speech and Hearing Research, 24,* 490–495.

Yairi, E. (1982). Longitudinal studies of disfluencies in two-year-old children. *Journal of Speech and Hearing Research, 25,* 155–160.

Yairi, E. (1983). The onset of stuttering in two- and three-year old children: A preliminary report. *Journal of Speech and Hearing Disorders, 48,* 171–178.

Yairi, E. (1997a). Early stuttering. In R.F. Curlee & G.M. Siegel (Eds.), *Nature and treatment of stuttering: New directions,* 2nd ed. Boston: Allyn & Bacon.

Yairi, E. (1997b). Home environment and parent-child interaction in childhood stuttering. In R.F. Curlee & G.M. Siegel (Eds.), *Nature and treatment of stuttering: New directions,* 2nd ed. Boston: Allyn & Bacon.

Yairi, E., & Ambrose, N. (1992a). A longitudinal study of stuttering in children: A preliminary report. *Journal of Speech and Hearing Research, 35,* 755–760.

Yairi, E., & Ambrose, N. (1992b). Onset of stuttering in preschool children: Selected factors. *Journal of Speech and Hearing Research, 35,* 782–788

Yairi, E., & Ambrose, N. (1996). *Disfluent speech in early childhood stuttering.* Unpublished manuscript. Stuttering Research Project, University of Illinois.

Yairi, E., Ambrose, N., & Cox, N. (1996). Genetics of stuttering: A critical review. *Journal of Speech and Hearing Research, 39,* 771–784.

Yairi, E., Ambrose, N., & Niermann, R. (1993). The early months of stuttering: A developmental study. *Journal of Speech and Hearing Research, 36,* 521–528.

Yairi, E., Ambrose, N., Paden, E., & Throneburg, R.N. (1996). Predictive factors of persistence and recovery: Pathways of childhood stuttering. *Journal of Communication Disorders, 29,* 51–77.

Yairi, E., & Lewis, B. (1984). Disfluencies at the onset of stuttering. *Journal of Speech and Hearing Research, 27,* 154–159.

Yaruss, J.S., & Conture, E.G. (1995). Mother and child speaking rates and utterance lengths in adjacent fluent utterances: Preliminary observations. *Journal of Fluency Disorders, 20*(3), 257–278.

Young, M.A. (1981). A reanalysis of "Stuttering therapy: The relation between attitude change and long-term outcome." *Journal of Speech and Hearing Disorders, 46,* 221–222.

Young, M.A. (1984). Identification of stuttering and stutterers. In R.F. Curlee & W.H. Perkins (Eds.), *The nature and treatment of stuttering: New directions.* (pp. 13–30). San Diego: College-Hill Press.

Zebrowski, P. (1991). Duration of the speech disfluencies of beginning stutterers. *Journal of Speech and Hearing Research, 34*(3), 483–491.

Zebrowski, P. (1995). Temporal aspects of the conversations between children who stutter and their parents. *Topics in Language Disorders, 15*(3), 1–17.

Zenner, A.A., Ritterman, S.I., Bowen, S.K., & Gronhovd, K.D. (1978). Measurement and comparison of anxiety levels of parents of stuttering, articulatory defective, and normal-speaking children. *Journal of Fluency Disorders, 3,* 273–283.

Zimbardo, P.G. (1985). *Psychology and life,* 11th ed. Glenview, IL: Scott, Foresman & Company.

Zimmerman, G.N. (1980). Articulatory dynamics of fluent utterances of stutterers and nonstutterers. *Journal of Speech and Hearing Research, 23,* 95–107.

Names Index

References followed by "n" denote footnotes.

Subject Index

Page numbers in italics denote figures; those followed by a "t" denote tables.